PULMONARY DISEASES
AND DISORDERS

Second Edition

Companion Handbook

NOTICE

Medicine is an ever-changing science. As new research and clinical experience broaden our knowledge, changes in treatment and drug therapy are required. The editors and the publisher of this work have checked with sources believed to be reliable in their efforts to provide information that is complete and generally in accord with the standards accepted at the time of publication. However, in view of the possibility of human error or changes in medical sciences, neither the editors nor the publisher nor any other party who has been involved in the preparation or publication of this work warrants that the information contained herein is in every respect accurate or complete. Readers are encouraged to confirm the information contained herein with other sources. For example and in particular, readers are advised to check the product information sheet included in the package of each drug they plan to administer to be certain that the information contained in this book is accurate and that changes have not been made in the recommended dosages or in the contraindications for administration. This recommendation is of particular importance in connection with new or infrequently used drugs.

PULMONARY DISEASES AND DISORDERS

Second Edition

Companion Handbook

Editor

ALFRED P. FISHMAN, M.D.
William Maul Measey Professor of Medicine
Department of Rehabilitation Medicine
University of Pennsylvania School of Medicine
Philadelphia, Pennsylvania

Contributing Editor

ROBERT M. KOTLOFF, M.D.
Assistant Professor of Medicine
Pulmonary and Critical Care Division
University of Pennsylvania School of Medicine
Philadelphia, Pennsylvania

McGRAW-HILL, INC.
Health Professions Division

New York   St. Louis   San Francisco   Auckland
Bogotá   Caracas   Lisbon   London   Madrid
Mexico City   Milan   Montreal   New Delhi   Paris
San Juan   Singapore   Sydney   Tokyo   Toronto

PULMONARY DISEASES AND DISORDERS, SECOND EDITION COMPANION HANDBOOK

Copyright © 1994 by McGraw-Hill, Inc. All rights reserved. Printed in the United States of America. Except as permitted under the United States Copyright Act of 1976, no part of this publication may be reproduced or distributed in any form or by any means, or stored in a data base or retrieval system, without the prior written permission of the publisher.

1234567890   DOCDOC   9876543

ISBN 0-07-021157-4

This book was set in Times Roman by ComCom. The editors were J. Dereck Jeffers and Susan Finn; the production supervisor was Clare Stanley; the cover designer was Ed Schultheis. R. R. Donnelley & Sons Company was printer and binder.

The book is printed on acid-free paper

Library of Congress Cataloging-in-Publication Data

Pulmonary diseases and disorders : companion handbook / Alfred P. Fishman [editor].—2d ed.
     p. cm.
   Includes bibliographical references and index.
   ISBN 0-07-021157-4 (acid-free paper)
   1. Lung—Diseases—Handbooks, manuals, etc. I. Fishman, Alfred P.
RC756.P826 1993
616.2'4—dc20   93-27563
                                                           CIP

CONTENTS

CONTRIBUTORS

Michael Beers, M.D., Assistant Professor of Medicine, Pulmonary and Critical Care Division, University of Pennsylvania School of Medicine, Philadelphia, Pennsylvania [13,15,17,48]

Patrick J. Brennan, M.D., Assistant Professor, Infectious Diseases; Director, Infection Control, Infectious Diseases Section, University of Pennsylvania School of Medicine, Philadelphia, Pennsylvania [39,43,46]

Peter E. Callegari, M.D., Assistant Professor of Medicine, Division of Rheumatology, University of Pennsylvania School of Medicine, Philadelphia, Pennsylvania [6]

John E. Connors, Pharm.D., Associate Professor of Clinical Pharmacy, Philadelphia College of Pharmacy and Science, Philadelphia, Pennsylvania; Adjunct Assistant Professor of Pharmacy in Medicine, Associated Faculty of the School of Medicine, University of Pennsylvania School of Medicine, Philadelphia, Pennsylvania [37]

Horace M. DeLisser, M.D., Assistant Professor of Medicine, Pulmonary and Critical Care Division, University of Pennsylvania School of Medicine, Philadelphia, Pennsylvania [4,51]

Deborah DeMarco, M.D., Assistant Professor of Medicine; Director of Medical Specialties Clinic, Department of Rheumatology, University of Massachusetts Medical Center, Worcester, Massachusetts [20]

Paul E. Epstein, M.D., Chief, Pulmonary Division, Graduate Hospital, Philadelphia, Pennsylvania; Clinical Professor of Medicine, University of Pennsylvania School of Medicine, Philadelphia, Pennsylvania [16]

Stanley Fiel, M.D., Professor of Medicine; Chief, Pulmonary and Critical Care Medicine, Medical College of Pennsylvania, Philadelphia, Pennsylvania [24]

Alfred P. Fishman, M.D., William Maul Measey Professor of Medicine, Department of Rehabilitation Medicine, University of Pennsylvania School of Medicine, Philadelphia, Pennsylvania [12,18,29,31,34,54]

Neil O. Fishman, M.D., Assistant Professor of Medicine, Infectious Diseases Section, University of Pennsylvania School of Medicine, Philadelphia, Pennsylvania [44,45]

John Hansen-Flaschen, M.D., Associate Professor of Medicine; Director, Pulmonary and Critical Care Division, University of Pennsylvania School of Medicine, Philadelphia, Pennsylvania [49]

Abby Huang, M.D., Attending Physician, Infectious Diseases Section, Grandview Hospital, Sellersville, Pennsylvania [41]

Jay R. Kostman, M.D., Assistant Professor of Medicine, Division of Infectious Diseases, Cooper Hospital University Medical Center, Robert Wood Johnson Medical School at Camden, Camden, New Jersey [38,47]

Robert M. Kotloff, M.D., Assistant Professor of Medicine, Pulmonary and Critical Care Division, University of Pennsylvania School of Medicine, Philadelphia, Pennsylvania [5,8,10,11]

Aili Lazaar, M.D., Research Fellow, Pulmonary and Critical Care Division, University of Pennsylvania School of Medicine, Philadelphia, Pennsylvania [28]

Mitchell Margolis, M.D., Associate Professor of Medicine, Division of Pulmonary Medicine, Medical College of Pennsylvania, Philadelphia, Pennsylvania; Chief, Pulmonary and Critical Care Medicine, Philadelphia VA Medical Center, Philadelphia, Pennsylvania [35]

Ignacio Mendiguren, M.D., Research Associate, Pulmonary and Critical Care Division, University of Pennsylvania School of Medicine, Philadelphia, Pennsylvania [50]

Stephen Mette, M.D., Director, Medical Intensive Care Unit, Graduate Hospital, Philadelphia, Pennsylvania; Clinical Assistant Professor of Medicine, University of Pennsylvania School of Medicine, Philadelphia, Pennsylvania [2]

Wallace T. Miller, Jr., M.D., Assistant Professor of Radiology, Department of Radiology, University of Pennsylvania School of Medicine, Philadelphia, Pennsylvania [36]

David Murphy, MB, BAO, BcH, MRCP, Chairman, Pulmonary Medicine, Deborah Heart and Lung Center, Browns Mill, New Jersey [14]

Richard K. Murray, M.D., Assistant Professor of Medicine, Pulmonary and Critical Care Division, University of Pennsylvania School of Medicine, Philadelphia, Pennsylvania [22,23]

Harold I. Palevsky, M.D., Associate Professor of Medicine, Pulmonary and Critical Care Division, University of Pennsylvania School of Medicine, Philadelphia, Pennsylvania [18,19,53]

Reynold A. Panettieri, Jr., M.D., Assistant Professor of Medicine, Pulmonary and Critical Care Division, University of Pennsylvania School of Medicine, Philadelphia, Pennsylvania [22,23]

Joseph Pilewski, M.D., Research Fellow, Pulmonary and Critical Care Division, University of Pennsylvania School of Medicine, Philadelphia, Pennsylvania [28]

Paul Richman, M.D., Assistant Professor of Medicine, Central Emek Hospital, Israel [9,33]

Michael Scharf, M.D., Consultant in Pulmonary Diseases, Jeanes Hospital, Philadelphia, Pennsylvania; Consultant in Pulmonary Diseases, American Oncologic Hospital, Philadelphia, Pennsylvania [1]

Mindy G. Schuster, M.D., Assistant Professor of Medicine, Infectious Diseases Section, University of Pennsylvania School of Medicine, Philadelphia, Pennsylvania [40]

Richard J. Schwab, M.D., Assistant Professor of Medicine, Pulmonary and Critical Care Division, University of Pennsylvania School of Medicine, Philadelphia, Pennsylvania [27,52,55]

William Sexauer, M.D., Assistant Professor of Medicine; Director, Pulmonary Rehabilitation Program, Pulmonary and Critical Care Medicine, Medical College of Pennsylvania, Philadelphia, Pennsylvania [26]

Randi Silibovsky, M.D., Assistant Professor of Medicine, Infectious Diseases Section, Temple University Medical Center, Philadelphia, Pennsylvania; Attending Physician, Infectious Diseases Section, Albert Einstein Medical Center, Philadelphia, Pennsylvania [42]

Gregory Tino, M.D., Assistant Professor of Medicine, Pulmonary and Critical Care Division, University of Pennsylvania School of Medicine, Philadelphia, Pennsylvania [13,15,17]

Kenneth A. Tolep, M.D., Assistant Professor of Medicine, Division of Pulmonary and Critical Care Medicine, Temple University School of Medicine, Philadelphia, Pennsylvania [3]

Gregory Underwood, M.D., Pulmonologist, Charlotte Medical Clinic, Charlotte, North Carolina [7]

Robert L. Vender, M.D., Assistant Professor of Medicine, Division of Pulmonary and Critical Care Medicine, Medical College of Pennsylvania, Philadelphia, Pennsylvania [21]

Joan Marie von Feldt, M.D., Assistant Professor of Medicine, Division of Rheumatology, University of Pennsylvania School of Medicine, Philadelphia, Pennsylvania [6]

Robert E. Walker, M.D., Senior Investigator, Laboratory of Immunoregulation, National Institute of Allergy and Infectious Diseases, National Institutes of Health, Bethesda, Maryland [30,32]

Gerald Weinhouse, M.D., Pulmonary Fellow, Pulmonary and Critical Care Division, University of Pennsylvania School of Medicine, Philadelphia, Pennsylvania [25]

Jerry M. Zuckerman, M.D., Attending Physician, Infectious Diseases Section, Albert Einstein Medical Center, Philadelphia, Pennsylvania [43]

PREFACE

In bygone days, when physicians still made house calls, they carried along a little black bag that contained the tools of the trade. Invariably, alongside of the stethoscope and flashlight was a small inconspicuous volume, an epitome of medical diagnosis and treatment. After completing the physical examination, the physician would consult the small volume—usually in the privacy of the bathroom after hand washing—before delivering the diagnostic verdict to the family and handing over the prescription. Reassured by the compendium, physicians could complete their appointed rounds, confident that they, at least, had done no harm. Back at the office after completing the circuit, there would be opportunity to peruse larger tomes for fuller expositions, to ferret out greater detail, to consult edifying illustrations, and to refer to a more comprehensive bibliography.

This small volume is intended to provide the reader with a compendium of pulmonary medicine, to provide in a nutshell both a summary and an overview of the essential ingredients of pulmonary medicine. The prospective users are pictured as house officers, fellows, and practitioners. To reach this audience, contributors were sought from among pulmonary physicians who are regularly obliged to make on-the-spot decisions about diagnosis and patient care. Those chosen were then advised to draw heavily on the three-volume tome *"Pulmonary Diseases and Disorders"* and the more recent *"Update."* They were also urged to provide a brief supplementary bibliography to ensure timeliness.

This is what the book is about. Now it is time to recognize those who made it possible. At the very beginning, Dr. Reynold Panettieri's energy and enthusiasm set the process into motion. Dr. Robert Kotloff subsequently pitched in, devoting considerable time and energy to activating the contributors and to orchestrating the first phase of the editorial review. His catalytic and editorial activities are recognized in the designation "Contributing Editor." For directing the flow of manuscripts and for the editorial process, per se, I am indebted to Ms. Alice K. Glover, without whose help the book would have been long delayed, mired in sluggish revisions, and anachronistic bibliographies. I also owe a great debt to Ms. Betsy Ann Bozzarello, who continually freed up time by sparing me many of the daily demands and distractions of academic life. Another individual who played a major role in the genesis of this book was Mr. Dereck Jeffers, editor-in-chief at McGraw-Hill, whose gentle, but relentless prodding of the editor from the time of conception to delivery, ensured that the idea would be brought to fruition. Last, but not least, I must tip my hat to the folks at home: without the understanding, forebearance, and encouragement of my wife Linda and my daughter Hannah, this book would not have been possible.

PULMONARY DISEASES AND DISORDERS

Second Edition

Companion Handbook

I | APPROACH TO THE PATIENT

1 | Cough, Dyspnea, and Wheezing

Michael Scharf

COUGH

Definition

Cough is an explosive expiration following inspiration and closure of the glottis, which may be automatic or deliberate and protects and cleanses the airways. It does so by directing tracheobronchial secretions and particulate matter cephalad toward the mouth. It is an essential defense against aspiration.

A cough may be acute in onset or chronic. A cough of unknown cause generally comes to the attention of the chest physician when it persists unabated for more than a month or so, after failing to respond to empirical treatment.

Mechanism

A cough may be voluntary or involuntary. It can be visualized as occurring in a stepwise fashion: (1) inspiration; (2) closure of the glottis; (3) contraction of the expiratory muscles (raises intrathoracic pressure); (4) sudden opening of the glottis; and (5) expulsion of air through airways narrowed by the raised intrathoracic pressures, carrying with it the offending particulate matter. The effectiveness of a cough in dislodging particles from the airways depends on the forceful compression of the intrathoracic airways and the increase in the linear velocity of gas molecules in the air stream.

A variety of mechanisms can evoke cough: (1) *mechanical,* such as stimulation of "irritant" receptors in the epithelial lining of the airways by inhaled dusts or smoke or by distortion of the airways by pulmonary fibrosis, atelectasis, or intrabronchial masses; (2) *inflammatory processes,* such as postnasal drip, gastroesophageal reflux syndromes, laryngitis or tracheobronchitis; and (3) *psychogenic stimuli.* A psychogenic cough is generally a dry cough brought about by anxiety. Psychogenic stimuli can aggravate a cough that originates in mechanical or inflammatory mechanisms.

Etiology

In Table 1-1, the causes of cough are sorted into five broad categories: (1) infectious—acute and chronic; (2) parenchymal and airways inflammation, including asthma; (3) tumor; (4) foreign body; and (5) cardiovascular.

Diagnostic Tests

Evaluation of cough (Table 1-2) begins with a thorough history and physical examination, paying special attention to the naso-

TABLE 1-1 Some Causes and Characteristics of Coughs

Cause	Characteristics
Infectious Processes	
Acute	
Tracheobronchitis	Cough associated with sore throat, running nose and eyes.
	Cough often preceded by symptoms of upper respiratory infection: cough dry, painful at first; later becomes productive.
Bronchopneumonia	Usually begins as acute bronchitis: dry or productive cough.
Mycoplasma and viral pneumonia	Paroxysmal cough, productive of mucoid or blood-stained sputum associated with flulike syndrome.
Exacerbation of chronic bronchitis	Cough productive of mucoid sputum becomes purulent.
Chronic	
Bronchitis	Cough productive of sputum on most days for > 3 consecutive months and for > 2 successive years. Sputum mucoid until acute exacerbation, when it becomes mucopurulent.
Bronchiectasis	Cough copious, foul, purulent, often since childhood; forms layer on standing.
Tuberculosis or fungus	Persistent cough for weeks to months often with blood-tinging of sputum.
Inflammatory Processes (Parenchymal and Airways)	
Asthma	Cough which may or may not occur with wheezing.
Interstitial fibrosis and infiltrations	Cough nonproductive, persistent, depends on etiology.
Postnasal drip, with or without sinusitis	Cough which may be associated with dripping sensation in throat.
Reflux esophagitis	May be productive or nonproductive and typically occurs when in a supine position.
Smoking	Cough usually associated with injected pharynx; persistent, most marked in morning, usually only slightly productive unless succeeded by chronic bronchitis.
Tumors	
Bronchogenic carcinoma	Nonproductive to productive cough for weeks to months: recurrent small hemoptysis common.
Alveolar cell carcinoma	Cough similar to bronchogenic carcinoma except in occasional instance when large quantities of watery, mucoid sputum are produced.
Benign tumors in airways	Cough nonproductive, occasionally hemoptysis.

TABLE 1-1 Some Causes and Characteristics of Coughs (*Continued*)

Cause	Characteristics
Mediastinal tumors	Cough, often with breathlessness, caused by compression of trachea and bronchi.
Aortic aneurysm	Brassy cough.
Foreign body	
Immediate, while still in upper airway	Cough associated with progressive evidence of asphyxiation.
Later, when lodged in lower airway	Nonproductive cough, persistent, associated with localizing wheeze.
Cardiovascular	
Left ventricular failure	Cough intensifies while supine along with aggravation of dyspnea.
Pulmonary infarction	Cough associated with hemoptysis, usually with pleural effusion.

SOURCE: Modified after Table 26-3. Szidon PJ, Fishman AP: Approach to the pulmonary patient with respiratory signs and symptoms, in Fishman AP (ed), *Pulmonary Diseases and Disorders*, 2d ed. New York, McGraw-Hill, 1988, p 345.

pharyngeal and oropharyngeal airways and lungs, followed by a chest radiograph. If infection or malignancy is suspected, sputum should be collected for Gram stain culture and cytology. A complete blood count may help in distinguishing between infectious and allergic disorders.

The decision to initiate any of the "special" diagnostic tests outlined in Table 1-2 begins with the clinical impression. If the etiology of the cough remains unclear, lung spirometry may be helpful in suggesting either obstructive pulmonary disease, caused by asthma or chronic bronchitis, or restrictive disease caused by pulmonary fibrosis. If spirometry is normal but obstructive airway disease is still suspected, bronchoprovocational testing, using inhaled methacholine, carbachol, or histamine, may help to uncover

TABLE 1-2 Cough: Diagnostic Tests

General	1.	History and physical examination
	2.	Chest radiograph, posteroanterior and lateral
	3.	Sputum examination, Gram stain and culture, cytology
	4.	Complete blood count with differential leukocyte count
Special	1.	Lung spirometry
	2.	Broncho provocational, using methacholine, carbachol, or histamine
	3.	Sinus radiography
	4.	Bronchoscopy
	5.	Esophageal dysmotility tests
		a. Esophageal contrast study
		b. 24-h monitoring of esophageal pH

bronchial hyperreactivity. Sinus radiographs may disclose a sinusitis that is accompanied by a postnasal drip.

If the etiology of the cough remains enigmatic, bronchoscopy should be done in an attempt to detect lesions of the larynx, trachea, or large bronchi that are inapparent on the chest radiograph. If bronchoscopy is unrevealing, then a search can be made for gastroesophageal reflux; either esophageal swallowing studies using radiopaque contrast material or the monitoring of esophageal pH over a 24-h period may be useful.

Posttussive Syncope

Ordinarily, intrathoracic pressure increases by 50 to 100 mmHg during a cough; occasionally, pressures as high as 300 to 400 mmHg may be reached. The abrupt increase in intrathoracic pressure decreases pulmonary venous pressure which, in turn, reflexly elicits systemic vasodilation. If marked, the resultant drop in arterial blood pressure can evoke syncope. Syncope sometimes occurs within a few seconds after the onset of a paroxysm of coughing followed by prompt return to full consciousness when coughing stops. This posttussive syncope occurs predominantly in men; it can occur in either the supine or upright position. The mechanism responsible for posttussive syncope is a considerable decrease in cardiac output and cerebral blood flow caused by the reflex systemic vasodilation.

Treatment

Treatment begins by addressing the underlying condition, e.g., antibiotics for infection, bronchodilator and anti-inflammatory therapy for asthma. Cigarette smoking should be stopped. Antihistamines or decongestants are useful in symptomatic sinusitis or postnasal drip. H_2-blockers and metoclopramide HCl may improve cough due to gastroesophageal reflux.

Treatment of a cough may be directed either at suppression or at increasing effectiveness. When coughing is inadequate to clear the airways properly, protussive therapy should be considered. Unfortunately, the value of protussive agents, such as guaiacol glycerol (guaifenesin), in enhancing cough effectiveness is questionable even though many patients feel they are helpful.

DYSPNEA

Definition

Dyspnea denotes a sensation of breathlessness. To determine the clinical significance of dyspnea, a careful history and physical examination are essential not only for insight into etiology, but also to direct specialized examinations.

Assessment

One etiology for dyspnea is pulmonary parenchymal or airway disease. However, dyspnea may also have other causes, e.g., ischemic heart disease, deconditioning, or anxiety. Objective evidence in support of the complaint of dyspnea (a subjective complaint) may be found in a disproportionately high minute ventilation or respiratory rate with respect to the level of activity.

Etiology

The common denominators in the etiology of cardiac or pulmonary diseases are usually an increase in the work (and energy cost) of breathing or a heightened ventilatory drive. Less common and more obscure are stimuli from receptors in the respiratory muscles and airways. Three causes of dyspnea are generally identified: pulmonary disease, cardiac disease, and others.

Pulmonary Of the pulmonary causes, the three most common are chronic obstructive pulmonary disease (COPD), widespread pulmonary fibrosis, and asthma.

In COPD, the work and oxygen cost of breathing are abnormally high, especially during exercise. The relationship between the maximum voluntary ventilation (MVV) and the ventilation at rest or during maximum exercise can be willfully correlated with dyspnea. For example, in the "pink puffer," the reduction in the MVV correlates well with the severity of the airway obstruction and dyspnea. This relationship does not apply as well to the "blue bloater" even though the degree of pulmonary function abnormality may be the same, presumably because of the chronic hypercapnia which blunts the urge to breathe and is accompanied by a more modest increase in $\dot{V}_E$ during exercise.

In widespread pulmonary fibrosis, the MVV is usually well maintained. However, at rest and during exercise, tachypnea and the increased work of ventilating stiff lungs contribute to the development of dyspnea.

In asthma, the characteristic feature of dyspnea is an exacerbation in chest tightness. The intensity of the dyspnea is influenced by the severity of the airway obstruction, the acuity of onset, and by emotional factors. Bronchoprovocation tests may be helpful in demonstrating hyperreactive airways. Spirometry, before and after exercise, is useful in demonstrating exercise-induced bronchoconstriction as a cause of exercise-induced asthma.

Cardiac The cardiac causes of dyspnea may be subdivided according to the stiffness of the lungs, i.e., low or normal lung compliance.

In cardiac disease associated with a *low pulmonary compliance,* tachypnea, fatigue, and dyspnea are especially prominent during exercise. In this category are chronic pulmonary venous hypertension due to left ventricular dysfunction, aortic or mitral valvular disease, or primary venous hypertension. In these disorders, pulmonary compliance is reduced due to congestion, edema, and fibrosis, and is often accompanied by arterial hypoxemia that generally intensifies during exercise, by an increase in the work of breathing, and by a low cardiac output.

In *cardiac disease with normally compliant lungs,* e.g., congenital heart disease such as pulmonic stenosis, dyspnea may be due to a drop in arterial oxygenation during exercise or to a low cardiac output.

Others Severe anemia, because of the low O_2-carrying capacity of the blood, is commonly associated with dyspnea. Severe pulmonary hypertension, acting by some obscure mechanism, also evokes dyspnea. So does circulatory collapse, not only because of the metabolic acidosis, but also because of obscure mechanisms.

WHEEZING

Definition

Wheezing is a whistling sound during breathing. The musical pulmonary sounds characteristic of wheezing are produced by oscillation of the narrowed airways as air exits and enters the lungs.

Etiology

Wheezing may occur because of narrowing of the upper airway, e.g., laryngotracheal injury, or of the lower respiratory tree, e.g., asthma. *Stridor* designates a loud constant-pitched wheezing that may signal laryngotracheal dysfunction caused by laryngospasm, laryngeal edema, obstruction due to a large foreign body, or hysteria. Bronchial or tracheal narrowing may be due to extrinsic compression, stricture, or an endotracheal mass. Most often, wheezing is caused by bronchial hyperreactivity and associated bronchoconstriction.

Eight major types of stimuli can provoke wheezing by inducing acute bronchoconstriction:

1. *Inhaled allergens* may stimulate the release of chemical mediators of airway inflammation, i.e., leukotrienes, prostaglandins, and platelet-activating factor. Airway obstruction usually occurs within minutes, followed by gradual spontaneous regression over the next 30 to 60 min.
2. *Exercise* may produce wheezing ("exercise-induced asthma"); characteristically it occurs within the first 15 to 20 min after

exercise and regresses spontaneously. The inhalation of warm, humid air during exercise seems to decrease the occurrence of "exercise-induced asthma"; cold air typically promotes its development.

3. *Upper respiratory tract infections,* primarily due to viruses, enhance bronchial responsiveness.
4. *Wheezing* may develop in the workplace in response to exposure to certain products, e.g., metal salts; wood and vegetable dusts; pharmaceutical agents; industrial chemicals; plastics; biologic enzymes; and animal, bird, and fish proteins.
5. *Environmental pollutants,* such as sulfur dioxide, ozone, and nitrogen dioxide, may evoke wheezing by enhancing bronchial hyperreactivity.
6. *Pharmacologic agents* sometimes provoke bronchospasm; among the more common are aspirin, drug additives such as tartrazine, and food preservatives such as metabisulfite and β-adrenergic antagonists (see Chapter 12).
7. *Psychological factors* may contribute to the development of wheezing.
8. *Acute or chronic left heart failure* accompanied by pulmonary venous hypertension may be associated with "cardiac asthma"; the basis for this "cardiac asthma" is an increase in the transudation of plasma across the endothelium of distended bronchial venules which, in turn, leads to submucosal airway edema.

Treatment

The treatment of wheezing depends on its etiology. In the case of endotracheal or endobronchial obstruction, removal of the obstructing body, either bronchoscopically or surgically, may be required. Wheezing due to extrinsic compression by neoplasm may respond to irradiation or chemotherapy. Wheezing due to inhalation of an agent which enhances bronchial reactivity is best managed by avoiding the agent. Pharmacologic treatment of asthma is considered elsewhere in this book.

BIBLIOGRAPHY

For a more detailed discussion, see McFadden ER Jr: Asthma: General features, pathogenesis, and pathophysiology, in Fishman AP (ed), *Pulmonary Diseases and Disorders,* 2d ed. New York, McGraw-Hill, 1988, pp 1295–1310.

Irwin RS, Corley FJ: The treatment of cough: A comprehensive review. Chest 99:1477–1484, 1991.

McFadden ER Jr: Asthma: Acute and chronic therapy, in Fishman AP (ed), *Pulmonary Diseases and Disorders,* 2d ed. New York, McGraw-Hill, 1988, pp 1311–1323.

Murray RK, Panettieri RA Jr: Management of asthma: The changing approach, in Fishman AP (ed), *Update: Pulmonary Diseases and Disorders.* New York, McGraw-Hill, 1992, pp 67–82.

Poe RH, Varder RV, Israel RH, Kallay MC: Chronic persistent cough. Experience in diagnosis and outcome using an anatomic diagnostic protocol. Chest 95:723–728, 1989.

Stephen Mette

DEFINITION

The coughing up of blood, regardless of the quality and quantity, is defined as *hemoptysis*. This may range from scant amounts of blood-streaked sputum to the expectoration of gross blood. *Life-threatening* or *massive hemoptysis* has a distinct prognostic connotation and has been defined as the expectoration of frank blood at the rate of 300 to 600 ml/24 h. Unfortunately, this definition often relies on quantification by the patient of the volume of expectorated blood. Because asphyxiation is the usual cause of death related to massive hemoptysis, any amount of blood which cannot be cleared from the anatomic dead space, usually about 150 ml, should be considered as life-threatening.

ETIOLOGY

Table 2-1 lists the diverse etiologies of hemoptysis. The etiology seems to influence whether the hemoptysis is ordinary or massive; certain etiologies, such as tuberculosis, aspergilloma, and bronchiectasis, have a propensity to cause massive bleeding. In the United States, bronchogenic carcinoma, a common cause of hemoptysis, is infrequently associated with massive hemoptysis. Occasionally, fiberoptic bronchoscopy or a flow-directed pulmonary artery catheter may cause life-threatening hemoptysis.

If the reason for hemoptysis is not evident after physical examination, chest radiography, and bronchoscopy, it is unlikely that the etiology will be uncovered. The prognosis for patients with so-called idiopathic or cryptogenic hemoptysis is generally favorable, with a high likelihood of spontaneous resolution.

PATHOGENESIS

Hemoptysis usually stems from lesions that receive their blood supply from the bronchial circulation. However, other systemic vessels may contribute, at least in part, to the bleeding source. For example, the internal mammary artery, the long thoracic artery, an intercostal artery, or a diaphragmatic artery may be the source of bleeding in such lesions as lung cancer, pulmonary tuberculosis, lung abscess, necrotizing pneumonias, and other pulmonary inflammatory processes. The pulmonary circulation may be responsible for bleeding from pulmonary artery embolism, trauma from flow-directed pulmonary artery catheters, chest trauma, and some arteriovenous malformations. The vascular supply of other bleeding lesions can be more complex because some arteriovenous malfor-

TABLE 2-1 Causes of Hemoptysis
_____
Infections
  Bronchitis
  Tuberculosis*
  Necrotizing pneumonia*
  Lung abscess*
  Mycetoma (aspergillus)*
Neoplasm
  Bronchogenic carcinoma
  Bronchial adenoma
Cardiovascular disorders
  Pulmonary infarction
  Mitral stenosis
  Severe chronic congestive heart failure
Trauma
  Penetrating
  Blunt
Alveolar hemorrhage syndromes
  Goodpasture's syndrome
  Lupus erythematosus
  Wegener's granulomatosis
Miscellaneous
  Cystic fibrosis/bronchiectasis*
  Foreign body
  Pulmonary artery catheter trauma
  Procedure related (fiberoptic bronchoscopy)
  Arteriovenous malformations
  Bronchial telangiectasia
  Thrombocytopenia/coagulopathy
  Idiopathic (cryptogenic)
_____
*Common causes of massive hemoptysis

mations, bronchiectasis, lung sequestration, and chronic infection may involve communications between the pulmonary and bronchial circulations. In mitral stenosis and chronic severe congestive heart failure, hemoptysis originates in bronchial venous engorgement.

CLINICAL MANIFESTATIONS

History Certain features in the history of the patient with hemoptysis can direct the search for an etiology. A history of underlying chest disease can often be elicited for the more frequent causes of hemoptysis. The patient's smoking history and age can also be helpful. Lung cancer rarely occurs before the age of 40 years; it is even more unusual in the nonsmoker. A chronic cough which changes its character often occurs in the patient with a carcinoma of the lung. Expectoration of large amounts of purulent sputum in the febrile patient suggests a lung abscess or necrotizing pneumonia. Massive hemoptysis sometimes occurs without premonitory hemoptysis. Although patients often have difficulty in quantifying the amount of hemoptysis, they usually can distinguish between coughed up or vomited blood. A history of prior vomiting or esophageal varices can help in directing attention to the upper gastrointestinal tract as the source rather than to the lungs. Alternatively, the history can point to a nasopharyngeal source.

Physical examination Patients with hemoptysis are usually hemodynamically stable even though they are apt to be anxious, tachycardic, and tachypneic. Examination of the oropharynx and nasopharynx usually suffices to rule out a supraglottic source of blood. Sometimes the presence of unilateral rales, rhonchi, or consolidation points to the lung from which the blood is coming. However, aspirated blood can be misleading. Careful cardiac examination occasionally discloses unsuspected mitral stenosis or left heart failure.

USUAL DIAGNOSTIC TESTS

Chest radiography The chest radiograph is the single most important test in localizing and defining an etiology for hemoptysis. Neoplasms, necrotizing pneumonias, and aspergillomas are usually obvious on the posteroanterior and lateral projections of the chest film. The same is true for severe left ventricular failure or mitral stenosis. Diffuse bilateral alveolar infiltrates raise the possibility of alveolar hemorrhage syndrome, e.g., Goodpasture's.

Some important causes of bleeding, such as endobronchial adenomas and bronchiectasis, may not be evident on the chest radiograph. Also, the distinctive radiographic features of the primary etiology may be obscured during an acute episode of blood, e.g., the infiltrate produced by aspirated blood can resemble that of a pneumonia or pulmonary edema. Aspiration of blood into the contralateral lung may further complicate attempts to localize the site of bleeding.

Bronchoscopy Bronchoscopy is the major tool for expeditiously localizing and diagnosing the source of bleeding. Fiberoptic bronchoscopy is most useful for direct visualization of the lesion when the bleeding site is in the major airways; frequently it identifies a peripheral lesion as the source by disclosing blood emerging from a segmental bronchus. However, rigid bronchoscopy is used when bleeding is brisk because the aspiration channel of the fiberoptic bronchoscope is too narrow to evacuate clot and blood rapidly and effectively. Precisely when bronchoscopy should be done in non–life-threatening hemoptysis is debatable, but there is general agreement that it should be done within 24 h of the onset of bleeding. In contrast, when hemoptysis is massive, bronchoscopic evaluation should be done immediately.

SPECIFIC DIAGNOSTIC TESTS

Computed tomography (CT) High-resolution CT scanning has proved valuable in the noninvasive diagnosis of bronchiectasis and of arteriovenous malformations as the source of hemoptysis.

Angiography This technique can be helpful in localizing the bleeding site and defining the vascular anatomy. It is the "gold standard" in the diagnosis of pulmonary embolism and arteriovenous malformations.

DIFFERENTIAL DIAGNOSIS

The differential diagnosis includes all the etiologies listed in Table 2-1. Epistaxis, hematemesis, and factitious sources are important etiologies that have to be excluded. A coagulopathy can be the primary or confounding reason for hemoptysis. In searching for the cause, the clinical situation must be fully considered. For example, as noted above, in the patient with an indwelling, flow-directed catheter in the pulmonary artery, the search for the cause of massive hemoptysis begins with the possibility of a pulmonary arterial perforation.

NATURAL HISTORY AND PROGNOSIS

The natural history and prognosis of hemoptysis that is not life-threatening depends on the underlying condition. In contrast, the course and prognosis of patients with massive hemoptysis are often linked to the ability to control the bleeding swiftly. Mortality rates from massive hemoptysis range from 50 to 100 percent when definitive therapy is withheld or delayed; patients die either from asphyxiation or from complications arising from their underlying disease. Early aggressive and definitive therapy can reduce mortality to 10 to 20 percent, depending on the underlying disease, the patient's general condition, and the ability of the patient to withstand pulmonary resection.

TREATMENT

The management of ordinary or nonmassive hemoptysis depends on the disease. For example, antibiotics usually suffice to handle infectious causes of hemoptysis. Hemoptysis due to mitral stenosis requires valve repair or replacement. Management of non–life-threatening bleeding from a neoplasm depends on the extent of the tumor and the pulmonary function of the patient. Surgical resection should be undertaken when feasible, but radiation, chemotherapy, and laser therapy are options in the patient who is not a candidate for surgery.

The management of massive hemoptysis involves clearing the airways, protecting the uninvolved lung, controlling bleeding, and instituting therapy directed at arresting the primary cause. Treatment can be divided into medical, surgical, endobronchial, and endovascular categories.

Medical Medical therapy is directed at stabilizing the patient before definitive therapy is started. Endotracheal intubation should be considered in any patient who is at risk of asphyxiation. Isolation of the bleeding lung with a double-lumen tube for intubation is often necessary in ongoing hemoptysis to protect the contralateral lung. However, this procedure may not be feasible because (1) it is technically difficult and requires expert placement to avoid atelectasis or main-stem bronchial injury; and (2) the small diameter of each channel of the double-lumen tube limits the ability to suction the airway free of blood clots and secretions and precludes diagnostic bronchoscopy. Consequently, some prefer a single-lumen, large-bore tube.

The patient who does not undergo endotracheal intubation is placed either in the sitting position or with the bleeding side down to promote clearing of the airways and aid in avoiding aspiration of blood into the contralateral lung. Narcotics or cough suppressants are avoided to preserve the cough reflex; a benzodiazepine may be helpful in comforting the patient without suppressing the cough. Sufficient supplemental oxygen is provided to ensure adequate oxygenation. Large-bore intravenous lines are placed for fluid and blood administration. A coexisting coagulopathy is corrected quickly. Although it is important to start antibiotics for infectious etiologies, they will have no immediate effect and will not affect the short-term prognosis from the hemoptysis. Pitressin (vasopressin; 0.2 to 0.4 units per min), administered intravenously, may decrease or stop bleeding from bronchial venous sources.

Surgical Lung resection is considered in patients who can tolerate surgery and whose prognosis from their underlying disease is reasonably good. For example, resection of a lung carcinoma responsible for hemoptysis may not increase the patient's life expectancy but may prevent death from aspiration of blood. Massive hemoptysis from aspergillomas is not easily arrested and the affected lobe should be resected if the patient's lung function permits. Surgical intervention should also be considered in patients with recurrent hemoptysis from focal bronchiectasis, arteriovenous malformations, trauma, and foreign bodies.

Endobronchial Bronchoscopy is used to identify the source of bleeding, to determine its course and rate, and to slow or arrest the bleeding before surgery. As indicated above, choosing between rigid and fiberoptic bronchoscopy depends on the magnitude of the bleeding, the location of the lesion, and the experience of the bronchoscopist.

Fiberoptic bronchoscopy can be useful in different ways to slow bleeding: topical placement of epinephrine (1:20,000) at the bleeding site, installation of fibrin precursors to promote endobronchial coagulation, and tamponade of the airway using a Fogerty catheter balloon.

Rigid bronchoscopy, the instrument of choice in massive bleeding, enables more effective lavage with saline (iced or at room temperature), and aspiration of large quantities of blood and clots. It also can be used to ensure ventilation (ventilating bronchoscope), for packing of the airway, and for safer access to the bleeding site when laser photocoagulation is to be used. Laser photocoagulation can be regarded as definitive therapy for endobronchial neoplasms in patients who are not surgical candidates.

Endovascular Angiographic identification and embolization of the bronchial or other systemic arteries has been used successfully to treat life-threatening hemoptysis. The best results are obtained in patients in whom the etiology of the hemoptysis is tuberculosis, bronchogenic cancer, bronchiectasis, abscess, or an arteriovenous malformation. Recurrent bleeding is particularly common with aspergillomas. Embolization calls for considerable technical skill and has been complicated by inadvertent spinal artery embolization, retrograde systemic embolization, and bronchial infarction.

SPECIAL CONSIDERATIONS

Aspergilloma Transthoracic, intracavitary instillation of amphotericin B has been used successfully to arrest bleeding in patients who are not candidates for surgical extirpation.

Alveolar hemorrhage syndromes The treatment of diffuse alveolar hemorrhage associated with a number of immune-mediated disorders, including Goodpasture's syndrome, lupus erythematosus, and granulomatous or necrotizing vasculitis, involves the use of high-dose corticosteroids and cytotoxic agents (cyclophosphamide or azathioprine). Plasmapheresis is added to this regimen in patients with Goodpasture's syndrome.

BIBLIOGRAPHY

For a more detailed discussion, see Szidon JP, Fishman AP: Approach to the pulmonary patient with respiratory signs and symptoms, in Fishman AP (ed), *Pulmonary Diseases and Disorders,* 2d ed. New York, McGraw-Hill, 1988, pp 346–351, 451–452.

Fraser RS: Pulmonary aspergillosis: Pathologic and pathogenetic features. Pathol Annu 28 Pt 1:231–277, 1993.

Goldman JM: Hemoptysis: Emergency assessment and management. Emerg Med Clin North Am 7:325–338, 1989.

Johnston H, Reisz G: Changing spectrum of hemoptysis. Arch Intern Med 149:1666–1668, 1989.

Thompson AB, Teschler H, Rennard SI: Pathogenesis, evaluation and therapy for massive hemoptysis. Clin Chest Med 13:69–82, 1992.

Ken Tolep

DEFINITION

Solitary pulmonary nodule (SPN) is the term used to describe the radiographic finding of a small (usually ≤ 4 cm) round density surrounded by normal lung parenchyma, without intrathoracic adenopathy or associated atelectasis. The nodule may be calcified or noncalcified, and its borders may be either sharp or irregular.

INCIDENCE

Based on recent data from the American Cancer Society, approximately 135,000 new SPNs are discovered in this country each year. One radiologic series found SPNs in 1:500 consecutive chest radiographs.

ETIOLOGY

There are many causes of SPNs. However, by far, the most common causes are granulomas (due to prior infections such as histoplasmosis and tuberculosis) and neoplasms (either bronchogenic carcinoma or metastases from extrathoracic malignancies). Although the relative frequency of the various etiologies varies widely among series, bronchogenic carcinoma seems to account for approximately one third of SPNs (Table 3-1). Several reasons account for the variability among series, including different criteria for the definitions of a nodule, differences in the populations studied, and differences in the nature of the series (surgical or radiologic).

INITIAL DIAGNOSTIC EVALUATION

The major goal in the evaluation of a patient with an SPN is to distinguish a benign lesion from an early bronchogenic carcinoma. Although the 5-year survival rate for lung cancer overall is < 15 percent, resection of a stage I lung cancer (tumor ≤ 3 cm with no involved lymph nodes) may result in a 5-year survival rate of up to 70 percent. After identifying the SPN on the chest radiograph, evaluation of its nature begins with a search for possible etiology in the history, physical examination, and tuberculin skin testing. Subsequently, more definitive studies, such as computed tomography (CT), biopsy, and in some instances, thoracotomy, may be indicated.

History

Two characteristics affect the likelihood that an SPN is malignant: the age of the patient and a history of cigarette smoking. Cancer is

TABLE 3-1 Incidence of Various Disease Processes as Causes of
Solitary Pulmonary Nodules

Etiology	Incidence %
Malignant nodules	40
Bronchogenic carcinoma	30
Bronchial adenoma (usually carcinoid)	2
Solitary metastatic lesions	8
Benign nodules	60
Infectious granulomas	50
Tuberculoma	
Histoplasmoma	
Coccidioidoma	
Cryptococcoma	
Aspergilloma	
Noninfectious granulomas	3
Rheumatoid granuloma	
Wegner's granulomatosis	
Paraffinoma	
Sarcoidosis	
Benign tumors	3
Hamartoma	
Others	
Miscellaneous	4
Rounded atelectasis	
Pulmonary infarct	
Amyloidoma	
Hematoma	
Dirofilaria nodule	
Pseudotumors (loculated fluid in fissure)	
Spherical pneumonia	
Bronchopulmonary sequestration	

Figures are based on multiple reported series. The criteria for inclusion in
these series were not uniform.
SOURCE: Modified from Lillington GA: Systematic diagnostic approach to
pulmonary nodules, in Fishman AP (ed), *Pulmonary Diseases and Disorders*, 2d ed. New York, McGraw-Hill, 1988, p 1945.

a rare cause of SPN in patients under age 35 (reported incidence 1
to 3 percent). Also, an SPN is much less likely to be malignant in
a life-long nonsmoker than in a smoker.

The patient should be questioned about prior history of tuberculosis or contact with an infected individual. Additionally, a detailed
travel history should be elicited to determine if the patient ever
traveled to or resided in an area endemic for histoplasmosis or
coccidioidomycosis.

Radiography

The first question to be answered is whether the presumed SPN is
within the lung parenchyma. Other possibilities include a lesion

within the pleura or chest wall or an artifact. Additional radiographic views, such as lateral and oblique projections, can be used to confirm that the nodule is real and that it is within the lung itself.

Many radiographic criteria have been suggested for distinguishing benign from malignant nodules, including size, shape, contour of borders, growth rate, and calcification. Although nodules that are small (≤ 3 cm) and have smooth borders are more likely to be benign, many exceptions occur to these generalizations. Attempts have also been made to use the growth rate (expressed as *doubling time*) of a nodule in distinguishing benign from malignant processes. The time needed for a nodule to double in volume based on serial chest radiographs can be determined by changes in the radius of the nodule (volume of a sphere is equal to $4/3 \times \pi \times r^3$). Both the insensitivity of standard radiographs in detecting small changes in the radius of nodules ≤ 2 cm in size and interobserver variability in measurements have limited the usefulness of this technique. Nonetheless, a nodule which has shown no growth on serial radiographs separated by at least 2 years *can* safely be considered to be benign.

Calcification in a nodule greatly increases the probability that a nodule is benign (< 1 percent of pulmonary malignancies appear calcified on chest radiographs). However, calcification in a nodule may not be visible on the chest radiograph because of the high kilovoltage used to take conventional chest radiographs. If calcification is seen, additional information can be gained from its pattern. Nodules that contain a central focus of calcification or in which the pattern is either laminated or homogeneous can be considered to be a healed granuloma. Although "popcorn-type calcification" is virtually pathognomonic of a hamartoma, most hamartomas do not display this feature. When the focus of calcification is eccentric, the lesion may not be benign. For example, in a lung carcinoma that arises from calcified granulomatous disease ("scar carcinoma"), the calcification is usually eccentric. Also, metastatic lesions from extrathoracic primary malignancies often contain calcification.

Tomography

Both conventional and computed tomography are more accurate than standard chest radiographs in assessing the presence and pattern of calcification within a pulmonary nodule. Although conventional tomograms are much less expensive and usually suffice for diagnosis, CT has several important advantages. For example, CT, using thin sections (1 to 5 mm) is useful in quantifying the density of a pulmonary nodule (measured in Houndsfield units). By using the "phantom" technique, the density of the pulmonary nodule in question is compared with that of a calcium carbonate "phantom" nodule within a model thorax. Although many lesions can accurately and noninvasively be diagnosed by this technique as benign, false negatives do occasionally occur. These can be minimized by considering other radiographic criteria, e.g., size, borders, and clinical circumstances, such as the presence of an extrathoracic neoplasm.

CT is much more sensitive than conventional radiographs and tomograms for detecting other pulmonary nodules. This can be important in the patient with lung cancer who is being considered for resection of an apparently solitary lung nodule (an estimated 1 percent of lung cancers are multiple and synchronous).

CT can also help in selecting the diagnostic procedure to perform. If a nodule is shown to be contiguous with a bronchus, the yield of bronchoscopy may rise dramatically (up to 90 percent if the nodule has an endobronchial component). CT can identify bullae that are not evident on the standard chest radiograph, thereby helping to select the approach that will be used during transthoracic needle aspiration biopsy.

Sputum Cytology

Because this method is noninvasive, it should be performed even though the diagnostic yield is low. For lung cancers overall, the diagnostic yield is approximately 10 to 20 percent. It is greater for tumors that are centrally located and have an endobronchial component (both of these features are more common with squamous cell carcinoma).

APPROACH TO THE PATIENT WITH AN INDETERMINATE LESION

Until a few years ago, patients with a pulmonary nodule that did not satisfy the radiologic criteria of benignity either underwent thoracotomy or serial radiography to determine the stability or growth pattern of the lesion. The approach to these patients has recently been broadened as a result of technical improvements in bronchoscopy and needle biopsy and the widespread introduction of thoracoscopic biopsy.

The selection of which diagnostic procedure to perform is dictated by a number of factors: the a priori likelihood that the SPN is malignant, i.e., the presence of risk factors for bronchogenic carcinoma, characteristics of the nodule (size and location), the patient's ability to tolerate surgical intervention, and the familiarity and competence of the operator with the various technical procedures.

Serial Chest Radiographs

The most conservative approach involves expectant management with serial chest radiographs; thoracotomy is then reserved for those cases where growth of the nodule is demonstrated. The greatest concern about this approach is that delaying resection of a bronchogenic carcinoma will adversely affect survival, though insufficient data are available to substantiate this fear. Nonetheless, this approach is probably only appropriate for patients with very low probability of having a malignant process, e.g., patients under 35 years old without evidence of an extrathoracic malignancy. It is also reserved for patients in whom surgery is contraindicated because of serious concurrent cardiopulmonary disease.

Bronchoscopy

One favorable feature of bronchoscopy is its extremely low morbidity. Estimates of the ability of bronchoscopy to identify malignant nodules vary from 20 to 70 percent. Factors which affect the yield include size of the nodule (the yield is only 20 percent of nodules $\leq$ 2 cm), location (low yield if the SPN is in the extreme periphery of the lung), and the existence of an endobronchial component (yield is up to 90 percent if present). Transbronchial (Wang) needle can be used to sample lesions which may not be accessible to bronchial brush biopsy or transbronchial biopsy. Bronchoscopy can be useful in staging bronchogenic carcinoma by excluding synchronous endobronchial lesions and enlarged nodes which may compress central airways. Bronchoscopy may be useful in diagnosing benign nodules, but the yield is even lower than for malignant ones.

Transthoracic Needle Aspiration (TNA)

This technique has a much higher diagnostic yield than does bronchoscopy for SPNs. Some studies have reported that up to 95 percent of malignant nodules can be correctly identified. However, to replicate such results, it is often necessary to make multiple passes through the nodule to provide the cytologist with sufficient material. It is helpful to have the cytologist available during the procedure so that the adequacy of the sample can be assessed and the need for additional passes determined. The yield for the diagnosis of benign nodules is less than that of malignant nodules because benign lesions are more difficult to enter and because histopathologic and not cytologic specimens are frequently required. Use of a large-bore biopsy needle which provides a core of tissue successfully diagnoses nearly 70 percent of benign lesions but runs a high risk of pneumothorax. The absence of malignant cells in a sample does not establish that a nodule is benign. However, some clinicians claim that a lesion may be presumed to be benign if adequate material other than normal lung tissue is obtained; it can be verified (radiographically) that the nodule was sampled; no cells suspicious of malignancy are obtained; and no endobronchial lesions are seen during bronchoscopy.

The technique used is simple. Needles of 18 to 24 gauge are passed through the chest wall under fluoroscopic or CT guidance under local anesthesia. The majority of the aspirate is submitted for cytologic evaluation. Small quantities are sent for fungal and mycobacterial stains and cultures. If larger fragments (> 2 mm) are obtained, they may be used for histologic evaluation.

The major complications of TNA are pneumothorax and hemoptysis. A pneumothorax occurs in 10 to 20 percent of patients who undergo TNA; most of these can be managed conservatively. Fewer than 10 percent of cases require tube thoracostomy. Hemoptysis is usually mild although bleeding can be brisk in acute inflammatory lesions and metastatic renal carcinomas. Despite these complications, the procedure is safe if it is not performed in patients with bleeding diatheses, those with severe pulmonary dysfunction (FEV_1 < 1 L), and if the needle does not traverse bullae to reach the nodule.

Thoracoscopy

Thoracoscopically directed lung biopsy is becoming increasingly popular as a minimally invasive alternative to thoracotomy for the diagnosis of SPNs. Peripherally situated nodules are particularly well-suited for thoracoscopically guided biopsy; in contrast, centrally located lesions deep within the lung parenchyma may not be accessible.

The procedure is usually performed under general anesthesia. A double-lumen endotracheal tube is used and the lung to be biopsied is partially deflated. Two small incisions are required—one to introduce the thoracoscope equipped with a video camera and high-intensity light source and a second for the biopsy instrument. A chest tube is left in place after the biopsy and is removed once the lung has fully sealed, usually within 12 to 24 h. Recovery time is brief and postoperative pain is readily controlled with oral analgesics. Complications of thoracoscopy occur infrequently; they include bleeding, subcutaneous emphysema, and persistent bronchopleural fistula.

Although ideally suited as a diagnostic technique, it must be emphasized that the role of thoracoscopically directed wedge resection as definitive treatment for malignant nodules remains uncertain. In most cases, formal thoracotomy and lobectomy are carried out if biopsies demonstrate malignancy, though thoracoscopic wedge resection alone is used in those patients with extremely marginal pulmonary function.

Thoracotomy

As discussed above, the advent of thoracoscopic biopsy can be expected to greatly decrease the reliance on thoracotomy for diagnostic and, possibly, therapeutic purposes. Immediate thoraco-

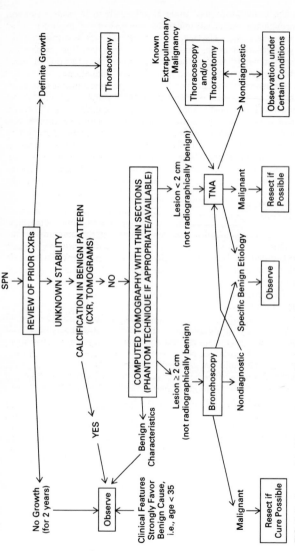

FIG. 3–1 Approach to the management of a solitary pulmonary nodule.

tomy, in the absence of less invasive attempts at tissue diagnosis, remains an appropriate approach for patients who are good surgical candidates and for whom the likelihood of cancer is high, i.e., smokers over the age of 45 with a new or enlarging nodule. A number of assumptions underlie the *early* use of thoracotomy. First, operative mortality from the procedure must be low; in general, mortality related to surgery is < 1 percent. Second, most nodules are resectable at the time of thoracotomy; indeed, between 80 and 90 percent of lesions are found to be resectable. Finally, early thoracotomy should increase survival; while intuitively correct, this assumption remains difficult to substantiate. In one study using decisional analysis, a marginal survival advantage was found when the results of immediate surgery were compared with those of "wait and watch," i.e., thoracotomy only after serial radiographs demonstrate growth of the nodule. In this study, immediate surgery was of the greatest value when the likelihood of cancer was high.

SUMMARY

By considering clinical characteristics of the patient and radiographic characteristics of the nodule, a sensible approach to the management of a solitary pulmonary nodule is possible. This is illustrated in Figure 3-1.

BIBLIOGRAPHY

For a more detailed discussion, see Lillington GA: Systematic diagnostic approach to pulmonary nodules, in Fishman AP (ed), *Pulmonary Diseases and Disorders,* 2d ed. New York, McGraw-Hill, 1988, pp 1945–1954.

Mack MJ, Gordon MJ, Postma TW, Berger MS, Aronoff RJ, Acuff TE, Ryan WH: Percutaneous localization of pulmonary nodules for thoracoscopic lung resection. Ann Thorac Surg 53:1123–1124, 1992.

Miller DL, Allen MS, Deschamps C, Trastek VF, Pairolero PC: Video-assisted thoracic surgical procedure: management of solitary pulmonary nodules. Mayo Clin Proc 67:462–464, 1992.

Viggiano RW, Swensen SJ, Rosenow EC III: Evaluation and management of solitary and multiple pulmonary nodules. Clin Chest Med 13:83–95, 1992.

Zwirewich CV, Vedal S, Miller RR, Muller NL: Solitary pulmonary nodule: High resolution CT and radiologic-pathologic correlation. Radiology 179:469–476, 1991.

In evaluating a patient for any type of surgery involving anesthesia, it is essential to keep in mind that even an uncomplicated operation has pulmonary consequences. These can be sorted into four general categories: lung volumes, gas exchange, control of breathing, and pulmonary defense mechanisms (Table 4-1).

Lung volumes Following thoracic and abdominal surgery, the pattern of restrictive lung disease is seen, i.e., moderate-to-severe reduction in the vital capacity (VC) and smaller, but more significant reductions in the functional residual capacity (FRC). In the 24 h immediately after upper abdominal surgery, the VC and FRC may be greatly reduced, i.e., more than 70 percent and 50 percent respectively; values for these parameters generally remain low for more than a week. In contrast, large and persistent changes in lung volumes are not seen after superficial surgery or after surgery involving the extremities. Postoperative pain and muscle splinting play a role in reducing lung volumes. However, diaphragmatic dysfunction secondary to a decrease in central nervous system (CNS) output to the phrenic nerves may be the predominant process.

Gas exchange Postoperatively, after thoracic or abdominal surgery, arterial hypoxemia is common. Two phases can be identified. (1) Hypoxemia during the hours immediately after surgery is due largely to residual effects of anesthesia; this phase resolves within 24 h. (2) Persistent hypoxemia lasts for days or weeks; this phase is due primarily to the restrictive defect described above.

Control of breathing Respiratory depression is common after surgery. Two processes are involved. Residual effects of preanesthetic and anesthetic medications may blunt the inherent respiratory drive as well as the ventilatory responses to acidemia, hypercapnia, and hypoxia. Hypoxic and hypercapnic ventilatory drives are inhibited by narcotics given for analgesia; narcotics also reduce (or eliminate) the number of sighs.

Lung defenses Two major defense mechanisms, i.e., cough and mucociliary clearance, are impaired postoperatively. Pain or excessive use of narcotics may inhibit coughing. Additionally, the expulsive force generated by each cough is reduced as a result of impaired lung mechanics. Mucociliary clearance is decreased for up to 6 days following upper abdominal surgery due to the impaired cough; damage to cilia; presence of the endotracheal tube; anesthetic and preanesthetic agents; and atelectasis.

TABLE 4-1 Changes in Pulmonary Function after Thoracic and Abdominal Surgery

Reduction in lung volumes (restrictive defect)
Diaphragm dysfunction
Impaired gas exchange, including hypoxemia
Respiratory depression secondary to residual effects of anesthesia or postoperative narcotics
Impaired cough and mucociliary clearance

RISK FACTORS FOR PULMONARY COMPLICATIONS

These factors can be separated into two categories: preoperative and intraoperative.

Preoperative Factors

Chronic lung disease Most attention has been paid to the risk associated with chronic obstructive pulmonary disease (COPD). Depending on the type of surgery, the extent of preexisting lung disease, and the definitions used to define complications, postoperative respiratory problems in these patients have been reported to range from 25 to 75 percent. The idea of an arbitrary level of pulmonary function, e.g., forced expiratory volume in 1s (FEV_1) < 1 L, which would automatically deny surgery, has gradually given way to more liberal criteria. However, the general rule still applies that the more severely compromised the pulmonary function, the greater the risk from anesthesia and surgery. This general rule applies to other pulmonary conditions, e.g., restrictive or pulmonary vascular disease.

Smoking Smoking, independent of COPD, increases the risk of postoperative pulmonary morbidity. The risk arising from cigarette smoking becomes particularly appreciable when the use of tobacco exceeds 20 pack-years. Eight weeks of smoking cessation is required for a statistically significant reduction in complications.

Obesity Obese individuals are somewhat at increased risk for postoperative pulmonary complications primarily because obesity favors the development of atelectasis. It may also predispose to pulmonary aspiration.

Age Not long ago, advanced age was considered to be a major risk factor. More recently, the magnitude of risk attributed to advanced age has been downgraded as long as due regard is paid to the variety of factors in the elderly that may compromise postoperative recovery.

Malnutrition Malnutrition and starvation can have deleterious effects on the respiratory system. However, it is not clear that aggressive preoperative nutritional support improves pulmonary outcome.

Intraoperative Factors

Type of anesthesia General anesthesia impairs oxygenation and carbon dioxide elimination. Although these changes may contribute to postoperative respiratory problems, in general, the effects resolve within 24 h. Epidural anesthesia is generally considered to be safer than general anesthesia. Probably its greatest advantage is in reducing the incidence of thromboembolic problems.

The anatomic site of operation Complication rates are several times higher for patients who undergo thoracic or abdominal surgery than for those who undergo surgery on the extremities. Also, more complications are seen after upper abdominal surgery than after lower abdominal procedures.

Duration of surgery The incidence of postoperative respiratory complications increases significantly for operations that last longer than 3 to 4 h.

Type of surgical incision For abdominal procedures, vertical incisions are associated with a higher incidence of postoperative pulmonary problems than are horizontal incisions.

EVALUATION OF THE PATIENT FOR SURGERY

The four basic components of preoperative pulmonary evaluation are history and physical examination, chest radiography, arterial blood-gas analysis, and pulmonary function tests.

History and physical examination The following issues warrant special attention: (1) the extent of preexistent lung disease; (2) the smoking history; and (3) a history of respiratory symptoms, e.g., cough, chest pain, dyspnea, or the recent respiratory infection.

When the history is unrevealing, the physical examination is usually also unremarkable. However, exceptions do occur. Moreover, the physical examination provides a baseline for postoperative evaluation.

Chest radiography A preoperative chest radiograph should be obtained when new or unexplained respiratory symptoms or signs appear, when the history of chronic lung disease is unaccompanied by recent chest radiographs, or when thoracic surgery is undertaken.

Arterial blood-gas analysis Arterial blood-gas analysis is indicated in patients who have underlying lung disease, or who, by history or physical examination, have new pulmonary pathology.

Pulmonary function tests In evaluating the risk of postoperative pulmonary complications, spirometry is all that is generally used. In patients with COPD, the degree of obstruction (as determined by spirometry) correlates with the risk of postoperative pulmonary complications. Correlations between pulmonary function tests and outcome in other types of pulmonary disease are not available.

Pulmonary function testing should be done in the following settings: (1) a history of chronic lung disease; (2) cigarette smoking history > 20 pack-years; (3) history of unexplained dyspnea or cough, especially if the cough is productive; and (4) planned lung resection. There is no evidence to support routine preoperative pulmonary function testing in the elderly, the obese, or in individuals who are to undergo abdominal surgery.

EVALUATION FOR LUNG RESECTION

Preoperative evaluation for pulmonary resection is designed to ensure that the patient will be left without serious respiratory disability if a pneumonectomy has to be performed. The evaluation consists of two steps. As a start, pulmonary function tests are obtained. If the FEV_1 is > 2 L or than 80 percent predicted, the patient is cleared for a pneumonectomy and no further testing is required. However, if the FEV_1 is < 2 L or than 80 percent predicted, the predicted *postpneumonectomy* FEV_1 should be calculated. A quantitative perfusion scan of the lung is done and the percent of perfusion to the lung that will remain after the resection is determined. The predicted postpneumonectomy FEV_1 is then calculated using the following formula:

$$\text{Predicted postpneumonectomy } FEV_1 = \text{preoperative } FEV_1 \times \% \text{ of perfusion to remaining lung}$$

If the predicted postpneumonectomy FEV_1 is $\geq$ 800 cc or 40 percent of predicted, then the patient is cleared for a pneumonectomy; if not, then the patient is not a candidate for pneumonectomy. As a rule, even though a lesser operative procedure is anticipated, a patient who is being considered for pulmonary resection should be evaluated as though being considered for a pneumonectomy.

However, if the patient will be unable to tolerate a pneumonectomy but appears to be a good candidate for a lobectomy, then the predicted postlobectomy FEV_1 should be calculated using the above equation. Clearly, the patient may prove to be inoperable if the findings at the time of surgery disclose the need for a more extensive procedure than removal of a single lobe. For the borderline patient, the diffusing capacity (DL_{CO}) and exercising testing may be used to gain further insight into operability.

PREOPERATIVE PREPARATION

In patients undergoing elective surgery, the following preoperative prophylactic measures should be undertaken: (1) cessation of smoking for at least 8 weeks before surgery; (2) optimization of pulmonary function in individuals with COPD; therapy should be initiated 48 to 72 h before surgery, and the possible interventions include the use of bronchodilators, corticosteroids, and antibiotics (if indicated), and chest physical therapy (when excessive secretions are present); (3) weight loss in obese patients; and (4) instruction of patient with respect to the importance of coughing and either deep breathing exercises or the proper use of the incentive spirometer. Time spent in preparing the patient along these lines is of great value in shaping postoperative recovery.

POSTOPERATIVE PROPHYLACTIC MEASURES

Several interventions can be helpful postoperatively in preventing pulmonary complications: early patient mobilization and ambulation; prophylactic maneuvers to promote lung expansion, i.e., incentive spirometry or deep breathing exercises; adequate analgesia; prophylaxis for thromboembolism; careful monitoring for respiratory complications. Adequate control of pain is essential: not only analgesics in adequate dosage, but also regional anesthesia, e.g., epidural anesthesia, intercostal nerve blocks may be required.

PULMONARY COMPLICATIONS

Four major groups of pulmonary complications can be identified: atelectasis; infection (tracheobronchitis and pneumonia); exacerbation of underlying lung disease; and inability to wean from assisted ventilation. In addition, the possibilities of thromboembolic lung disease and permeability pulmonary edema have to be kept in mind. Finally, several unique respiratory complications can occur in patients undergoing thoracic surgery (Table 4-2). Nonetheless, as a rule, a healthy nonsmoker who undergoes nonthoracic or nonabdominal surgery, runs a low risk of postoperative pulmonary

TABLE 4-2 Pulmonary Complications Associated with Thoracic Surgery

Procedure	Complication	Incidence
Coronary artery bypass surgery	Phrenic nerve damage	10%
	Late pleural effusion*	unclear
Thoracotomy with lung resection	Bronchopleural fistula and/or empyema	5–20%†
Median sternotomy	Sternal wound infection (mediastinitis and/or osteomyelitis)	1–2%
Esophagectomy and/or gastrectomy	Anastomotic leak	3–6%

*Pleural effusions occurring after hospital discharge.
†Higher for patients with sarcoidosis and aspergilloma.
SOURCE: Modified from DeLisser HM, Grippi MA: in press.

complications, i.e., of the order of 1 percent, primarily related to anesthesia.

BIBLIOGRAPHY

For a more detailed discussion, see Olsen GN: Pre- and postoperative evaluation and management of the thoracic surgical patient, in Fishman AP (ed), *Pulmonary Diseases and Disorders,* 2d ed. New York, McGraw-Hill, 1988, pp. 2413–2432.

DeLisser HM, Grippi MA: Preoperative evaluation and preparation of the patient with pulmonary disease, in Goldmann D, Brown F, Guarnieri D (eds), *Perioperative Medicine.* New York, McGraw-Hill (in press).

Markos J, Mullan BP, Hillman DR, Musk AR, Antico VF, Lovegrove FT, Carter MJ, Finucane KE: Preoperative assessment as a predictor of mortality and morbidity after lung resection. Am Rev Respir Dis 139:902–910, 1989.

Zibrack JD, O'Donnell CR, Morton K: Indications for pulmonary function testing. Ann Intern Med 112:703–771, 1990.

II | INTERSTITIAL LUNG DISEASE

Robert M. Kotloff

DEFINITION

Sarcoidosis is a multisystem granulomatous disorder of unknown etiology which principally affects the lungs and intrathoracic lymph nodes. Although no single feature of the disease is pathognomonic, certain clinical constellations, e.g., bilateral hilar adenopathy and erythema nodosum or uveitis, are strongly suggestive. The diagnosis rests on two key elements: (1) the demonstration of noncaseating granulomas in a patient with compatible clinical and radiographic features; and (2) the exclusion of other known causes of granulomatous inflammation.

ETIOLOGY

The cause of sarcoidosis remains unknown. The presence of epithelioid granulomas and the accumulation of CD4+ helper T lymphocytes within the lung strongly suggest that sarcoidosis represents the end result of activation of the cellular arm of the immune system. It remains to be determined whether this activation is endogenously triggered or, more likely, is the result of challenge with one or more as yet unidentified exogenous antigens.

The increased incidence of sarcoidosis among certain ethnic groups and the occasional occurrence of familial clustering suggest that genetic factors may play a role in predisposition to sarcoidosis.

PATHOLOGY

The hallmark of sarcoidosis is the noncaseating epithelioid granuloma comprised of a central core of epithelioid cells and multinucleated giant cells, surrounded by a rim of mononuclear inflammatory cells and occasional fibroblasts. The epithelioid cells and giant cells sometimes contain cytoplasmic inclusion bodies referred to as Schaumann bodies (calcium- and iron-containing lamellar concretions) and asteroid bodies (star-shaped structures composed of lipoprotein metabolic products). Granulomas may be found in virtually any organ or tissue, although the lung, liver, spleen, and lymph nodes are most commonly involved. In the lung, granulomas tend to localize to subpleural, interstitial, and peribronchial regions. Involvement of the bronchial mucosa is common. Granulomas may be preceded by or occur concomitantly with an interstitial pneumonitis or "alveolitis," comprised of mononuclear inflammatory cells. Most granulomas gradually resolve completely, leaving the underlying lung parenchyma undisturbed. However, in approximately 20 percent of patients, granulomas heal by fibrosis which, if extensive, can lead to distortion of alveolar and bronchiolar architecture, obliteration of pulmonary vasculature, and end-stage honeycomb lung.

EPIDEMIOLOGY

Sarcoidosis is worldwide in distribution. In the United States, the overall prevalence is estimated to be 10/100,000; however, the prevalence among African Americans in the United States is 10 to 17 times that among whites. A slight female predominance has been suggested. Onset of disease occurs most commonly in the third and fourth decades of life. Despite occasional reports of familial clustering, the great majority of cases appear to be sporadic.

ABNORMAL PHYSIOLOGY

Abnormalities in pulmonary function stem from the presence of interstitial inflammation or fibrosis or both. Extensive parenchymal involvement leads to a decrease in diffusing capacity, a concentric decrease in lung volumes, and a decrease in lung compliance. Airflow obstruction, due either to granulomatous involvement of the bronchial mucosa or to distortion of airways resulting from peribronchial fibrosis, occurs in a minority of patients. Arterial hypoxemia is common, occurring during exercise in mild cases, but also at rest in patients with more advanced disease. Hypocapnia often accompanies the arterial hypoxemia; it is due to reflex stimulation of breathing both by the arterial hypoxemia (via peripheral chemoreceptors) and by the stiff lungs. Respiratory failure, pulmonary hypertension, and right ventricular failure are complications of far-advanced disease.

CLINICAL MANIFESTATIONS

Because of the systemic nature of the disease and the potential to involve any organ or tissue, the clinical manifestations of sarcoidosis are protean. These manifestations are summarized in Table 5-1.

History Up to one third of patients are asymptomatic at the time of diagnosis, with the disease being detected as an incidental finding on a chest radiograph obtained for unrelated reasons. Constitutional complaints including fever, night sweats, and weight loss, occur in 25 to 40 percent of patients. More specific complaints reflect the particular pattern of organ involvement in a given patient, but even extensive organ involvement may be clinically silent. Pulmonary symptoms, most commonly cough, dyspnea, and chest pain, occur in one third of patients. Wheezing may be noted by patients with extensive endobronchial disease. Hemoptysis is uncommon; it

TABLE 5-1 Clinical Manifestations of Sarcoidosis

Organ or system	Manifestations
Lungs	Interstitial lung disease, bronchial stenosis, bronchiectasis, pleural effusion (rare), pneumothorax, aspergilloma
Lymph nodes	Hilar/mediastinal adenopathy, peripheral adenopathy
Skin	Erythema nodosum, lupus pernio, papules, nodules, plaques, enlargement and tenderness of previous traumatic or surgical scars
Eyes	Uveitis, scleral and conjunctival lesions, lacrimal gland enlargement, optic neuritis, papilledema, keratoconjunctivitis sicca syndrome
Liver	Asymptomatic abnormalities in liver function studies, hepatomegaly, cirrhosis and portal hypertension, intrahepatic cholestasis
Endocrine	Hypercalcemia, hypercalciuria, panhypopituitarism
Musculoskeletal	Arthralgias, acute and chronic arthritis, osseous lesions, granulomatous myopathy
Heart	Cor pulmonale, arrhythmias, heart block, congestive cardiomyopathy, mitral regurgitation
CNS	Chronic basilar meningitis, space-occupying lesions, hydrocephaly, increased intracranial pressure, peripheral and cranial neuropathies, diabetes insipidus secondary to hypothalamic involvement, pituitary involvement
Kidney	Nephrolithiasis, interstitial nephritis, glomerulonephritis

is most apt to occur in patients with advanced disease who develop bronchiectasis or an aspergilloma.

Patients may also seek medical attention because of extrapulmonary involvement. Cutaneous involvement is common and may produce a variety of lesions (see below). Among these, the most distinctive is erythema nodosum, which presents as painful, red nodules usually on the lower extremities. Ocular symptoms (photophobia, redness, and blurred vision) occur in 25 percent of patients and generally signify the presence of uveitis. A minority of patients present with neurologic, musculoskeletal, and cardiac symptoms.

Physical examination A thorough physical examination is essential to determine the extent of involvement. Skin lesions vary from nonspecific papules, nodules, or plaques to the more characteristic lesions of lupus pernio (large, violaceous nodules in a malar distribution) or erythema nodosum. Examination of the eyes should include the use of a slit lamp and will reveal evidence of ocular involvement in 25 percent of patients. The most common lesion is granulomatous uveitis, but abnormalities of the conjunctiva, cornea, retina, or lacrimal gland can also be detected. Examination of the lungs is often surprisingly normal even with extensive radiographic abnormalities. Wheezes are heard in a few patients and suggest bronchial narrowing or distortion. Evidence of cor pulmonale (right ventricular heave, a loud pulmonic component of the second heart sound, increased jugular venous pressure, lower extremity edema) is common in patients with severe and extensive fibrotic disease. Other physical findings sometimes encountered are peripheral adenopathy, enlargement of the parotid glands, hepatosplenomegaly, and cranial or peripheral nerve palsies. Clubbing is distinctly unusual.

USUAL DIAGNOSTIC TESTS

Chest radiography The chest radiograph is abnormal in 90 percent of patients. Most characteristic is the presence of bilateral hilar adenopathy, often accompanied by right paratracheal adenopathy. Parenchymal infiltrates are present in approximately 50 percent of patients; they usually occur in conjunction with hilar adenopathy but may be present independently. Infiltrates are most commonly reticular or reticulonodular, bilateral, and distributed in the mid and upper lung zones. Occasionally, parenchymal involvement may assume the form of multiple nodular densities, mimicking metastatic malignancy. In far-advanced cases, extensive fibrotic changes, with honeycombing, upward retraction of the hila, and cystic areas, may be seen. Pleural effusions occur in < 5 percent of cases, and, when present, should not be ascribed to sarcoidosis until other possibilities have been excluded.

A staging system is commonly used to classify the chest radiographic abnormalities (Table 5-2). This staging system has been useful in management (see below).

Pulmonary function tests Pulmonary function tests may be entirely normal despite extensive radiographic evidence of interstitial disease. When abnormal, pulmonary function tests do not distinguish between granulomatous inflammation and irreversible fibrosis nor do they correlate well with the presence or extent of radiographic abnormalities. A low diffusing capacity, often associated with

TABLE 5-2 Radiographic Staging of Sarcoidosis

Stage	Description	% of Patients at presentation
0	Normal	8
I	Bilateral hilar adenopathy	43
II	Bilateral hilar adenopathy + infiltrates	35
III	Infiltrates	14

SOURCE: Data derived from Siltzbach LE: Sarcoidosis: Clinical features and management. Med Clin North Am 51:483, 1967.

diminished lung volumes (restrictive pattern), is characteristic. An obstructive pattern is noted in some patients and suggests extensive narrowing of the airways due to endobronchial inflammation or peribronchial fibrosis. Arterial blood gases characteristically reveal hypoxemia, occurring only with exercise in mild cases and at rest in association with more advanced disease. Hypocapnia occurs in the majority of patients, but is succeeded by eucapnea and then hypercapnia in the few patients who progress to respiratory failure.

Blood studies Hypercalcemia occurs in up to 11 percent of patients. Hepatic involvement is often accompanied by an increase in the serum alkaline phosphatase and, less commonly, by increased levels of transaminases or bilirubin or both. Hypergammaglobulinemia is a common but nonspecific feature.

SPECIAL DIAGNOSTIC EVALUATION

Biopsy Confirmation of the diagnosis of sarcoidosis requires the demonstration of noncaseating epithelioid granulomas on tissue biopsy. When present, skin lesions (except erythema nodosum), conjunctival lesions, or palpable peripheral lymph nodes provide easily accessible sites for biopsy. In their absence, bronchoscopy for obtaining transbronchial biopsy specimens is generally considered to be the procedure of choice. Noncaseating granulomas have been recovered in 75 to 90 percent of patients, even in the absence of radiographically apparent parenchymal abnormalities. Liver biopsy is occasionally helpful in situations where transbronchial biopsies are negative. The yield from liver biopsy is high (75 percent) but the utility of this procedure is limited by the large number of diseases that can produce hepatic granulomas. If all other attempts to establish a diagnosis prove unsuccessful, mediastinoscopy or open lung biopsy may be required, with the yield of the latter procedure approaching 100 percent.

Bronchoalveolar lavage (BAL) An increased absolute number of cells recovered by BAL accompanied by an increased percentage of lymphocytes supports the diagnosis of sarcoidosis. However, these findings are nonspecific and can occur in hypersensitivity pneumonitis, berylliosis, lymphoma, and tuberculosis.

Gallium scan Avid uptake of gallium in the lungs often occurs in patients with widespread pulmonary involvement and suggests ongoing inflammation. This finding, in itself, is not diagnostic because it also occurs in other infectious, inflammatory, and neoplastic pulmonary disorders. Nonetheless, the association of considerable uptake of gallium in the lungs accompanied by appreciable uptake in the parotid or lacrimal glands and hilar lymph nodes is highly suggestive of sarcoidosis.

Angiotensin-converting enzyme (ACE) Elevated serum ACE levels are seen in 50 to 80 percent of patients. This finding is not specific for sarcoidosis and therefore is of limited diagnostic value.

Kveim reaction This test involves the intradermal injection of a sterile suspension of splenic material obtained from patients with active sarcoidosis. A positive result consists of the development of a papule 4 to 6 weeks after injection which, on histologic examination, reveals noncaseating granulomas. Because of the lack of standardized preparations, the prolonged period of time involved, and the health risks posed by use of human material, this test has fallen into disuse.

DIFFERENTIAL DIGANOSIS

The diagnosis of sarcoidosis is made by excluding other diseases that can present with histologically and, in some instances, radiographically identical findings. These include mycobacterial and fungal infections, berylliosis, hypersensitivity pneumonitis, granulomatous vasculitides, talc granulomatosis, primary biliary cirrhosis, and regional enteritis. On occasion, granulomas identical to those of sarcoidosis may be found in association with certain malignancies, particularly lymphoma. This so-called sarcoid reaction is usually confined to draining lymph nodes, but may, on occasion, occur within the tumor itself.

NATURAL HISTORY AND PROGNOSIS

For the majority of patients with sarcoidosis, the disease follows a relatively benign course with a high rate of spontaneous resolution. Permanent impairment of pulmonary function as a result of irreversible interstitial fibrosis or airway narrowing occurs in approximately 20 percent of patients. The reported mortality rate is between 2 and 8 percent; respiratory failure, cor pulmonale, and aspergillus-associated massive hemoptysis account for the majority of deaths.

Although the course of sarcoidosis varies from patient to patient, several prognostic features have emerged. Patients in whom the disease is acute in onset tend to do better than those in whom the onset is insidious. This is especially true of patients who present with Lofgren's syndrome (acute onset of erythema nodosum and arthritis in association with a stage I radiograph) for whom complete resolution is likely. In African Americans, pulmonary involvement tends to be more severe, extrathoracic manifestations are more common, and irreversible organ damage (both pulmonary and extrapulmonary) is more likely. The radiographic stage of disease at the time of presentation is of prognostic import. In 50 to 80 percent of patients with stage I disease, the pulmonary disease undergoes spontaneous resolution, whereas only 40 to 60 percent with stage II and only 20 percent with stage III disease do so.

TREATMENT

Systemic corticosteroids are the mainstay of therapy for patients with active sarcoidosis. However, the extremely variable natural history and the lack of reliable criteria for predicting outcome in a particular patient make it difficult to set rigid guidelines for when to institute steroid therapy. Despite these uncertainties, it is generally agreed that patients with posterior uveitis, clinically evident cardiac involvement, symptomatic liver involvement, overt central nervous system disease, and hypercalcemia unresponsive to dietary manipulation should be treated.

With respect to pulmonary involvement, patients with stage I disease do not require corticosteroids unless the disease remains active and progresses. Patients with stage II and III disease are usually treated with corticosteroids, but some who are asymptomatic and in whom pulmonary function tests are only mildly impaired may be managed expectantly.

The usual starting dose of corticosteroid therapy is 40 mg prednisone daily or on alternate days depending on the severity of disease. Serial pulmonary function tests and chest radiographs are obtained as objective gauges of response to treatment. Monitoring of gallium scans, BAL cell populations, and serum ACE levels does not offer any advantage over chest radiographs and pulmonary function tests. After a favorable response has been achieved, the dose of prednisone is gradually tapered over several months in an attempt to eventually withdraw the drug or to continue it at the lowest dose that will maintain a remission. Relapse during tapering or after withdrawal of steroid therapy is common and long-term treatment is often required. In some patients with severe or progressive disease in whom steroids have proven unsuccessful or intolerable due to significant side effects, immunosuppressive agents such as methotrexate, chlorambucil, or azathioprine have been tried with anecdotal reports of success.

BIBLIOGRAPHY

For a more detailed discussion, see Johns CJ: Sarcoidosis, in Fishman AP (ed), *Pulmonary Diseases and Disorders,* 2d ed. New York, McGraw-Hill, 1988, pp 619–644.

Kotloff RM, Rossman MD: Sarcoidosis. Immunol Allergy Clin North Am 12:421–449, 1992.

Lynch JP, Stricter RM: Sarcoidosis, in DeRemee RA, Lynch JP (eds), *Immunologically Mediated Pulmonary Diseases,* Philadelphia, JB Lippincott, 1991, pp 189–216.

Joan Marie von Feldt   Peter E. Callegari

The collagen vascular diseases are multisystem inflammatory disorders in which autoimmune disturbances feature prominently. The lungs are often involved in these disorders, and the manifestations may be exceedingly diverse, i.e., pleural, parenchymal, airways, or vascular (Table 6-1).

RHEUMATOID ARTHRITIS

Although rheumatoid arthritis (RA) is primarily an articular disease, extra-articular manifestations are common. These include ocular (episcleritis), neurologic (peripheral neuropathy), lymphatic (lymphadenopathy, splenomegaly), hematologic (anemia, thrombocytopenia), pericardial, and pulmonary.

Rheumatoid factor (RF), an autoantibody reactive with IgG, is present in 75 percent of patients with chronic RA. However, this serologic parameter is not specific for RA. Other laboratory features of RA can include antinuclear antibody (ANA), circulating cryoglobulins, and low serum complement (usually seen in patients with associated vasculitis).

Rheumatoid nodules Microscopic lesions, identical histologically with subcutaneous rheumatoid nodules, are common in the lungs. However, the lesions are usually too small to be evident on the chest radiograph. When they are visible, they usually appear as single or multiple nodules, generally subpleural in location from a few millimeters to several centimeters in size; occasionally they are cavitary. As a rule, these nodules are harmless and significant only because of the diagnostic confusion they pose with other causes of nodular and cavitary lesions, e.g., malignancy, infection. Commonly, biopsy is required to exclude these other possibilities. A cavitary lesion occasionally either becomes secondarily infected or ruptures into the pleural space, causing a pneumothorax.

Caplan's syndrome Caplan's syndrome was originally described in coal miners as a triad consisting of pulmonary necrobiotic nodules, RA, and coal miner's pneumoconiosis (silicosis). More recently, pneumoconioses other than coal miner's pneumoconiosis, e.g., asbestosis, have been associated with this syndrome. Histologically, the pulmonary lesions are identical with rheumatoid nodules elsewhere except for the presence of mineral dust in the macrophages. RF is detectable in virtually all patients with Caplan's syndrome.

Interstitial lung disease Histologic evidence of interstitial lung disease can be found in up to 60 percent of patients with RA, even

TABLE 6-1 Pulmonary Manifestations of Collagen Vascular Diseases

Manifestations	RA	SLE	PM/DM	PSS	Sjögren's	AS
Pleural	++	++	0	0	0	0
Parenchymal						
Acute pneumonitis	0	++	0	+	+	0
Interstitial fibrosis	++	+	++	++	++	+
Nodules	++	0	0	0	0	0
BOOP	+	+	+	0	0	0
Airways	+	0	0	0	+	0
Malignancy						
Carcinoma	0	0	+	+	0	0
Lymphoma	0	0	0	0	+	0
Mechanical						
Aspiration	0	0	++	+	0	0
Ventilatory insufficiency	0	+	++	0	0	+
Vascular						
1° Pulmonary vasculopathy	+	+	0	++	0	0
Thromboembolism	0	+	0	0	0	0

0 = absent or extremely rare; + = uncommon; ++ = common; RA = rheumatoid arthritis; SLE = systemic lupus erythematosis; PM/DM = polymyositis and dermatomyositis; PSS = progressive systemic sclerosis; AS = ankylosing spondylitis; BOOP = bronchiolitis obliterans with organizing pneumonia.
SOURCE: Modified from Table 43-2, in Fishman AP (ed), *Pulmonary Diseases and Disorders*, 2d ed. New York, McGraw-Hill, 1988, p 646.

though abnormalities on the chest radiograph or in pulmonary function can be found in only 20 percent. The predominant form of interstitial disease is pulmonary fibrosis. Clinical manifestations include dyspnea and a nonproductive cough. The chest radiograph demonstrates bilateral reticular or reticulonodular infiltrates with a predilection for the lower lung fields. Pulmonary function tests reveal a restrictive pattern in which lung volumes and the diffusing capacity are decreased. The pulmonary disease usually progresses insidiously. It is poorly responsive to corticosteroids or cytotoxic agents.

In addition to pulmonary fibrosis, RA of the lungs is sometimes manifested histologically by either bronchiolitis obliterans with organizing pneumonia (BOOP), or cellular interstitial pneumonitis, or widespread interstitial deposition of rheumatoid nodules. In patients with RA who have been treated with gold, penicillamine, or methotrexate (see below), the possibility of drug-induced pneumonitis must be considered.

Pleural disease Pleural effusions occur in about 5 percent of patients with RA. As a rule, the effusion is unilateral and small to moderate in size. It may be asymptomatic or manifested by dyspnea or pleuritic chest pain. The pleural fluid is an exudate that contains high concentrations of protein and lactic dehydrogenase (LDH); lymphocytes are the predominant cells. Particularly characteristic of RA-associated effusions is a very low concentration of glucose and a low pH. Closed pleural biopsies show only nonspecific inflammation and fibrosis; they are primarily helpful in excluding malignancy and tuberculosis. Most rheumatoid effusions are self-limited and do not require therapy. Occasionally, tube thoracostomy is required for persistent, symptomatic effusions. Rarely is decortication required to deal with residual pleural thickening.

Obliterative bronchiolitis Obliterative bronchiolitis is characterized histologically by inflammation of the bronchioles leading to progressive fibrosis and obliteration of the small airways. Some reports have implicated penicillamine (administered therapeutically) as the cause of this complication.

Clinically, the patients complain of dyspnea. Pulmonary function studies demonstrate airflow obstruction and air trapping. The disease is generally refractory to treatment and often fatal. Anecdotal reports exist of improvement in response to corticosteroids or cyclophosphamide.

Upper airway involvement In up to 10 percent of patients with RA, cricoarytenoid arthritis produces hoarseness and cough. On rare occasion, cricoarytenoid involvement produces upper airway obstruction. Even rarer is upper airway obstruction caused by rheumatoid nodules on the vocal cords.

SYSTEMIC LUPUS ERYTHEMATOSUS

Eleven diagnostic criteria for systemic lupus erythematosis (SLE) have been set forth by the American College of Rheumatology (Table 6-2); the presence of four of these is required for definitive diagnosis.

The incidence of SLE in the general population is approximately 50/100,000. An SLE syndrome, predominantly manifest as a polyserositis, can be induced by a variety of agents including hydralazine, procainamide, quinidine, isoniazid, and diphenylhydantoin.

Pleurisy Pleurisy develops in one third of patients with SLE at some time during the course of their disease; it is the initial manifestation in 5 percent. Chest pain, worsened by inspiration, is the cardinal symptom of pleural involvement; cough, dyspnea, and fever frequently accompany the chest pain.

Pleural involvement is frequently, but not invariably, marked by the presence of pleural effusions. These effusions are usually small and bilateral; when unilateral, they occur more commonly on the left. The pleural fluid is exudative with few inflammatory cells. The glucose level and pH are usually normal, helping to distinguish

TABLE 6-2 American College of Rheumatology Criteria for the Diagnosis of Systemic Lupus Erythematosus

1. Malar rash
2. Discoid rash
3. Photosensitivity
4. Oral ulcers
5. Arthritis
6. Serositis (pleuritis or pericarditis)
7. Renal disorder (proteinuria or cellular casts)
8. Neurologic disorder (seizures or psychosis)
9. Hematologic disorder (hemolytic anemia or leukopenia or lymphopenia or thrombocytopenia)
10. Immunologic abnormality (positive lupus erythematosus prep or anti-dsDNA antibody or anti-Smith antibody or false-positive syphilis serology)
11. Antinuclear antibody

*Criteria for the diagnosis of SLE include the presence of four or more of the above.

lupus-related effusions from those associated with RA. Pleural fluid complement levels are often low. Although no feature of the pleural fluid is pathognomonic, the presence of lupus erythematosus cells in the pleural fluid, or a titer of ANA in pleural fluid that is greater than that of serum, is highly suggestive of lupus pleurisy.

Treatment of symptomatic patients usually begins with nonsteroidal anti-inflammatory drugs (NSAIDs). For more severe cases, systemic corticosteroids are used. Response to systemic corticosteroids is usually prompt and dramatic.

Pneumonitis Acute pneumonitis is a rare complication of SLE. It is characterized clinically by hypoxemia, dyspnea, fever, and diffuse pulmonary infiltrates. The infiltrates have a predilection for the bases and a pattern of alveolar consolidation. The lung injury is widespread and diffuse, and often mimics the adult respiratory distress syndrome both clinically and histologically. Immunoglobulins, immune complexes, and complement are deposited in the pulmonary capillaries, suggesting that the injury is immunologically mediated.

The treatment entails supportive care (the hypoxemia is difficult to correct), high doses of corticosteroids administered intravenously, and immunosuppressives, e.g., cyclophosphamide. Despite treatment, the mortality rate approaches 50 percent.

Pulmonary alveolar hemorrhage Pulmonary alveolar hemorrhage is another uncommon, but potentially life-threatening, complication of SLE. The syndrome begins with the abrupt onset of fever, cough, and dyspnea. Hemoptysis is common but rarely massive; the degree of hemoptysis often understates the severity of alveolar hemorrhage. Indeed, life-threatening alveolar hemorrhage can occur without hemoptysis. The chest radiograph reveals bilateral fluffy infiltrates. An otherwise unexplained drop in the hematocrit provides a valuable clue to the diagnosis. Bronchoscopic lavage yields bloody fluid; hemosiderin-laden macrophages are seen microscopically. High-dose corticosteroids are the mainstay of therapy; some clinics advocate the addition of a cytotoxic agent, e.g., cyclophosphamide. Despite intervention, the mortality rate is up to 70 percent.

Chronic interstitial pneumonitis Chronic interstitial lung disease is uncommon (incidence of < 5 percent) in the course of SLE. It is usually the sequel to a bout of acute lupus pneumonitis. Pulmonary function studies reveal a restrictive process in up to 50 percent of patients. However, often the impairment is due to respiratory muscle dysfunction rather than to interstitial lung disease itself. Dyspnea on exertion, basilar rales, and radiographic evidence of a bibasilar reticulonodular pattern are characteristic. Because chronic interstitial pneumonitis is so rare in SLE, its presence should prompt consideration of either an overlap syndrome or a mixed connective tissue disorder.

Diaphragmatic weakness/shrinking lung syndrome Some individuals with SLE develop a radiographic picture of progressively diminishing lung volumes and basilar atelectasis, without radiographic evidence of parenchymal lung disease. This entity, called *shrinking lung syndrome,* appears to be caused by diaphragmatic weakness which is unrelated to peripheral muscle dysfunction. The diagnosis is based on the demonstration of a restrictive defect on pulmonary function testing in association with a decrease in peak inspiratory and expiratory pressures. A reduction in the vital capacity of 25 percent or greater in moving from a seated to recumbent position provides additional support for diaphragmatic dysfunction. In case of doubt, measurement of transdiaphragmatic pressures by means of a double-lumen tube ending in esophageal and gastric balloons is required to establish diaphragmatic weakness. Treatment is reserved for patients with clinically significant compromise, i.e., dyspnea, impaired cough, or hypoxemia from atelectasis. Although corticosteroids and β-adrenergic agents have been used, reports of success are anecdotal.

Pulmonary hypertension The syndrome of primary pulmonary hypertension, both clinical and histologic, occasionally occurs in patients with proven SLE. An unexplained high incidence of positive ANA has been found in patients with primary pulmonary hypertension who have no other manifestations of SLE.

The incidence of pulmonary thromboembolic disease is high in patients with SLE and circulating antiphospholipid antibodies ("lupus anticoagulant"). In turn, recurrent or nonresolving pulmonary thromboembolism may lead to the development of pulmonary hypertension and cor pulmonale.

SCLERODERMA

In scleroderma, involvement of connective tissue can be widespread (progressive systemic sclerosis or PSS) or limited (CREST syndrome). Patients with CREST (*C*alcinosis, *R*aynaud's phenomenon, *E*sophageal dysmotility, *S*clerodactyly, and *T*elangiectasia) have a more favorable prognosis.

The skin often manifests thickening, fibrosis, hypo- and hyperpigmentation, telangiectasis, and cutaneous calcinosis. Ninety percent of the patients manifest Raynaud's phenomenon. The gastrointestinal tract, kidney, heart, and lungs may be involved.

Interstitial pulmonary fibrosis Radiographically, approximately 50 percent of patients with diffuse scleroderma manifest evidence of interstitial fibrosis; the incidence appears to be somewhat lower in patients with the CREST variant. The clinicoradiographic features are identical to those of idiopathic pulmonary fibrosis—insidious onset of dyspnea and cough associated with reticulonodular infiltrates that favor the lower lobes. Pulmonary function studies demonstrate a decrease in lung volumes and in diffusing capacity. The interstitial process tends to be slowly progressive, not infrequently culminating in honeycombing and respiratory failure.

Treatment of the interstitial fibrosis complicating scleroderma has been disappointing. Corticosteroids and cytotoxic agents have been of no benefit. A possible role for D-penicillamine has been suggested, but several clinical trials have failed to support this approach.

Pulmonary hypertension Pulmonary hypertension, *without* parenchymal lung disease, is a common, and often lethal, manifestation of scleroderma. Pulmonary hypertension has been found in up to 50 percent of patients with scleroderma, and even more in patients with CREST syndrome. Histologically, the disorder is indistinguishable from that of primary pulmonary hypertension. Initial suspicion that vasospasm of the pulmonary vasculature, akin to the peripheral vasospasm of Raynaud's phenomenon, contributes to the development of pulmonary hypertension has not withstood closer scrutiny.

The prognosis for patients with scleroderma who develop pulmonary hypertension is poor. A marked decrease in diffusing capacity (of ≤ 40 percent of predicted) portends a particularly poor prognosis, i.e., a 5-year survival rate of only 9 percent in one study. In general, pulmonary vasodilator agents, such as nifedipine, are not effective in scleroderma-associated pulmonary hypertension. In a few patients with severe pulmonary hypertension due to scleroderma who were free of clinical evidence of disease of other organs, lung transplantation has been successfully performed.

Other associated disorders   The incidence of bronchogenic carcinoma appears to be increased in patients with scleroderma. This incidence has been attributed to "scar carcinomas" arising in pulmonary fibrosis. Curiously, bronchoalveolar cell carcinoma predominates.

On rare occasion, restrictive lung disease has resulted from limitation of thoracic expansion by extensive skin involvement of the trunk.

Esophageal dysfunction, a common manifestation of scleroderma, predisposes to aspiration. This complication should be suspected when recurrent episodes of pneumonia involve the dependent segments of lung.

POLYMYOSITIS AND DERMATOMYOSITIS

Polymyositis and dermatomyositis (PM/DM) are inflammatory myopathies of unknown etiology characterized clinically by muscle weakness of the proximal limbs, neck, and pharyngeal muscles. Laboratory abnormalities include increased serum creatinine kinase, aldolase, LDH and transaminases, and frequently, autoantibodies. The electromyographic (EMG) pattern is one of spotty muscle necrosis, regeneration, and inflammation. Muscle biopsy reveals diffuse inflammatory infiltrates of lymphocytes and macrophages surrounding muscle fibers with evidence of muscle cell degeneration, variation in fiber size, and perifascicular atrophy. The diagnostic criteria include four of the following: proximal muscle weakness, increased concentrations of muscle enzymes in the serum, suggestive EMG findings, muscle biopsy, and characteristic skin findings.

The cutaneous manifestations of dermatomyositis may assume several characteristic forms: (1) an erythematous, scaly rash over the upper trunk and extensor surface of the extremities; (2) violaceous papules over the dorsal surface of the interphalangeal joints (Gottron's rash); and (3) a heliotrope rash over the eyelids.

Interstitial fibrosis   Approximately 5 to 10 percent of patients with PM/DM demonstrate radiographic evidence of interstitial lung disease. Lung disease usually occurs concurrently, or shortly after, the development of myopathy. However, in up to one third of patients, lung disease antedates muscle involvement. Dyspnea and nonproductive cough are typical symptoms. Although the onset is usually insidious, the presentation is sometimes fulminant. On the chest radiograph, the pattern is usually reticulonodular.

In patients with PM/DM, the presence of anti-Jo-1 antibody, an autoantibody directed against histidyl-tRNA-synthetase, correlates strongly with the presence of interstitial lung disease. In one large clinical series, anti-Jo-1 antibody was detected in 70 percent of patients with PM/DM who had interstitial lung disease, whereas it was found only in 7 percent of patients with PM/DM alone.

Histologically, the interstitial lung disease usually resembles idiopathic pulmonary fibrosis. However, in some patients with PM/DM, the histologic patterns are those of BOOP or widespread alveolar damage.

In contrast to the collagen vascular diseases discussed above, in up to 50 percent of patients with PM/DM and interstitial lung disease, the interstitial disease is responsive to corticosteroids. The more acute the onset of the lung disease, the more likely a favorable response. The likelihood of a favorable response is also greater in those with biopsy-demonstrated cellularity or BOOP.

Aspiration pneumonitis Aspiration pneumonitis is the most common pulmonary complication of PM/DM. It occurs in patients whose swallowing function is impaired because of weakness of the striated muscles of the soft palate, pharynx, and esophagus. Weakness of the expiratory muscles of respiration, with resultant diminution in the protective cough reflex, increases the likelihood of aspiration.

Respiratory muscle weakness Although diaphragmatic involvement is often documented at autopsy or biopsy, ventilatory insufficiency due to diaphragmatic dysfunction occurs in < 10 percent of patients. Those who do progress to respiratory failure usually have severe generalized weakness, dysphagia, and dysphonia. Overt respiratory failure is often preceded by the development of atelectasis and recurrent pneumonias; the latter is attributable to the combined effects of aspiration and the impaired ability to clear secretions. On pulmonary function testing, a restrictive pattern is found; a reduction in the maximum inspiratory pressure and a relatively normal diffusing capacity (corrected for lung volume) suggest that respiratory muscle weakness, and not the interstitial lung disease, is the root cause of the restrictive pattern. In addition, the occurrence of hypercapnia (generally in the preterminal stage of the disease) is often accompanied by weakness of the respiratory muscles.

Lung cancer PM/DM is associated with neoplasia in up to 10 percent of patients. Lung cancer is one of the more commonly associated malignancies.

SJÖGREN'S SYNDROME

Sjögren's syndrome is a chronic inflammatory disorder characterized by lymphocytic infiltration of the lacrimal and salivary glands. In > 50 percent of the patients, Sjögren's syndrome is associated with another connective tissue disease (secondary Sjögren's). RF is present in 90 percent of patients, even in the absence of RA. Ten percent of patients with Sjögren's syndrome have some clinical evidence of pulmonary involvement, most often either xerotrachea, obstructive airway disease, or interstitial lung disease.

Airway disease Desiccation of the tracheobronchial tree, resulting in a chronic dry cough, is a common pulmonary manifestation of Sjögren's syndrome. Biopsy of the airway, though rarely undertaken for diagnostic purposes, shows lymphocytic infiltration of the bronchial mucous glands. Desiccation of respiratory secretions and consequent impaired clearance mechanisms may account for the high incidence of bronchiectasis, bronchitis, and pneumonia.

Airflow obstruction, usually affecting the small airways, is common in patients with Sjögren's syndrome. Lymphocytic infiltration of the small airways, frequently demonstrated on biopsy of the airways, has been invoked to account for the increased resistance to airflow.

Interstitial lung disease Interstitial lung disease occurs radiographically in 4 percent of patients. Two distinct histologic patterns are seen: lymphocytic interstitial pneumonia (LIP) and interstitial fibrosis. LIP is characterized histologically by peribronchial, perivascular, and interstitial infiltration with lymphocytes and plasma cells. The natural history of this lesion is poorly defined; corticosteroid therapy is said to have promoted resolution in some patients. Lung biopsy is required to distinguish LIP from interstitial fibrosis because these two processes share common clinical, radiographic, and physiologic features.

Other manifestations In addition to LIP, two other lymphoproliferative disorders involving the lung may occur: pseudolymphoma and malignant lymphoma.

Pseudolymphoma, considered to be a premalignant lesion, is comprised of nodular aggregates of mature lymphocytes forming germinal centers; it does not involve regional lymph nodes.

Malignant lymphoma also presents as one or more nodular lesions; it is distinguished histologically from pseudolymphoma by the presence of immature lymphocytes, the absence of germinal centers, and the tendency to involve regional lymph nodes. The incidence of malignant lymphoma is 40 times greater in patients with Sjögren's syndrome than in the population at large.

ANKYLOSING SPONDYLITIS

Ankylosing spondylitis (AS) is one of the seronegative, i.e., RF negative, spondyloarthropathies affecting the sacroiliac joints and axial skeleton, as well as peripheral joints. A strong association exists between AS and HLA B27. Chest wall expansion is severely restricted in these patients because of fusion of the costovertebral joints impairing the normal bucket handle movement of the ribs. Despite this restriction, lung volumes tend to be relatively well preserved due to compensatory enhancement of diaphragmatic excursion.

Parenchymal lung involvement, in the form of apical fibrobullous disease, affects 1 percent of patients with AS, usually late in the course of the disease. Radiographically, these lesions often mimic tuberculosis. Although harmless, apical fibrobullous lesions often become the nidus for aspergilloma formation or for atypical mycobacterial infection.

PULMONARY COMPLICATIONS OF ANTIRHEUMATIC DRUGS

In approaching the patient with collagen vascular disease and an associated pulmonary complication, the possibility of drug-induced lung disease should be entertained. As shown in Table 6-3, a number of the agents commonly used to treat collagen vascular disease are associated with lung disease that often mimics that associated with the underlying disorder.

TABLE 6-3 Pulmonary Complications of the Antirheumatic Drugs

Drug	Interstitial pneumonitis/ fibrosis	Bronchio- litis obliterans	Noncardio- genic pulmonary edema	Alveolar hemorrhage
Gold	+	+	–	–
Penicillamine	+	+	–	+
Methotrexate	+	–	+	–
Cyclophospha- mide	+	–	+	–
Azathioprine	+	–	–	–
NSAIDs	–	–	+	–

BIBLIOGRAPHY

For a more detailed discussion, see Dickey BF, Myers AR: Pulmonary manifestations of collagen-vascular diseases, in Fishman AP (ed), *Pulmonary Diseases and Disorders,* 2d ed. New York, McGraw-Hill, 1988, pp 645–666.

King TE, Mortenson RL: Bronchoalveolar lavage in patients with connective tissue disease. J Thorac Imaging 7:20–40, 1992.

Lynch JP, Hunninghake CW: Pulmonary complications of collagen vascular disease. Annu Rev Med 43:17–35, 1992.

Pronk LC, Swaak AJ: Pulmonary hypertension in connective tissue disease. Report of three cases and review of the literature. Rheumatol Int 11:83–86, 1991.

Weidemann HP, Matthay RA: Pulmonary manifestations of the collagen vascular diseases. Clin Chest Med 10:677–722, 1989.

Gregory Underwood

DEFINITION

Hypersensitivity pneumonitis is a descriptive term characterizing a group of immunologically mediated granulomatous and interstitial lung diseases caused by inhalation of organic dust antigens. Depending on the source of the antigen, the disease may be referred to by any number of colorful names (Table 7-1). In Great Britain, this group of diseases is referred to as extrinsic allergic alveolitis. Recently, exposure to certain simple inorganic chemicals, such as isocyanates, has also been shown to produce this disease.

ETIOLOGY

Inhalation of antigenic particles, usually organic, is necessary for the development of hypersensitivity pneumonitis. Although these particles must be in the respirable range (1 to 5 μm aerodynamic diameter), surprisingly little is known about the components of these agents that render them antigenic. The list of agents implicated in causing hypersensitivity pneumonitis is continuously expanding (see Table 7-1).

Thermophilic actinomycetes, fungal antigens, and bird proteins are the most important etiologic agents implicated in hypersensitivity pneumonitis. The usual sources of exposure are moldy hay, silage, or grain; cooling and humidification systems; and bird droppings. However, any environment that promotes inhalation of appropriately sized antigenic particles can lead to this disease.

Exposure to antigens alone is not sufficient for disease to develop. Host factors are also important in the pathogenesis of hypersensitivity pneumonitis. For all causes of hypersensitivity pneumonitis, most individuals exposed to antigenic material remain disease free. For example, fewer than 10 percent of farmers exposed to thermophilic actinomycetes develop farmer's lung. The host factors responsible for induction of clinical disease in exposed individuals remain poorly defined. However, the disease is not related to atopy or HLA haplotype.

Curiously, cigarette smoking seems to offer some protection against developing hypersensitivity pneumonitis. Most patients with this disease are nonsmokers, and smoking is less common in exposed subjects who have the disease than in exposed subjects who do not have the disease. The reasons for this phenomenon are unknown. However, they may relate to the increased numbers of activated macrophages seen in the alveoli of smokers, which may contribute to more rapid and efficient clearance of antigenic particles from the lung.

TABLE 7-1 Hypersensitivity Pneumonitis (Extrinsic Allergic Alveolitis)

Disease	Antigen	Source of particles
Farmer's lung	Thermophilic actinomycetes	Moldy hay, grain, silage
Bird fancier's, breeder's, or handler's lung	Parakeet, budgerigar, pigeon, chicken, turkey proteins	Avian droppings or feathers
Humidifier or air conditioner lungs	Thermophilic actinomycetes, *Aureobasidium pullulans,* or other	Contaminated water in humidification and air conditioning systems
Bagassosis	Thermophilic actinomycetes	Moldy bagasse (sugar cane)
Malt worker's lung	*Aspergillus fumigatus* or *A. clavatus*	Moldy barley
Mushroom worker's lung	Thermophilic actinomycetes	Mushroom compost
Sequoiosis	*Pullularia, Graphium* species	Redwood sawdust
Maple bark disease	*Cryptostroma corticale*	Maple bark
Woodworker's lung	Wood dust; *Alternaria*	Oak, cedar, and mahogany dusts; pine and spruce pulp
Cheese washer's lung	*Penicillium casei*	Moldy cheese
Suberosis	Cork dust mold	Cork dust
Sauna taker's lung	Unknown	Contaminated sauna water
Pituitary snuff taker's lung	Animal proteins	Heterologous pituitary snuff
Coffee worker's lung	Coffee bean dust	Coffee beans
Miller's lung	*Sitophilus granarius* (wheat weevil)	Infested wheat flour
Fish meal worker's lung	Fish meal dust	Fish meal
Furrier's lung	Animal fur dust	Animal pelts
Lycoperdonosis	Puffball spores	*Lycoperdon* puffballs
Chemical worker's lung	Isocyanates	Polyurethane foam, varnishes, lacquer, foundry casting

SOURCE: Adapted from Richerson HB: Hypersensitivity pneumonitis (extrinsic allergic alveolitis), in Fishman AP (ed), *Pulmonary Diseases and Disorders,* 2d ed. New York, McGraw-Hill, 1988, p 668.

PATHOLOGY

In the acute stages of hypersensitivity pneumonitis, the typical histologic changes are a granulomatous interstitial pneumonitis composed of lymphocytes, macrophages, epithelioid cells, and a few giant cells with variable degrees of interstitial fibrosis. The granulomas are noncaseating and are generally confined to the acute and subacute phases of the disease. Lymphocytes are numerous as are large macrophages with foamy or finely vacuolated cytoplasm. Bronchiolitis obliterans frequently accompanies the interstitial pneumonitis but usually is not a predominant feature. Vasculitis is virtually never observed. Differentiation of the histopathology of hypersensitivity pneumonitis from infectious fungal diseases or sarcoidosis can sometimes be difficult.

In chronic hypersensitivity pneumonitis, histologic examination generally reveals interstitial fibrosis with focal collections of mononuclear cells. Granulomas are infrequent.

CLINICAL MANIFESTATIONS

Hypersensitivity pneumonitis may present in acute, subacute, or chronic forms.

Acute hypersensitivity pneumonitis is temporally related to exposure to the antigen. Coughing is frequently the initial complaint, occurring on exposure and often clearing when the patient leaves the area of antigenic contact. However, 4 to 12 h later, transient dyspnea, generalized malaise, myalgias, fevers, and chills may develop. These symptoms generally resolve spontaneously after a few hours to days, only to recur with each subsequent exposure to the antigen. Systemic manifestations usually do not progress, but dyspnea frequently worsens with each episode of antigen exposure.

The major physical findings in acute hypersensitivity pneumonitis are tachypnea, tachycardia, cyanosis, rales with wheezes, and fevers as high as 40°C (104°F). Chest radiographs typically reveal miliary nodules, 1 to 3 mm in diameter, in the lower lung fields. Leukocytosis, with predominance of polymorphonuclear cells, is present in most instances. Pulmonary function tests typically reveal a reduction in lung volumes, compliance, and diffusing capacity for carbon monoxide. In general, pulmonary function abnormalities return to normal within a few weeks to months if further antigen exposure is avoided.

Subacute hypersensitivity pneumonitis may resemble progressive chronic bronchitis and is not as clearly related to discrete episodes of antigen exposure. A productive cough, dyspnea, easy fatigability, and weight loss may be present. Pulmonary function tests may show both restrictive and obstructive abnormalities. Hypoxemia may be absent at rest but may become severe during exercise.

Chronic hypersensitivity pneumonitis occurs after prolonged exposure to organic dust antigens. This typically results in the gradual development of disabling pulmonary symptoms of dyspnea, cough, and weight loss. Chest radiographs tend to show interstitial fibrosis predominating in the upper lobes. This fibrosis may progress even though the antigen is avoided and despite corticosteroid therapy.

In chronic disease, the signs and symptoms that accompany discrete exposures may be lacking, making the diagnosis difficult.

Unlike other granulomatous lung diseases, hypersensitivity pneumonitis is confined to the lung and is not associated with extrapulmonary abnormalities. Additionally, pleural effusions, pleural thickening, hilar adneopathy, calcification, cavitation, atelectasis, and coin lesions are rarely, if ever, seen in hypersensitivity pneumonitis.

DIAGNOSIS

The diagnosis of hypersensitivity pneumonitis depends on a high degree of suspicion and eliciting a history that relates symptoms to exposure. A careful clinical history is essential and is often the first clue to the diagnosis. The typical history reveals symptoms of acute disease that begin 4 to 6 h after exposure to large quantities of causative antigens, such as moldy hay or birds. A history of exposure may be more difficult to establish in situations involving domestic exposures, such as to humidifiers or air conditioners. A history of exposure may be particularly difficult to unearth when chronic symptoms arise from low-level, long-term exposures.

Serum precipitins A precipitating antibody against the offending organic dust antigen is usually found in patients with hypersensitivity pneumonitis. However, the presence of precipitins is not pathognomonic. They may be present in up to 50 percent of exposed but disease-free people; in addition, precipitins are not demonstrable in all patients with disease. These false-negative results may be due to the wrong choice of antigen or to poor preparation of the antigen for testing.

Skin testing Skin test antigens are generally crude and nonspecifically irritating. For this reason, skin testing currently has no role in the diagnosis of hypersensitivity pneumonitis.

Inhalation challenge Inhalation challenge using isolated antigens may produce typical signs and symptoms of acute hypersensitivity pneumonitis. These symptoms typically occur 4 to 12 h following the challenge and conclusively implicate the tested antigen in the disease process. However, no standardized antigens or techniques exist, and the challenge may produce severe symptoms and hypoxemia in the tested patient. Consequently, inhalation challenge testing should not be performed without careful consideration of potential risks.

Bronchoalveolar lavage Bronchoalveolar lavage may aid in diagnosing hypersensitivity pneumonitis. Lavage fluid typically reveals large numbers of lymphocytes, most of which are T lymphocytes. The predominant T-cell subset is T8$^+$ (suppressor-cytotoxic subset).

Lavage fluid may also contain significantly increased levels of IgG, IgM, and total protein. Although lavage fluid may be informative, the results are nonspecific.

Lung biopsy Open lung biopsy is sometimes undertaken in patients from whom a classic history cannot be obtained. Transbronchial lung biopsy samples are generally of insufficient size for adequate histopathologic assessment. Although the pathologic findings seen at lung biopsy can be helpful, particularly in excluding other disease entities, no pathognomonic characteristics of hypersensitivity pneumonitis are known.

DIFFERENTIAL DIAGNOSIS

Acute hypersensitivity pneumonitis is most often confused with infectious pneumonias. In chronic forms of the disease, the differential diagnosis includes many causes of diffuse interstitial fibrosis including idiopathic pulmonary fibrosis, eosinophilic pneumonia, collagen vascular diseases, and bronchiolitis obliterans with organizing pneumonia (BOOP). Sarcoidosis may present with a similar clinical and histopathologic picture. However, as a rule, sarcoidosis causes hilar adenopathy or involves other organ systems.

TREATMENT

Avoidance of further antigen exposure is the only established treatment of hypersensitivity pneumonitis. In acute disease, avoidance of the antigen is often all that is necessary for complete remission of symptoms and return to normal pulmonary function. Although the efficacy of corticosteroids is unproven, they are often used for acute exacerbations and also to inhibit pulmonary fibrosis in the chronic disease state. The usual treatment regimen for acute disease involves prednisone at doses of 40 to 60 mg daily for 1 to 2 weeks followed by 1 to 2 weeks of tapering doses. Bronchodilators are indicated only if a component of airway obstruction is present. Hyposensitization therapy is not indicated in the management of hypersensitivity pneumonitis.

BIBLIOGRAPHY

For a more detailed discussion, see Richerson HB: Hypersensitivity pneumonitis (extrinsic allergic alveolitis), in Fishman AP (ed), *Pulmonary Diseases and Disorders,* 2d ed. New York, McGraw-Hill, 1988, pp 667–674.
Adler BD, Padley SP, Muller NL, Remy-Jardin M, Remy J: Chronic hypersensitivity pneumonitis: High-resolution CT and radiographic features in 16 patients. Radiology 185:91–95, 1992.
Fink JN: Hypersensitivity pneumonitis. Clin Chest Med 13:303–309, 1992.

Gurney JW: Hypersensitivity pneumonitis. Radiol Clin North Am 30:1219–1230, 1992.

Kokkarinen JI, Tukiainen HO, Terho EO: Recovery of pulmonary function in farmer's lung. Am Rev Respir Dis 147:793–796, 1993.

Teschler H, Pohl WR, Thompson AB, Konietzko N, Mosher DF, Costabel U, et al: Elevated levels of bronchoalveolar lavage vitronectin in hypersensitivity pneumonitis. Am Rev Respir Dis 147:332–337, 1993.

Robert M. Kotloff

DEFINITION

Originally, the term *Goodpasture's syndrome* was used to describe
the clinical syndrome of diffuse alveolar hemorrhage and glomerulonephritis without regard to the initiating mechanism. It has since
been recognized that the clinical presentation of alveolar hemorrhage and glomerulonephritis may occur in association with a
number of distinct disorders. Use of the term Goodpasture's
syndrome is now commonly restricted to those cases in which
anti-glomerular basement membrane (GBM) antibodies can be
detected in serum or by immunofluorescent staining of lung or renal
biopsy specimens. To avoid confusion, some authors have advocated the use of the more specific term *anti-GBM disease* to denote
this subset of patients.

Most patients with anti-GBM disease present with both pulmonary hemorrhage and glomerulonephritis (the classic combination
of Goodpasture's syndrome). However, approximately 20 percent
of patients present with glomerulonephritis alone. Although it is
rare for patients to present with alveolar hemorrhage without
clinically overt glomerulonephritis, kidney biopsies in these patients
invariably demonstrate the characteristic linear deposition of immunoglobulin along the GBM.

ETIOLOGY AND PATHOGENESIS

Although the stimulus for production of anti-GBM antibodies
remains unknown, it is clear that these autoantibodies play a central
role in the pathogenesis of Goodpasture's syndrome. Circulating
anti-GBM antibodies are detected in over 90 percent of patients,
and immunofluorescent staining of kidney tissue demonstrates
linear deposition of antibody along the glomerular basement membrane in virtually all patients. Although less commonly looked for
in the clinical setting, linear deposition of antibody has also been
demonstrated along the alveolocapillary basement membrane in
some cases. Passive transfer of anti-GBM antibodies from affected
patients to experimental animals results in glomerulonephritis but
does not produce linear deposition of antibody in the alveolocapillary membrane unless the lungs are first exposed to the toxic effects
of hyperoxia or hydrocarbons. This suggests that alteration of
alveolocapillary permeability is first required to permit access of
antibody to the basement membrane. Lending further support for
this mechanism is the clinical observation that nonspecific pulmo-

nary insults such as smoking, fluid overload, hydrocarbon exposure, and respiratory infections can precipitate alveolar hemorrhage in patients with anti-GBM disease.

Recently, the antigen against which the anti-GBM antibodies are directed has been identified as a constituent of the type IV collagen molecule. Although type IV collagen is a component of basement membranes throughout the body, the tissue-specific heterogeneity in its structure may account for the selective targeting of alveolar and glomerular basement membrane by the antibodies responsible for Goodpasture's syndrome.

Genetic factors may play a role in predisposition to the development of Goodpasture's syndrome. The incidence of the histocompatibility antigens HLA-DRw2 and HLA-B7 is higher than in the population at large. In addition, familial clustering of cases has been reported.

PATHOLOGY

Microscopic examination of lung tissue reveals evidence of diffuse alveolar hemorrhage, with filling of the alveolar spaces by hemosiderin-laden macrophages. The interstitium is widened due to accumulation of neutrophils. Evidence of vasculitis is notably absent.

Microscopic examination of renal tissue usually demonstrates a necrotizing, proliferative glomerulonephritis with extensive crescent formation. Less commonly, the proliferative process is only mild and focal. Importantly, by light microscopy the renal lesions of Goodpasture's syndrome are indistinguishable from other glomerulonephritides. The hallmark of Goodpasture's syndrome is the demonstration by immunofluorescent staining of linear deposition of immunoglobulin, usually IgG, along the glomerular and alveolocapillary basement membranes. In approximately two thirds of cases, a similar pattern of complement (C3) deposition is seen.

EPIDEMIOLOGY

Anti-GBM disease, involving both the lungs and kidneys (i.e., classic Goodpasture's syndrome), most commonly affects young men, with the peak incidence in the second to fourth decades of life. Renal involvement alone is more commonly seen in older women.

The incidence of cigarette smoking is higher in patients presenting with both alveolar hemorrhage and glomerulonephritis than in patients who present with glomerulonephritis alone, suggesting that smoking may be a risk factor for lung involvement in patients with anti-GBM disease.

ABNORMAL PHYSIOLOGY

A reduction in lung volumes is seen due to filling of alveolar air spaces with blood. During an acute episode of hemorrhage, the diffusing capacity for carbon monoxide is often abnormally high because of the uptake of carbon monoxide by red blood cells in the alveoli. Alveolar filling with blood leads to the development of low ventilation-perfusion areas or shunt or both, resulting in arterial hypoxemia.

CLINICAL MANIFESTATIONS

History The most common presenting complaint is hemoptysis, which may vary in severity from mild blood-streaked sputum to massive bleeding. The magnitude of the hemoptysis does not necessarily reflect the extent of alveolar hemorrhage so that life-threatening bleeding may occur in the absence of gross hemoptysis. Other respiratory complaints include dyspnea, cough, and chest discomfort. A flulike illness often precedes the onset of hemoptysis. Symptoms referable to renal involvement are usually absent, but gross hematuria and abdominal or flank pain may rarely occur.

Physical examination With extensive alveolar hemorrhage, patients may present in marked respiratory distress. Rales or rhonchi are heard in one third to one half of patients. Pallor may be present if the anemia is severe.

USUAL DIAGNOSTIC TESTS

Chest radiography During episodes of acute alveolar hemorrhage, the chest radiograph typically demonstrates diffuse, bilateral alveolar infiltrates. After the bleeding stops, the alveolar infiltrates quickly resolve; residual reticulonodular infiltrates sometimes persist for up to 2 weeks. After chronic, recurrent hemorrhage, interstitial changes may persist indefinitely.

Pulmonary function tests The most useful pulmonary function test in determining the presence of alveolar hemorrhage is the diffusing capacity for carbon monoxide. As noted above, the diffusing capacity is abnormally high due to the uptake of carbon monoxide by intra-alveolar erythrocytes. A value for the diffusing capacity that is > 30 percent above baseline strongly suggests acute hemorrhage and is a more sensitive indicator than the chest radiograph. The diffusing capacity usually returns to baseline within 48 h after bleeding stops. Lung volumes decrease after alveolar hemorrhage. Arterial hypoxemia and hypocapnia frequently are present.

Routine laboratory evaluation Anemia, characteristically microcytic and hypochromic, is a feature of Goodpasture's syndrome. If otherwise unexplained, a decrease in hemoglobin concentration of at least 2 g in 24 h suggests fresh alveolar bleeding. Azotemia is present in more than two thirds of patients at the time of presentation. In the great majority of patients, gross or microscopic hematuria and proteinuria are present; some patients have red blood cell casts in their urine.

SPECIAL DIAGNOSTIC EVALUATION

Detection of circulating anti-GBM antibodies Circulating anti-GBM antibodies can be demonstrated by either a radioimmunoassay or enzyme-linked immunosorbent assay (ELISA). When performed by an experienced laboratory, these assays are both highly sensitive and specific for anti-GBM disease. Serial measurements of anti-GBM antibodies can be used to monitor response to therapy.

Renal biopsy Although renal biopsy is invasive, it provides the most expeditious means of establishing a diagnosis of Goodpasture's syndrome. Immunofluorescent staining of renal tissue reveals the characteristic linear deposition of immunoglobulin along the GBM. Renal biopsy should be used when results of anti-GBM antibody assays cannot be promptly obtained or are equivocal.

Bronchoscopy When the etiology of diffuse alveolar infiltrates remains in doubt, e.g., when hemoptysis is absent or scant, the presence of diffuse alveolar hemorrhage can be confirmed by demonstration of hemosiderin-laden macrophages in sputum and in bronchoalveolar lavage fluid. Although the diagnosis of Goodpasture's syndrome can sometimes be made by immunofluorescent staining of transbronchial biopsy specimens, the diagnostic yield from transbronchial biopsies is far less than that of renal biopsy.

DIFFERENTIAL DIAGNOSIS

It is important to note that a third or more of patients presenting with pulmonary hemorrhage and glomerulonephritis have etiologies other than anti-GBM diseases (Table 8-1).

THERAPY AND PROGNOSIS

The treatment of Goodpasture's syndrome involves the combined use of plasmapheresis, cytotoxic agents (cyclophosphamide or azathioprine), and corticosteroids. Plasmapheresis is used for the initial 2-week period to effect a rapid reduction in the level of circulating anti-GBM antibodies. Cytotoxic agents and corticosteroids are used to suppress antibody formation. They are given for 2 to 3 months or until anti-GBM antibodies are no longer detectable in the blood.

TABLE 8-1 Diverse Etiologies of Pulmonary Hemorrhage and
Glomerulonephritis

Goodpasture's syndrome (anti-GBM disease)
Systemic lupus erythematosus
Wegener's granulomatosis
Mixed essential cryoglobulinemia
Polyarteritis nodosa
Lymphomatoid granulomatosis
Allergic angiitis and granulomatosis (Churg-Strauss)
Hypersensitivity angiitis
Henoch-Schönlein purpura
D-Penicillamine toxicity
Idiopathic

SOURCE: Modified from Wilson CB: Immunological diseases of the lung and kidney (Goodpasture's syndrome), in Fishman AP (ed), *Pulmonary Diseases and Disorders*, 2d ed. New York, McGraw-Hill, 1988, p 675.

In most patients, this combined therapy appears to be beneficial in controlling alveolar hemorrhage. Response of the renal disease to therapy varies and depends on how severely the kidneys have been damaged by the time treatment is initiated. Even though oliguric renal failure is regarded as a poor prognostic indicator, striking improvement in renal function has occurred in some instances, favoring an aggressive therapeutic approach to renal failure. Nonetheless, in patients who present with anuric renal failure or in whom renal biopsy shows more than 90 percent crescents, irreversible renal failure is inevitable. In these patients, treatment is indicated only if concurrent alveolar hemorrhage is present.

In addition to the therapeutic regimen outlined above, attempts should be made to identify and correct factors which may have contributed to the precipitation of alveolar hemorrhage. Among these are fluid overload, infection, exposure to toxic fumes, and smoking. Ventilatory support is indicated for patients with severe hypoxic respiratory failure. High concentrations of inspired oxygen have been implicated in the precipitation of alveolar hemorrhage; efforts should be made to minimize the fraction of inspired oxygen, using positive end-expiratory pressure if necessary.

Despite current therapy, the 2-year mortality rate for Goodpasture's syndrome is about 50 percent. Because of the ability of dialysis to support patients with renal failure, the major cause of death now is alveolar hemorrhage. Patients who survive the initial episode of bleeding may experience recurrent episodes after therapy is withdrawn.

BIBLIOGRAPHY

For a more detailed discussion, see Wilson CB: Immunological diseases of
the lung and kidney (Goodpasture's syndrome), in Fishman AP (ed),

Pulmonary Diseases and Disorders, 2d ed. New York, McGraw-Hill, 1988, pp 675–682.

Hudson BG, Kalluri R, Gunwar S, Noelken ME, Mariyama M, Reeders ST: Molecular characteristics of the Goodpasture autoantigen. Kidney Int 43:135–139, 1993.

Leatherman JW: Diffuse alveolar hemorrhage in immune and idiopathic disorders, in Lynch JP, DeRemee RA (eds), *Immunologically Mediated Pulmonary Diseases.* Philadelphia, JB Lippincott, 1991, pp 473–498.

Weber MF, Andrassy K, Pullig O, Koderisch J, Netzer K: Antineutrophil-cytoplasmic antibodies and antiglomerular basement membrane antibodies in Goodpasture's syndrome and in Wegener's granulomatosis. J Am Soc Nephrol 2:1227–1234, 1992.

Wiseman KC: New insights on Goodpasture's syndrome. ANNA J 20:17–26, 1993.

Young KR: Pulmonary-renal syndromes. Clin Chest Med 10:655–675, 1989.

Paul Richman

DEFINITION

The term *eosinophilic pneumonia* encompasses a variety of different syndromes of diverse etiologies, the common denominator of which is eosinophilic pulmonary infiltrates. Often, but not invariably, the pulmonary eosinophilia is accompanied by eosinophilia in the peripheral blood and sputum. In addition to eosinophils, the inflammatory process in the lungs usually includes many histiocytes and, to a lesser extent, other inflammatory cells. The association of eosinophilic pulmonary infiltrates and eosinophilia in the peripheral blood is also referred to as the *PIE (pulmonary infiltrates with eosinophilia) syndrome.*

Attempts to sort the eosinophilic pneumonias into separate groups based either on pathology, clinical features, or presumed etiology have achieved no consensus. A classification based on etiology (Table 9-1) has proved most acceptable. Included in the etiologic categorization of the eosinophilic pneumonias are such unrelated entities as parasitic infection, drug-induced pulmonary eosinophilia, PIE in association with preexisting asthma, Churg-Strauss syndrome, and chronic eosinophilic pneumonia. Conspicuously absent from this list are a number of common pulmonary diseases in which peripheral blood eosinophilia sometimes occurs, but without predominantly eosinophilic infiltrates. These include sarcoidosis, Hodgkin's disease, tuberculosis, and lung cancer. Also omitted is eosinophilic leukemia, a rare disorder which frequently involves lung tissue.

THE ROLE OF THE EOSINOPHIL

Eosinophils play a central role in two major immune responses: host defense against parasitic infiltration and immediate hypersensitivity to allergic stimuli. These cells are uniquely equipped to defend against helminths: major basic protein, the chief protein constituent in the core of the eosinophilic granules, promotes adherence to helminths, whereas cationic proteins in the granule matrix are strongly helminthicidal. In animals, selective depletion of eosinophils using antisera diminishes resistance to parasitic infection.

Through interactions with mast cells, eosinophils modulate type I immediate hypersensitivity, the presumed immunopathogenetic mechanism underlying a number of the PIE disorders, including those associated with asthma, *Aspergillus* colonization of the airways, and drug-induced reactions. Mast cells in the lung release a number of mediators which recruit and activate eosinophils; in turn,

TABLE 9-1 Etiologic Classification of Eosinophilic Pneumonia

Eosinophilic pneumonia due to parasitic infestation (Loeffler's syndrome)
Eosinophilic pneumonia induced by chemicals
Eosinophilic pneumonia associated with the asthmatic syndrome
  Bronchial asthma
  Mucoid impaction of bronchi
  Bronchopulmonary aspergillosis
Eosinophilic pneumonia seen with infections
Eosinophilic pneumonia in association with hypersensitivity disorders
and systemic angiitis
  Periarteritis nodosa
  Allergic angiitis and granulomatosis (Churg-Strauss syndrome)
Eosinophilic pneumonia of unknown etiology (chronic eosinophilic
pneumonia)

SOURCE: Table 46-1 from Mayock RL, Iozzo RV: The eosinophilic pneumonias, in Fishman AP (ed), *Pulmonary Diseases and Disorders,* 2d ed. New York, McGraw-Hill, 1988, p 684.

leukotrienes released by eosinophils are capable of inducing bronchoconstriction and bronchial gland hypersecretion while major basic protein is directly injurious to airway epithelial cells. Oppositely, eosinophils can down-regulate mast cell activity by releasing enzymes that degrade mast cell products including histamine, platelet activating factor, and leukotrienes. Thus, the eosinophil appears to be capable of both augmenting and inhibiting immediate hypersensitivity reactions; the factors which determine the balance between these offsetting influences are not well understood.

SPECIFIC DISEASES AND DISORDERS

Parasitic Infestation

Loeffler's Syndrome

In 1932, Loeffler recorded several cases of a mild transient illness that were due to the passage of *Ascaris lumbricoides* larvae through the lung. Other parasites may also cause Loeffler's syndrome. The syndrome is characterized by a mild cough, usually productive of sputum containing eosinophils, fever that resolves spontaneously in a week, and peripheral blood eosinophilia. Occasionally an adult worm is coughed up. The pulmonary infiltrates are patchy, occur most often at the lung bases, and clear in 2 weeks without treatment.

The peripheral blood eosinophilia can last longer than the pulmonary eosinophilia in keeping with the life cycle of the worm. The ingested eggs hatch into larvae in the bowel and then pass to the lungs via the portal circulation and mesenteric lymph channels; from the lung parenchyma they pass up the airway to the pharynx where they are swallowed and complete maturation to the adult stage in the gut. This sequence explains why ova and parasites are not found in the stool until approximately 2 months after pulmonary transit.

Because the disease runs a benign course, only few histologic examinations have been made. These have shown a patchy bronchopneumonia in which eosinophils and histiocytes predominate in association with a rare giant cell. Ascaris larvae are rarely found in the lungs, suggesting that hypersensitivity to the worm, rather than direct toxic effects, account for the pulmonary manifestations. Although heavy or repeated infestations can cause a chronic recurring course, as a rule, the disorder is self-limited. Specific antiparasitic drugs are required only to treat the consequences of a heavy intestinal infestation of worms, such as obstruction and malnutrition.

Tropical Eosinophilia

This parasitic PIE syndrome is distinct from Loeffler's syndrome and appears to be due to hypersensitivity to filarial worms. It is endemic in the tropical regions of Asia, South America, and Africa. Clinically, the disease is characterized by chronic symptoms of weight loss, fever, and nocturnal dyspnea. On physical examination, generalized lymphadenopathy is the most striking feature. Rales are usually heard at the lung bases; wheezing occurs in paroxysms, usually at night. In the acute form of the disease, pulmonary function tests characteristically demonstrate airflow obstruction; in the chronic form, a restrictive pattern may ensue. The chest radiograph usually shows a nodular interstitial infiltrate, most marked at the lung bases. Sometimes the hilar lymph nodes are enlarged.

Pertinent laboratory findings include a marked blood eosinophilia (the absolute count is sometimes as high as 20,000 mm³), increased IgE levels, and the presence of complement fixing antibodies to filaria; unfortunately, the latter are not specific. Histologically, the inflammatory process is characterized by peribronchial eosinophilia and mononuclear cell infiltrates.

If untreated, the disease often remits spontaneously. However, late relapses and a chronic course resulting in pulmonary fibrosis are not rare. For this reason, diethylcarbamazine is generally recommended (3 mg/kg tid for 2 weeks). A favorable clinical response to this agent, accompanied by improvement in the radiographic abnormalities, may take weeks.

Drug-Induced Pulmonary Eosinophilia

Many drugs and inorganic chemicals can induce a hypersensitivity response that presents clinically as the PIE syndrome. A partial list

TABLE 9-2 Partial List of Compounds and Elements Reported to be Associated with Eosinophilic Pneumonia

Acetylsalicylic acid	Methylphenidate
Aminosalicylic acid (PAS)	Nickel carbonyl
Amiodarone	Nitrofurantoin (Furandantin)
Azathioprine	Penicillins
Beclomethasone diproprionate inhaler	Poison ivy desensitization
Beryllium	Pollen inhalation
Bleomycin	Salazopyrin
Carbamazepine	Smoke inhalation
Chlorpropamide	Streptomycin
Chromoglycate	Sulfonamides
Clofibrate	Sulfonylureas
Desipramine	Talazamide
Gold salts	Tetracyclines
Isoniazid	Thiazides
Mecamylamine	Thiopramine
Mephenesin	Tolbutamide
Methotrexate	Tricyclic antidepressants

SOURCE: Table 46-3 from Mayock RL, Iozzo RV: The eosinophilic pneumonias, in Fishman AP (ed), *Pulmonary Diseases and Disorders,* 2d ed. New York, McGraw-Hill, 1988, p 687.

of these agents is given in Table 9-2. As a rule, acute dyspnea, fever, and cough become manifest within a week after exposure to the offending agent; in some instances, these symptoms may take up to 3 months to appear. The chest radiograph reveals diffuse or patchy infiltrates. Peripheral eosinophilia may be marked (up to 80 percent of the total leukocyte count). In one clinic, the diffusing capacity for carbon monoxide was the most common abnormality in pulmonary function. All manifestations usually resolve promptly after the drug is discontinued. One exception to this rule is nitrofurantoin, which may cause a subacute or chronic (> 6 months) PIE syndrome, even after the drug is withdrawn. In the chronic form of nitrofurantoin pulmonary disease, other systemic manifestations of allergic disease may coexist, including rash and a lupuslike syndrome. Anecdotal accounts suggest that corticosteroids may be beneficial in the treatment of the chronic phase of this disorder.

PIE with Preexisting Asthma

A small number (< 1%) of chronic asthmatics develop the PIE syndrome. This frequency is greater than that of PIE in the nonasthmatic population. In many of these patients the etiology is unclear. In those in whom the asthma is allergic in etiology, the eosinophilia is associated with mucous hypersecretion, mucous plugging, and postobstructive infiltrates on the chest radiograph.

Three distinct syndromes in which PIE occurs in patients with preexisting asthma warrant special attention: allergic bronchopulmonary aspergillosis, Churg-Strauss syndrome, and chronic eosinophilic pneumonia.

Allergic Bronchopulmonary Aspergillosis (ABPA)

ABPA is more common in Great Britain than in the United States. The inflammatory response to heavy *Aspergillus* colonization of the airway is important in the pathogenesis of this disorder. The major diagnostic criteria include (1) a history of asthma; (2) pulmonary infiltrates (often fleeting and migratory); (3) peripheral blood eosinophilia; (4) a positive immediate skin test; (5) serum IgG precipitins to *Aspergillus;* (6) an increased IgE level; and (7) proximal saccular bronchiectasis. Although not essential for the diagnosis, additional support can be provided by the demonstration of the characteristic fungal elements on staining of sputum or recovery of *Aspergillus* species on culture. Bronchiectasis occurs as a consequence of chronic plugging and inflammatory responses in the airways. It is often discernible on the conventional chest radiograph, but high-resolution CT may be required to disclose the less severe forms of this disease.

The goals of therapy for ABPA are to prevent irreversible changes in bronchial architecture as well as to control bronchospasm. Prednisone, at an initial dose of approximately 1 mg/kg daily, is the drug of choice. Prednisone decreases the frequency of subsequent pulmonary infiltrates, controls asthmatic symptoms, and possibly prevents the progression of the airway disease to parenchymal lung damage. Antibiotics directed at *Aspergillus* have not proved successful at eradicating the heavy fungal colonization.

Eosinophilia with Necrotizing Angiitis (Churg-Strauss Syndrome)

In this rare disorder, the PIE syndrome is simply a pulmonary manifestation of a systemic vasculitis; the syndrome is generally viewed as a variant of polyarteritis nodosa (PAN). Consistently, the patients are asthmatics who present with fever, weight loss, dyspnea, and cough. Aside from the lungs, the organ most often involved is the heart, causing acute coronary occlusion or pericardial effusion. The skin may be involved, characteristically with palpable purpura of the legs. Involvement of the prostate may cause urinary retention. Angiitis of the abdominal viscera may produce ulceration and bowel perforation.

On the chest radiograph, the most common abnormalities are migratory patchy infiltrates or large nodules which may cavitate. Peripheral eosinophilia is the rule; it is often marked. Histologic examination of an open lung biopsy is diagnostic: it shows necrotizing peribronchial granulomas and vasculitis of small arteries and veins with eosinophilic infiltration of the vascular walls. In the process of healing, the vasculitis culminates in progressive scarring and occlusion of vessels. This disease differs histologically from periarteritis nodosa in that the infiltrate in periarteritis nodosa is neutrophilic rather than eosinophilic, medium-sized (rather than small-sized) arteries are affected in periarteritis nodosa, and that the granulomas in periarteritis nodosa are confined to the vascular wall.

In many patients, the course is fulminant, ending in death. In some instances, corticosteroids or immunosuppressive therapy seem to ameliorate the course and to enable long-term survival.

Chronic Eosinophilic Pneumonia

This is a rare disorder originally described on the basis of a respiratory syndrome that featured a distinctive radiographic appearance of the chest in which dense peripheral infiltrates took the form of the "photographic negative" of pulmonary edema. Since then, patchy, randomly distributed infiltrates on the chest radiograph have proved to be just as common. Nonetheless, the entity has persisted on the basis of a distinctive clinical syndrome coupled with a characteristic histology.

Chronic eosinophilic pneumonia usually occurs in middle-aged women with preexisting asthma, often many years in duration. The clinical picture is characterized by a subacute respiratory illness consisting of fever, dyspnea, cough, and weight loss. Peripheral blood eosinophilia is not universally present. The histology, afforded either by bronchoscopy or surgery, reveals intra-alveolar and interstitial infiltration with eosinophils and histiocytes; bronchiolitis obliterans occurs in 25 percent of patients. The diagnosis is most firmly established on the basis of the presence of the distinctive histology, although a therapeutic trial with corticosteroids may suffice if the clinical picture is sufficiently distinctive: remarkably quick resolution of fever and cough (12 to 24 h) and clearing of the chest radiograph (1 to 2 weeks) are the rule. Although the course is usually benign, relapse is common if prednisone is discontinued before 6 months. Approximately 12 months of prednisone therapy is advisable, beginning at 40 to 60 mg daily for 2 weeks followed by gradual tapering.

Diagnostic Approach to the PIE Syndrome

Many instances of pulmonary infiltrates and peripheral eosinophilia occur as uncommon manifestations of common diseases, e.g., tuberculosis, sarcoidosis, and neoplasm. Once these diseases are excluded, then other conditions, such as drug-induced eosinophilia and asthma-associated PIE syndrome, become high in the differential diagnosis. A detailed history of current and previous medications is essential in diagnosing drug-induced eosinophilia. If ABPA is suspected, appropriate skin and serologic tests should be performed and the sputum sent for special stains and culture. Because patients may harbor an *Ascaris* infection without a history of travel to tropical regions, it is important to look for stool ova and parasites (repeatedly). The Churg-Strauss syndrome and chronic eosinophilic pneumonia are rare; the chest radiograph often gives strong clues to these entities and systemic symptoms are common. Lung biopsy should be performed to assess these possibilities especially when a course of corticosteroid therapy is being contemplated.

BIBLIOGRAPHY

For a more detailed discussion, see Mayock RL, Iozzo RV: The eosinophilic pneumonias, in Fishman AP (ed), *Pulmonary Diseases and Disorders,* 2d ed. New York, McGraw-Hill, 1988, pp 683–698.

Kay AB: The eosinophil, in Fishman AP (ed), *Pulmonary Diseases and Disorders,* 2d ed. New York, McGraw-Hill, 1988, pp 599–606.

Roig J, Romeu J, Riera C, Texido A, Domingo C, Morera J: Acute eosinophilic pneumonia due to toxocariasis with bronchoalveolar lavage findings. Chest 102:294–296, 1992.

Umeki S: Reevaluation of eosinophilic pneumonia and its diagnostic criteria. Arch Intern Med 152:1913–1919, 1992.

Robert M. Kotloff

DEFINITION

Idiopathic pulmonary fibrosis (IPF) is a chronic inflammatory disorder of the lung parenchyma which progresses at a variable pace to widespread interstitial fibrosis and irreversible destruction of normal lung architecture. IPF is referred to by some investigators as *cryptogenic fibrosing alveolitis,* a more descriptive term which highlights the inflammatory as well as the fibrotic nature of this disorder.

A distinction is made between IPF occurring as an isolated pulmonary process (so-called lone IPF) and IPF that occurs in association with a collagen vascular disease. Approximately 10 to 20 percent of patients who fulfill the criteria for IPF have, or will develop, an associated collagen vascular disease, most often rheumatoid arthritis, scleroderma, or polymyositis. The distinction between lone IPF and collagen vascular disease-associated IPF is, to a large extent, artificial because the clinical, radiographic, and histologic features of these two entities are identical, and ample evidence suggests common pathogenetic mechanisms.

ETIOLOGY AND PATHOGENESIS

The etiology of IPF is unknown and its pathogenesis is somewhat speculative. Nonetheless, the accumulation of immune and inflammatory effector cells within the interstitium and alveolar airspaces, i.e., an alveolitis, seems to be the precursor of both the parenchymal injury and the subsequent fibrosis. The numbers of macrophages and neutrophils in bronchoalveolar lavage fluid from patients with IPF are dramatically increased; the numbers of lymphocytes and eosinophils are also increased, but more modestly and less consistently. Activation of alveolar macrophages, possibly by locally formed immune complexes, appears to be a crucial step in triggering the inflammatory cascade; the release of neutrophil chemotactic factors by these activated macrophages attracts neutrophils to the lungs. Together, macrophages and neutrophils are capable of inducing tissue injury; oxygen radicals released by these cells are directly cytotoxic to the cellular constituents of the alveolar septae, whereas proteases elaborated by these cells degrade components of the interstitial matrix.

Mediators released by activated macrophages, notably platelet-derived growth factor, alveolar macrophage-derived growth factor, and fibronectin, also seem to have an essential role in modulating the fibrotic stage in IPF. These peptides orchestrate the recruitment and proliferation of lung fibroblasts, their attachment to the extracellular matrix, and the production of collagen.

PATHOLOGY

IPF principally affects the alveolar interstitium. The two histologic patterns associated with IPF are desquamative interstitial pneumonitis (DIP) and usual interstitial pneumonitis (UIP). The two patterns are not mutually exclusive and features of each may be found in the same biopsy specimens. The relationship between UIP and DIP is unsettled; although they may represent two distinct variants, most investigators view them as sequential stages of disease, with DIP representing the earlier, more inflammatory phase.

Desquamative interstitial pneumonitis is characterized by an inflammatory cell infiltration of the alveolar interstitium, comprised predominantly of lymphocytes with a smaller number of eosinophils, mast cells, and plasma cells. Despite the preponderance of neutrophils recovered by bronchoalveolar lavage, these cells are seen only occasionally on histologic examination. Most striking in DIP is the presence of a large number of cells filling the alveolar airspaces. Originally believed to be desquamated type II alveolar epithelial cells (thus the name), these cells are now recognized to be macrophages. Importantly, the alveolar architecture is relatively well preserved and fibrosis is minimal.

Usual interstitial pneumonitis is more commonly encountered than DIP. In contrast to DIP, the histologic picture of inflammation is less pronounced. Instead, the proliferation of fibroblasts and the deposition of collagen leads to progressive thickening and derangement of the alveolar walls. As the structural integrity of the alveolar wall is breached, the fibrotic process extends into the alveolar airspaces. Along with the interstitial fibrosis, characteristic changes occur in the alveolar epithelial cell lining. The flat, type I alveolar epithelial cells are replaced by cuboidal type II cells and by migrating bronchiolar epithelial cells, causing the alveolar wall to thicken further.

In the more advanced stage of UIP, the fibrotic process produces large cystic spaces that are lined by metaplastic bronchial epithelium. This *honeycomb lung* is nonspecific and represents the final common pathway of a number of inflammatory and fibrotic lung diseases.

PATHOPHYSIOLOGY

Mechanics The fibrotic process in the lungs produces characteristic abnormalities in pulmonary performance. Involvement of the alveolar walls by inflammation or fibrosis (or both) decreases the compliance of the lung. The lung volumes decrease and the work of breathing increases. In response to the increased work of breathing caused by the decreased distensibility of the lungs, the pattern of breathing in patients with IPF is rapid and shallow. Moreover, in contrast to the preferential increase in tidal volume that occurs in normal individuals during exercise, patients with IPF manifest a further increase in respiratory rate.

Airflow obstruction is not a feature of IPF. Indeed, expiratory flow rates at a particular lung volume are *increased* because of the increased elastic recoil of the lungs.

Gas exchange Arterial hypoxemia occurs at first only during exercise and later while at rest. Hypoxemia at rest is due predominantly to mismatching of ventilation and pulmonary blood flow. During exercise, impaired diffusion contributes to worsening hypoxemia; the transit time of blood through the capillary network quickens, leaving insufficient time for diffusion of oxygen through the thickened alveolar-capillary membrane.

Hyperventilation, a characteristic response to noncompliant lungs, maintains the alveolar and arterial P_{CO_2} at low levels through most of the course of IPF. In the advanced stages of disease, as ventilation-perfusion mismatching becomes extreme, hypercapnia supervenes.

Hemodynamics Pulmonary hypertension commonly occurs in the late stages of IPF and may lead to cor pulmonale. Factors contributing to the development of pulmonary hypertension include progressive obliteration of pulmonary vasculature by the fibrotic process and hypoxic vasoconstriction.

EPIDEMIOLOGY

IPF is a relatively uncommon disorder, with an estimated frequency of 3 to 5 cases per 100,000 population. It is, however, one of the more common causes of interstitial lung disease. IPF typically affects individuals in the 40- to 70-year age range. Men predominate by a slight margin. In the vast majority of cases the incidence is sporadic. A familial form, with an autosomal dominant pattern of inheritance also occurs, but its frequency is undetermined.

CLINICAL MANIFESTATIONS

History Dyspnea is the most common presenting symptom. It is typically insidious in onset and slowly progressive. Many patients also have a cough which is usually nonproductive. Less common symptoms include weight loss, fatigue, and arthralgias. In some patients, a flulike illness occurs at the start of the disease.

Physical examination The patients are frequently tachypneic, breathing rapidly and shallowly. A highly characteristic feature of IPF is the presence of fine end-inspiratory crackles ("Velcro" rales) that are best heard at the lung bases. Clubbing, encountered in 40 to 80 percent of patients, may provide another clue to the presence of IPF but typically occurs late in the course of disease. In the advanced stages of disease, findings suggestive of pulmonary hypertension (right ventricular heave, accentuated pulmonic component of S_2) and cor pulmonale (jugular venous distention, lower extremity edema, ascites) may be present. Central cyanosis accompanies profound hypoxemia.

DIAGNOSTIC EVALUATION

The diagnosis of IPF is based on identifying a characteristic constellation of clinical, radiographic, and histologic features. No single feature is pathognomonic (see Differential Diagnosis below).

Chest radiography The chest radiograph is normal in 10 to 15 percent of patients with IPF. The most common radiographic abnormality is a reticular or reticulonodular bilateral infiltrate that is most pronounced at the lung bases. Occasionally an alveolar filling pattern is seen; this pattern occurs in the early, cellular phase of disease. In the late stages of IPF, honeycombing occurs so that cystic spaces, 0.5 to 1.0 cm in diameter, are seen against the background of reticulonodular infiltrates.

High resolution computed tomography (HRCT) The 1- to 2-mm cuts afforded by this technique provide a detailed image of the lung parenchyma. IPF has a characteristic appearance on HRCT; the pulmonary involvement is patchy and reticular opacities are seen in a subpleural and basilar distribution. HRCT is also helpful in other ways in dealing with IPF. It is more sensitive than standard chest radiography in detecting interstitial lung disease and in defining the extent of involvement; it is more accurate in detecting the presence of honeycombing; and it assists in selection of suitable sites for biopsy.

Blood studies Laboratory studies are entirely nonspecific. The erythrocyte sedimentation rate and serum immunoglobulin levels are usually increased. Circulating autoantibodies (antinuclear antibody, rheumatoid factor) or immune complexes are detectable in up to 20 percent of patients; their presence alone does not signify that a collagen vascular disease is present.

Lung biopsy Histologic confirmation of suspected IPF is highly desirable both to enhance diagnostic certainty and to provide prognostic information. Unfortunately, transbronchial biopsy is not suitable for this purpose. The patchy nature of the pulmonary involvement in IPF, in combination with the small size of the specimens obtained, lead to a significant sampling error, i.e., the histologic features may be missed. Moreover, the finding of interstitial inflammation or fibrosis on transbronchial biopsy cannot be considered as diagnostic of IPF because the biopsy may not have included the histologic features diagnostic of another entity. Nonetheless, transbronchial biopsy does have a place in the diagnostic evaluation of patients with suspected IPF; it is done largely to exclude other entities that can be more readily diagnosed by this approach, e.g., sarcoidosis, malignancy, or infection.

Unless medically contraindicated, a surgical biopsy of the lung is recommended for all patients in whom bronchoscopy is nondiagnostic. Because of the patchy distribution of IPF, it is essential that the surgeon sample the more characteristic areas rather than areas that appear normal or extremely abnormal. Sampling from two sites is recommended. As noted above, HRCT may be useful preoperatively in guiding the surgeon to the optimal areas for biopsy. The recent introduction of thoracoscopy has greatly obviated the need for conventional thoracotomy. It permits surgical lung biopsies in patients who, only a short while ago, would have been considered too frail to undergo thoracic surgery.

DIFFERENTIAL DIAGNOSIS

The differential diagnosis of chronic interstitial lung disease is extensive (Table 10-1). A thorough and meticulous history, including occupational, environmental, and drug exposures, is essential in assessing the possibility of a number of these entities. Radiographic clues, e.g., pleural plaques, pleural effusions, hilar/mediastinal adenopathy, distribution and nature of parenchymal infiltrates, are frequently helpful in suggesting alternatives to IPF. Ultimately, distinction between many of these entities rests on histology.

NATURAL HISTORY AND PROGNOSIS

Although the natural history of IPF is somewhat variable, overall the prognosis is poor, with a median survival of only 5 years. Factors which portend a particularly poor prognosis include advanced age, long duration of symptoms (> 1 year), predominantly fibrosis on histologic examination, and lack of response to corticosteroids. Death is usually due to progressive respiratory failure, cor pulmonale, or a combination of the two. Complicating factors, such as infection, bronchogenic carcinoma, pulmonary embolism, and treatment-related side effects contribute importantly to morbidity as well as mortality.

TABLE 10-1 Diagnostic Considerations in Chronic Interstitial Lung Disease

I. Diseases of known etiology
Chronic congestive heart failure
Drug-induced lung disease (therapeutic and illicit)
Environmental lung disease
• Hypersensitivity pneumonitis
• Inhalation of irritant gases
• Pneumoconioses
Malignancy
• Lymphoma
• Lymphangitic carcinomatosis
Oxygen toxicity
Post ARDS* pulmonary fibrosis
Radiation fibrosis
II. Diseases of unknown etiology
Alveolar hemorrhage syndromes (chronic phase)
• Goodpasture's syndrome
• Idiopathic pulmonary hemosiderosis
Eosinophilic granuloma
Idiopathic pulmonary fibrosis (lone and associated with collagen vascular disease)
Lymphocytic interstitial pneumonitis
Lymphomatoid granulomatosis
Lymphangiomyomatosis
Sarcoidosis
Vasculitis
• Churg-Strauss
• Wegener's granulomatosis

*ARDS = acute respiratory distress syndrome.

TREATMENT

Unfortunately, attempts to modify the natural history of IPF by pharmacologic interventions have met with limited success. Medical treatment is aimed at suppressing the inflammatory component of the disease, dampening the mechanisms responsible for tissue injury, and minimizing fibrosis. Corticosteroids are the mainstay of therapy. There have been no randomized, placebo-controlled, prospective studies which would permit proper evaluation of their therapeutic efficacy. Instead, in a handful of studies treated patients were compared with historical controls. In contrast to the historical controls, who rarely undergo spontaneous improvement, 10 to 30 percent of corticosteroid-treated patients show objective evidence of improvement (pulmonary function tests and chest radiographs); subjective improvement occurs in a larger percentage. The patients most apt to respond to corticosteroids tend to be younger, with a shorter duration of symptoms, and with a more cellular histology on biopsy. Limited evidence suggests that an increased percentage of lymphocytes in bronchoalveolar lavage fluid is predictive of a favorable response to corticosteroid therapy. On casual inspection, early objective response appears to translate into improved survival. However, on closer scrutiny, this interpretation may be flawed by lead-time bias, i.e., by the likelihood that steroid responders are diagnosed at an earlier stage of their disease and that the survival from the time of onset of the disease is not altered by treatment.

Data concerning the use of other therapeutic agents are even sparser. Combination therapy, using corticosteroids and either cyclophosphamide or azathioprine, have failed to demonstrate a therapeutic advantage over the use of steroids alone. Nonetheless, these cytotoxic agents have been widely adopted as second-line therapy for patients who fail, or cannot tolerate, high-dose corticosteroid therapy.

Based on considerations such as those outlined above, current recommendations for the treatment of IPF vary from clinic to clinic. One relatively standard approach involves the use of high-dose oral prednisone (1 to 1.5 mg/kg per day) for 6 to 12 weeks followed by reassessment undertaken in the form of pulmonary function studies and chest radiography. For those who improve, the dose of prednisone is gradually tapered to the lowest dose that will maintain remission. For nonresponders, and for those who deteriorate while the dose of prednisone is tapered, cyclophosphamide (1 to 2 mg/kg per day) or azathioprine (1 to 3 mg/kg per day) is added. For those who exhibit a favorable response, treatment is continued for at least 1 year; frequently, lifelong maintenance therapy is required. Because of the potential for serious adverse effects, continued treatment of patients who fail to respond after several months of therapy is unjustified.

Single lung transplantation has recently emerged as an important therapeutic option for certain patients with IPF. This approach should be considered for patients with relentlessly progressive disease who are ambulatory but severely limited by their disease, and who do not have coexistent medical conditions that will compromise the results of surgery. The presence of cor pulmonale does not preclude successful single lung transplant because pulmonary artery pressures and right ventricular function rapidly normalize with implantation of the lung allograft. Successful transplantation results in marked improvement in pulmonary function, gas exchange, and exercise tolerance, and offers the potential for long-term survival.

BIBLIOGRAPHY

For a more detailed discussion, see Turner-Warwick M: Widespread pulmonary fibrosis, in Fishman AP (ed), *Pulmonary Diseases and Disorders,* 2d ed. New York, McGraw-Hill, 1988, pp 755–772.

Cherniak RM, Crystal RG, Kalica AR: Current concepts in idiopathic pulmonary fibrosis: A road map to the future. Am Rev Respir Dis 143:680–683, 1991.

Grossman RF, Frost A, Zamel N, Patterson GA, Cooper JD, Myron PR, Dear CL, Maurer J, and the Toronto Lung Transplant Group: Results of single-lung transplantation for bilateral pulmonary fibrosis. N Engl J Med 322:727–733, 1990.

Nishimura K, Kitaichi M, Izumi T, Nagai S, Kanaoka M, Itoh H: Usual interstitial pneumonia: Histologic correlation with high-resolution CT. Radiology 182:337–342, 1992.

Raghu G, Depaso WJ, Cain K, Hammar SP, Wetzel CE, Dreis DF, Hutchinson J, Pardee NE, Winterbauer RH: Azathiaprine combined with prednisone in the treatment of idiopathic pulmonary fibrosis: A prospective double-blind, randomized, placebo-controlled clinical trial. Am Rev Respir Dis 144:291–296, 1991.

Sheppard MN, Harrison NK: New perspectives on basic mechanisms in lung disease. 1. Lung injury, inflammatory mediators, and fibroblast activation in fibrosing alveolitis. Thorax 47:1064–1074, 1992.

Robert M. Kotloff

DEFINITION

Radiation pneumonitis is a complication of the use of ionizing radiation for the treatment of tumors within, or close to, the lung. It may be viewed as occurring in two sequential stages: (1) *radiation pneumonitis,* the acute phase of lung injury, which is characterized by dyspnea, radiographic infiltrates confined to the area of irradiated lung, and histologic evidence of alveolar epithelial and endothelial cell damage; and (2) *radiation-induced fibrosis,* which follows the acute injury and persists indefinitely.

PATHOGENESIS

Ionizing radiation causes tissue damage by several mechanisms. The predominant mechanism is the local generation of oxygen radicals by x-rays; in turn, the oxygen radicals directly damage DNA. The lethal effects of this damage are not immediate; instead, affected cells die during subsequent mitosis or produce nonviable daughter cells. The cells of the lung that have the highest mitotic rates, and therefore the greatest susceptibility to the damaging effects of radiation, are the airway epithelial cells, the type II alveolar epithelial cells, and the capillary endothelial cells. Because the latter two cell types have relatively slow turnover rates (1 to 2 months), a considerable delay is observed clinically between the delivery of radiation and appreciable parenchymal damage.

Free radicals can also directly damage nongenetic cellular constituents such as membrane proteins and polysaccharides, leading to immediate cell death. This mechanism is dose related and usually manifested only after large doses of radiation have been administered.

A third mechanism relates to the ability of ionizing radiation to evoke a brisk, lymphocyte-mediated inflammatory response in the lung.

EPIDEMIOLOGY

Radiation pneumonitis is most often associated with the treatment of breast cancer, lung cancer, Hodgkin's lymphoma, and non-Hodgkin's lymphoma. Although *radiographic* evidence of pneumonitis is common in patients undergoing treatment for these malignancies, only 5 to 15 percent of these patients develop *symptomatic* radiation pneumonitis. Radiation pneumonitis may also follow treatment of esophageal carcinoma and mediastinal tumors, e.g., thymoma, germinoma, as well as metastatic tumors of the lung, but the frequency of this complication is unknown. Patients who undergo whole body irradiation, including both lungs, before bone marrow transplantation are also at risk.

A number of factors influence the development and severity of radiation pneumonitis. The severity of injury is directly related to the volume of lung irradiated and the total dose administered and inversely related to the number of daily fractions into which the total dose is subdivided. Concurrent use of certain chemotherapeutic agents, including actinomycin D, cyclophosphamide, bleomycin, doxorubicin, and vincristine, can potentiate the damaging effects of radiation. In patients who are receiving high doses of corticosteroids, either as a component of chemotherapy or for an unrelated therapeutic purpose, abrupt discontinuation of the corticosteroids when radiotherapy is concluded may precipitate or exacerbate radiation pneumonitis. The incidence of clinically significant pneumonitis is higher after a second course of radiotherapy than after the first course.

PATHOLOGY

The *acute phase* of radiation injury is characterized by concurrent changes in the alveolar walls, air spaces, and vasculature. The histologic findings include capillary engorgement and thrombosis; alveolar epithelial cell atypia, hyperplasia, and desquamation; alveolar proteinosis and hyaline membranes; and interstitial edema and lymphocytic infiltration. Neutrophils are rare. Although none of these findings is specific for radiation pneumonitis, the combination of certain histologic features—alveolar epithelial cell hyperplasia, hyaline membrane formation, and vascular changes—and limitation of these changes to the area of lung that has been irradiated, strongly supports the diagnosis of radiation pneumonitis.

The *late stage* of radiation injury is characterized by extensive fibrosis that causes thickening of the alveolar septae and obliteration of alveolar spaces and pulmonary vasculature. These findings are entirely nonspecific and identical to those seen with end-stage pulmonary fibrosis from any cause.

ABNORMAL PHYSIOLOGY

The degree of impairment in lung function is directly related to the volume of lung irradiated. When only small volumes are damaged, lung mechanics and gas exchange are generally unaffected. A decrease in regional pulmonary perfusion, which can be demonstrated by radioisotopic perfusion techniques, is often the only detectable abnormality.

Involvement of larger volumes of lung causes a fall in static lung compliance without appreciable change in chest wall compliance. The decrease in static lung compliance accompanies the appearance of symptomatic pneumonitis and persists during the development of chronic fibrosis. A decrease in the production of surfactant, and the resultant increase in surface tension at the alveolar air-fluid interface, has been implicated as the major cause of the initial decrease in lung compliance. Interstitial fibrosis appears to be primarily responsible for the long-term persistence of the decreased lung compliance.

The decrease in static lung compliance is accompanied by a symmetrical decrease in static lung volumes and leads to an increase in the work of breathing. In turn, the increased work of breathing due to the "stiff lungs" causes a distinctive breathing pattern characterized by small tidal volumes, increased respiratory rate, and an increase in minute ventilation.

Gas exchange abnormalities are common in patients with symptomatic radiation pneumonitis. Obliteration of alveolar capillaries and thickening of the alveolar septae lead to a decrease in the diffusing capacity for carbon monoxide. Ventilation-perfusion mismatch results in mild-to-moderate arterial hypoxemia and an increase in the alveolar-arterial oxygen gradient. A decrease in arterial P_{CO_2} accompanies the hyperventilation caused by the stiff lungs and arterial hypoxemia. Hypercapnia and profound hypoxemia may occur as part of end-stage disease.

CLINICAL MANIFESTATIONS

History It is distinctly unusual for symptoms of radiation pneumonitis to appear sooner than 6 to 8 weeks after completion of radiotherapy. The development of a dry cough during or immediately after the completion of radiation is attributable to radiation-induced bronchitis and not to pneumonitis. The onset of pneumonitis is insidious and is usually heralded by the appearance of a cough 6 weeks to 3 months after the radiotherapy. Although the cough is dry at the onset, it often becomes productive of small amounts of whitish or pink sputum. Purulent sputum or hemoptysis should lead to a search for other causes, e.g., infection or recurrent tumor. Dyspnea is common, occurring only on exertion when pulmonary involvement is mild and at rest in those with extensive lung involvement. Progression to severe respiratory insufficiency that requires mechanical ventilation occurs only in the few patients who develop extensive pneumonitis. A low-grade fever is common, but temperatures as high as 40°C (104°F) may accompany severe and extensive pneumonitis.

In patients with mild-to-moderate lung injury induced by the radiation, the symptoms of acute pneumonitis gradually resolve as the acute inflammatory process is succeeded by fibrosis. However, if the pulmonary fibrosis is extensive or if lesser degrees of fibrosis are superimposed on preexisting lung disease, dyspnea and diminished exercise tolerance can persist indefinitely.

Physical examination Patients with radiation pneumonitis are frequently febrile and tachypneic. Examination of the chest is usually entirely normal. Occasionally, a pleural friction rub, rales, or signs of consolidation may be detected. In severe radiation pneumonitis, respiratory distress and central cyanosis occur.

Physical examination of patients with radiation fibrosis is usually unremarkable. With extensive unilateral fibrosis, evidence of volume loss on the affected side (tracheal deviation, diminished inspiratory excursion) may occur. Few patients develop signs of pulmonary hypertension and cor pulmonale. Rarely is finger clubbing present.

USUAL DIAGNOSTIC TESTS

Chest radiograph Radiographic evidence of pneumonitis generally appears 1 to 3 months after treatment and commonly precedes the onset of symptoms. As noted above, a distinctive feature of radiation pneumonitis is the limitation of the radiographic changes to the margins of the radiation portal. Therefore, definition of the treatment field is prerequisite for accurate diagnosis. Initially, the affected area appears as a diffuse haze or ground-glass opacification, and lung markings are indistinct. Later on, the infiltrate may become nodular or alveolar. In severe cases, dense consolidation with air bronchograms occurs. In some patients, evidence of pleural or pericardial effusions accompany the parenchymal changes. Adenopathy is not seen. Cavitation does not occur except in occasional instances of radiation-induced necrosis of the underlying tumor.

The radiographic changes of acute pneumonitis gradually progress to those of chronic fibrosis. This progression takes place over 1 to 2 years and thereafter remains stable. As the irradiated segment contracts, the infiltrate becomes denser and remains sharply demarcated from the surrounding uninvolved lung. Cystic or bronchiectatic changes sometimes occur within the fibrotic lung segment. When volume loss is extensive, tracheal deviation, mediastinal shift, and hilar retraction occur accompanied by elevation and tenting of the hemidiaphragm.

Pulmonary function tests The degree of impairment in pulmonary function correlates roughly with the extent of lung involvement. As pointed out above, pulmonary function tests and arterial blood gases remain normal when only small volumes are involved, e.g., the apex of one lung. With more extensive involvement, pulmonary function tests characteristically assume a restrictive pattern with decreased lung volumes and a low diffusing capacity. Arterial blood gases reveal mild-to-moderate hypoxemia and hypocapnia. The advent of hypercapnia is ominous and frequently preterminal.

Blood studies A mild leukocytosis and increase in the erythrocyte sedimentation rate are frequent, but nonspecific, findings.

SPECIAL DIAGNOSTIC EVALUATION

In many patients, the diagnosis of radiation pneumonitis can be made on the basis of characteristic clinical features and radiographic changes occurring at an appropriate interval after completion of radiotherapy. However, when other etiologies for the pulmonary findings enter into the differential diagnosis (see below), it may be helpful to obtain histologic samples from the involved segment of lung. Bronchoscopy, with transbronchial biopsy, affords the least invasive means of obtaining lung tissue. Rarely is open lung biopsy required.

DIFFERENTIAL DIAGNOSIS

The differential diagnosis of radiation pneumonitis includes infection, recurrent malignancy, drug-induced lung disease, and thromboembolism. The presence of purulent sputum, frank hemoptysis, or radiographic changes beyond the margins of the radiation portal should lead to consideration of diagnoses other than radiation pneumonitis.

NATURAL HISTORY AND PROGNOSIS

Most patients with radiation pneumonitis survive the acute episode. Spontaneous resolution of symptoms occurs gradually over several weeks to months. In a few patients with extensive pneumonitis, the manifestations progress from mild dyspnea to acute respiratory distress so that mechanical ventilation may become necessary. Death from radiation pneumonitis occurs in between 0.25 to 5 percent of patients. The development of hypercapnia or cor pulmonale is an especially ominous sign and usually portends a fatal outcome.

The patients who survive the acute episode invariably develop radiation fibrosis in the area of prior pneumonitis. Most patients with radiation fibrosis remain asymptomatic. Relatively few patients, particularly those with preexistent lung disease or those in whom the pneumonitis was extensive, develop chronic respiratory failure as a result of radiation fibrosis.

TREATMENT

In mild radiation pneumonitis, aspirin, cough suppressants, and restriction of activity usually suffice to ensure patient comfort. Patients with more extensive lung injury are treated with corticosteroids. Treatment is initiated with prednisone at a dose of 60 to 100 mg daily. Corticosteroids administered early in the course of pneumonitis sometimes produce dramatic improvement, with defervescence, relief of cough and dyspnea, and normalization of the chest radiograph, often within 24 to 72 h. Unfortunately, many patients with severe pneumonitis fail to respond to corticosteroid therapy. In those who demonstrate a favorable response, corticosteroids should be continued at the initial dose for several weeks and then tapered gradually. During steroid tapering, supervision should be close to avoid relapse. There is no role for the prophylactic use of corticosteroids, nor do corticosteroids have any place in the treatment of radiation fibrosis.

Supplemental oxygen is administered to patients with radiation pneumonitis who demonstrate significant hypoxemia ($P_{O_2} < 60$ mmHg). To minimize the risk of oxygen toxicity, needlessly high levels of oxygen should be avoided.

BIBLIOGRAPHY

For a more detailed discussion, see Phillips TL: Radiation fibrosis, in Fishman AP (ed), *Pulmonary Diseases and Disorders,* 2d ed. New York, McGraw-Hill, 1988, pp 773–792.

Gibson PG, Bryant DH, Morgan GW: Radiation-induced lung injury: A hypersensitivity pneumonitis? Ann Intern Med 109:288–291, 1988.

Gross NJ, Holloway NO, Narine KR: Effects of some nonsteroidal anti-inflammatory agents on experimental radiation pneumonitis. Radiat Res 127:317–324, 1991.

Roberts CM, Foulcher E, Zaunders JJ, Bryant DH, Freund J, Cairns D, et al: Radiation pneumonitis: A possible lymphocyte-mediated hypersensitivity reaction. Ann Intern Med 118:696–700, 1993.

Rosiello RA, Merrill WW: Radiation-induced lung injury. Clin Chest Med 11:65–72, 1990.

Alfred P. Fishman

All parts of the respiratory apparatus—from lungs and thorax to the respiratory centers in the brain—are vulnerable to toxic effects exerted by agents administered for therapeutic purposes. Some, such as respiratory depression due to narcotic overdosage, are predictable consequences of the pharmacologic effects of the drug. Others, such as abnormal immune or metabolic responses or direct cytotoxicity, are generally unpredictable. Bleomycin, which can cause pulmonary damage by a direct cytotoxic effect that is mediated by oxygen radicals, sometimes evokes a hypersensitivity reaction.

Some drugs can damage the lungs by more than one mechanism. Combinations of drugs, such as the combination of bleomycin, mitomycin, vincristine, and cisplatin, are more toxic to the lungs than any of these agents alone. Also, pulmonary irradiation enhances the pulmonary toxicity of many chemotherapeutic agents, e.g., cyclophosphamide, bleomycin, and vincristine.

Once an adverse reaction to a drug is suspected, the drug must be discontinued. One major problem in this regard is distinguishing between the adverse effect and the underlying disease, e.g., penicillamine-induced lesions versus rheumatoid arthritis (RA; see below). Although corticosteroids are widely used for drug-induced inflammatory disease, especially interstitial pneumonitis and drug-induced systemic lupus erythematosus (SLE), there is no consensus about their effectiveness. As a rule, corticosteroids are reserved for severe reactions because mild reactions usually resolve spontaneously once the drug is stopped. The dosage is then high, e.g., 80 mg prednisone daily or, if feasible, every other day, with tapering keyed to clinical improvement.

PULMONARY INTERSTITIAL DISEASE

Pulmonary interstitial disease, i.e., interstitial pneumonitis and fibrosis, is the most common manifestation of drug-induced pulmonary disease. As a rule, the inflammatory process that culminates in interstitial disease begins in the alveoli and spreads to the interstitium. When first seen by the physician, the disease may be acute or chronic. In the evolution of interstitial fibrosis, the original cellular infiltrate of macrophages, lymphocytes, and other inflammatory cells, is gradually succeeded by the deposition of fibrin within the alveoli and by interstitial fibrosis. After the drug is discontinued, the acute and subacute forms generally clear, whereas the chronic form may persist due to irreversible pulmonary fibrosis.

Diagnosis The presenting manifestations usually consist of dyspnea, especially on exertion, and a nonproductive cough. The onset of symptoms may be abrupt, as in hypersensitivity pneumonitis, or gradual, as in other causes of widespread interstitial pulmonary fibrosis.

History and physical examination A history of drug intake is critical both for diagnosis and management (Table 12-1). The *acute* reaction generally begins with fever and cough, sometimes associated with tachypnea and cyanosis. The *chronic* form is generally insidious in onset and the offending agent may be difficult to pinpoint. Without historical identification of the offending agent, the differential diagnosis is apt to be sidetracked into consideration of a host of other widespread interstitial diseases.

In addition to searching for an offending agent, the history should identify any underlying pulmonary disorder or other relevant information. For example, a history of treated rheumatoid disease is relevant not only in that rheumatoid disease can affect the lungs, but drugs used in its treatment, such as methotrexate, gold, and penicillamine, can evoke pulmonary lesions that can be confused with rheumatoid lung disease. Sulfasalazine, used in the treatment of inflammatory bowel disease, i.e., Crohn's disease, has been implicated in the pathogenesis of granulomatous interstitial pneumonitis and fibrosis. Recent exposure to cytotoxic drugs also raises the possibility of infection as a result of immunosuppression. On occasion, the offending agent can evoke associated extrapulmonary disease, e.g., penicillamine-associated Goodpasture's syndrome.

TABLE 12-1 Drugs That Cause Interstitial Infiltrates or Fibrosis

Cancer chemotherapy: cytotoxic agents	Miscellaneous
Azathioprine	Amiodarone
Bleomycin	Amphotericin B
Busulfan	Ampicillin
Chlorambucil	Carbamazepine
Cyclophosphamide	Chlorpropamide
Cytosine arabinoside	Cromolyn
Melphalan	Diphenylhydantoin
6-Mercaptopurine	Ergot derivatives
Methotrexate	Gold
Mitomycin-C	Hydralazine
Nitrosoureas, e.g., BCNU	Imipramine
Procarbazine	Isoniazid
Vinblastine	Nitrofurantoin
Vindesine	Para-aminosalicylic acid
	Penicillamine
	Penicillin

SOURCE: From Rosenow EC, Myers JL, Swensen SJ, Pisani RJ: Drug-induced pulmonary disease. An update. Chest 102:239–250, 1992.

The physical examination may strengthen the possibility that the pulmonary lesions are part of a systemic process, such as drug-induced SLE or bleomycin-induced lesions of the skin and mucus membranes. Examination of the chest is usually relatively nonspecific, e.g., dry rales over affected areas of the lungs or evidence of a pleural effusion.

Chest radiography Depending on the acuity of the process, the radiographic pattern can take different forms. In the *acute stage,* the picture is usually that of an extensive pneumonitis that may be sufficiently extensive to simulate pulmonary edema. Pleural effusions are common. In the *chronic stage,* the chest radiograph may show either a widespread increase in interstitial markings, often most apparent at the lung bases, or a mixed picture of diffuse reticulonodular infiltrates, interstitial fibrosis, and even honeycombing.

Computed tomography (CT) often discloses more subtle changes than can be visualized by chest radiography. However, interpretation can be complicated by lesions of the underlying disease, e.g., metastases from a neoplasm, such as a germ cell tumor, for which the patient is undergoing chemotherapy.

Laboratory studies Conventional laboratory studies are most informative in the hypersensitivity reactions, e.g., peripheral eosinophilia and increased serum IgE in gold-induced hypersensitivity pneumonitis. The test for antinuclear antibodies (ANA) is usually positive in drug-induced SLE and may become positive in the asymptomatic patient before the clinical picture evolves.

Pulmonary function tests Pulmonary function testing is usually reserved for patients with *chronic* pulmonary interstitial disease. The characteristic pattern of *chronic* pulmonary interstitial disease is that of restrictive lung disease: the forced vital capacity (FVC) and lung volumes are decreased; the forced expiratory volume in 1 s (FEV_1)/FVC ratio is preserved. The diffusing capacity of the lungs (DL_{CO}) is decreased. Arterial O_2 saturation, which is often normal at rest, decreases often strikingly, during exercise.

Unfortunately, interpretation of abnormal pulmonary function tests can be difficult, especially in patients undergoing chemotherapy for cancer, because concurrent anemia, weakness, pulmonary metastases, and intercurrent surgery can all influence the measurements.

Lung biopsy A tissue biopsy is usually more helpful in excluding a variety of possible etiologies of widespread interstitial pneumonitis and fibrosis, and in suggesting the diagnosis, than in proving that the disease is a drug reaction. Tissue can be obtained by transbronchial biopsy via bronchoscopy or by open lung biopsy. As a rule, open lung biopsy is apt to be more diagnostic. However, bronchoscopic biopsy can exclude certain widespread interstitial diseases such as sarcoidosis, eosinophilic granuloma, and alveolar proteinosis. In some instances, bronchoalveolar lavage is helpful in excluding pulmonary infection or neoplasm.

The histologic changes of drug-induced pulmonary interstitial disease depend on the stage of the disease. Early on, the picture is that of an alveolitis in which macrophages and lymphocytes predominate, sometimes accompanied by neutrophils or eosinophils. Although these changes are not specific for a drug reaction, they usually suffice to establish the diagnosis of a drug reaction when considered in light of the history of drug intake, the chest radiograph, and the exclusion of histologic evidence of other parenchymal diseases. In the more chronic stages, the predominant histologic appearance of an alveolitis is succeeded by that of an interstitial inflammatory process and fibrosis. In these stages, distinction from other etiologies of interstitial disease becomes more difficult.

ALVEOLAR DISEASE

Three types of drug-induced injury primarily affect the alveoli: edema, hemorrhage, and phospholipidosis. The chest radiograph is distinctive: widespread alveolar filling in association with a normal cardiac silhouette.

Pulmonary Edema

This is noncardiogenic in origin, presumably due to "leaky vessels" caused by widespread injury to the pulmonary capillaries; pulmonary capillary wedge pressures are normal.

Five categories of drugs, acting in different ways, are common causes of "permeability pulmonary edema."

Narcotics Overdosage with heroin, methadone, or propoxyphene can elicit acute pulmonary edema (within minutes to hours after overdosage). The pulmonary edema is accompanied by severe respiratory depression, alveolar hypoventilation; often it is complicated by aspiration. Treatment relies heavily on restoring alveolar ventilation toward normal, usually by mechanical ventilation.

Salicylates Aside from attempts at suicide, the pulmonary edema usually occurs in elderly individuals; as a rule, these are chronic users of salicylates who had been inadvertently overdosed. Although aspirin sensitivity is generally held to be immunologic, experience with other cyclooxygenase inhibitors suggests that in some instances, an arachidonic acid metabolite, such as a leukotriene, may be involved. The mainstays of treatment are gastric emptying followed by the administration of activated charcoal, ensuring airway patency and protection, and respiratory and circulatory support.

Chemotherapeutic agents Both cytotoxic agents (bleomycin, Ara-C, mitomycin, vinblastine) and noncytotoxic agents (amiloride and amiodarone) are implicated as causes of edema.

Sympathomimetics Agents used to treat premature labor (often in concert with glucocorticoids) are among the more common offenders of this type.

Miscellaneous Nonsteroidal anti-inflammatory drugs (NSAIDs), which sometimes cause hypersensitivity pneumonitis, more rarely evoke noncardiogenic pulmonary edema (Table 12-2). Also, in a few instances, chemotherapeutic agents, such as mitomycin alone or in combination with vinblastine, have caused noncardiogenic pulmonary edema, sometimes as part of a syndrome that included microangiopathic anemia and renal failure.

Pulmonary Hemorrhage

Bleeding into the alveoli generally arises from one of three mechanisms: (1) interference with normal clot formation, e.g., by anticoagulants (heparin and warfarin) and thrombolytic agents (streptokinase, urokinase, and tissue plasminogen activator); (2) thrombocytopenia induced by drugs; and (3) damage to the alveolar-capillary membrane, e.g., by pencillamine, which can elicit a nonimmunologic pulmonary-renal syndrome, or by cocaine, which can cause diffuse alveolar hemorrhage possibly due to direct toxicity of the drug on alveolar capillary membranes.

Phospholipidosis: Amiodarone Toxicity

Amiodarone, a powerful antiarrhythmic agent, produces a unique phospholipidosis in the lungs along with hepatic, cardiac, central nervous system, and endocrine function. Lung biopsy shows macrophages in alveoli with pale and foamy cytoplasm. In later stages, the macrophage-rich exudate can organzie to cause obliterative bronchiolitis. The patient manifests fever, nonproductive cough, dyspnea, and arterial hypoxemia. Chest radiographs usually show widespread interstitial infiltrates with patches of alveolar filling;

TABLE 12-2 Pulmonary Injury Caused by Anti-inflammatory and Antirheumatic Drugs

Syndrome	Drug
Hypersensitivity pneumonitis, pulmonary interstitial fibrosis	Penicillamine, gold, methotrexate, NSAIDs
Pulmonary-renal syndrome	Penicillamine
Bronchiolitis obliterans	Penicillamine, gold
Noncardiogenic pulmonary edema	Salicylates

upper lobes are often more affected than lower lobes. Usually the lungs clear slowly after the drug is stopped, but fibrosis may ensue. Pulmonary function tests show a restrictive pattern.

The *physical findings* are those of widespread pulmonary edema.

Laboratory features depend on the etiologic agent: arterial hypoxemia is a regular feature of narcotic overdosage; a mixed metabolic acidosis and respiratory alkalosis is common in salicylate toxicity.

AIRWAY DISORDERS

Bronchospasm is the predominant manifestation of drug-induced airway reaction. Cough is another common manifestation.

Bronchospasm

Drug-induced bronchospasm can be elicited by agents taken by mouth or given parenterally. Three categories of drugs are particularly noteworthy in this regard.

Cyclooxygenase inhibitors Patients with nasal polyps and asthma (and to a lesser extent, those who have a history of vasomotor rhinitis and/or eosinophilia) are particularly susceptible to bronchospasm induced by aspirin and NSAIDs.

β-*Blockers* Bronchospasm is apt to become evident or even life-threatening in patients with hyperreactive airways, e.g., with asthma or chronic bronchitis, but not in normal individuals.

Radiographic contrast media Following intravenous administration, nonimmunologically mediated anaphylactic reactions (anaphylactoid reactions) are caused by direct release of mediators. The newer low-osmolality radiocontrast media cause fewer anaphylactoid reactions. If repeat examination is necessary after an anaphylactoid reaction, steroids and H_1-antihistamines are generally used for premedication.

Other agents, such as vinblastine or vindesine, occasionally evoke bronchospasm as one of a variety of pulmonary toxic effects. Bronchospasm can also occur after the administration of neuromuscular blocking agents, e.g., D-tubocurarine, but the incidence is low.

Bronchiolitis Obliterans

The small airways have been the seat of bronchiolitis obliterans in patients with RA undergoing penicillamine therapy. Bronchiolitis obliterans has also occurred in patients undergoing gold therapy for RA. However, the role of penicillamine (or gold) is not easily distinguished from that of the RA itself. Clinically, the patient becomes dyspneic. The chest radiograph usually shows discrete nodular lesions or airway opacities. Treatment consists of discontinuing the potential offending agent.

Cough

Agents administered by airway can act as nonspecific bronchial irritants to evoke coughing. Metered-dose inhalers are a common cause of cough and bronchospasm. The reaction is due primarily to the inert propellants and dispersants.

Cough and bronchospasm are also frequent side effects of aerosolized pentamidine; the mechanism is unclear but bronchial hyperreactivity may be involved. One to 2 percent of individuals taking angiotensin-converting enzyme (ACE) inhibitors develop a dry, persistent, nonproductive cough. As a rule, the cough begins within days after the medication is begun, but sometimes the onset is delayed for months; the cough usually stops in a matter of weeks after the medication is stopped.

PLEURAL DISEASE

Diverse types of drugs can elicit pleural disease in the form of effusion or thickening (Table 12-3). Often, pleural effusions due to drug toxicity are associated with interstitial lung disease.

Systemic Lupus Erythematosus

Pleural effusion is particularly common as part of the syndrome of drug-induced SLE. Among the common inciting agents are procainamide, hydralazine, isoniazid, chlorpromazine, and diphenylhydantoin. The syndrome is apparently due to interaction of the drug or a reactive metabolite with nuclear material to form ANA. In common with SLE that is not drug-related, the serum ANA is almost invariably increased, and anemia, leukopenia, and thrombocytopenia are common. In contrast, SLE induced by these drugs is not accompanied by hypocomplementemia or a reactive VDRL.

Other agents, such as carbamazepine and methyldopa, are less common offenders and induce a lupuslike syndrome in which the

TABLE 12-3 Drugs That Cause Pleural Effusion or Thickening

Cancer chemotherapy	Miscellaneous
Bleomycin	Anticoagulants
Busulfan	Dantrolene
Methotrexate	Ergot derivatives
Mitomycin	Methysergide
Procarbazine	Bromocriptine
	Nitrofurantoin
Lupuslike syndrome	Oxyprenolol
Procainamide	Para-aminosalicylic acid
Hydralazine	Penicillin
Isoniazid	Practolol
Diphenylhydantoin	

ANA is not increased. The kidneys are less often involved in drug-induced SLE than in spontaneous SLE. The variety of agents that have been reported to cause pleural effusions underscore the importance of an adequate history in dealing with pleural effusions of uncertain cause. Also, pleural effusions in SLE may be due to a variety of causes other than drugs, e.g., nephrotic syndrome, congestive heart failure, pulmonary emboli.

In addition to the drugs that evoke pleural effusions as part of the syndrome of SLE, some drugs, such as nitrofurantoin, bromocriptine, and amiodarone, cause pleuropulmonary syndromes, whereas others, such as methysergide and dantrolene, affect only the pleura. Methysergide is notorious for causing retroperitoneal and mediastinal fibrosis, but pleural fibrosis or effusion generally occurs without evidence of fibrosis elsewhere. Discontinuance of the drug may cause complete resolution of the effusion or fibrosis.

ABNORMAL RESPIRATORY MUSCLES

A wide variety of drugs, notably muscle relaxants, can impair respiratory muscle function. The effects of muscle relaxants on the diaphragm are slower to develop, less severe, and quicker to resolve than on peripheral muscle. As a rule, single agents rarely depress respiratory function sufficiently to become clinically significant. However, combinations of drugs are more apt to interact adversely, e.g., muscle relaxants and antibiotics or neuromuscular blocking agents and high doses of corticosteroids.

As a rule, drugs are most likely to trigger respiratory failure in predisposed individuals, e.g., calcium channel blockers in Duchenne's muscular dystrophy or D-penicillamine in subclinical myasthenia gravis.

MEDIASTINAL ADENOPATHY AND DISEASE

Mediastinal lymphadenopathy (and hilar lymphadenopathy), lipomatosis, and fibrosis can be caused by drugs. The adenopathy and lipomatosis are manifested on the chest radiograph by mediastinal widening. Mediastinal fibrosis is usually much less overt. CT scanning is often helpful in unraveling a pathologic process in the mediastinum.

Mediastinal and Hilar Adenopathy

Mediastinal and hilar lymphadenopathy is a hypersensitivity reaction. It can be caused by diphenylhydantoin and methotrexate. The mediastinal lymphadenopathy, due to diphenylhydantoin, occurs within days to weeks after the start of therapy. It is accompanied by fever, rash, peripheral lymphadenopathy, hepatosplenomegaly, and eosinophilia. The entire syndrome resolves within weeks after the drug is discontinued.

Methotrexate can elicit hilar adenopathy, presumably also as a hypersensitivity reaction, early or late in the course of therapy, independent of dosage. Often it is accompanied by peripheral eosinophilia. Symptoms usually regress spontaneously after the drug is stopped. In some instances, corticosteroids may speed resolution.

Mediastinal Lipomatosis

Mediastinal widening on the chest radiograph due to lipomatosis occurs primarily in patients who are being maintained on doses of corticosteroids and are overtly cushingoid. The widening regresses gradually after the drug is stopped.

Mediastinal Fibrosis

A syndrome of mediastinal and retroperitoneal fibrosis occurs in some individuals who are ingesting methysergide, an ergot derivative, for migraine.

BIBLIOGRAPHY

For a more detailed discussion, see Fulkerson WJ Jr, Gockerman JP: Pulmonary disease induced by drugs, in Fishman AP (ed), *Pulmonary Diseases and Disorders,* 2d ed. New York, McGraw-Hill, 1988, pp 793–810.

Cooper JA (ed): Drug-induced pulmonary disease. Clin Chest Med 11:1–194, 1990.

Kaltreïder HB (ed): Immunologically mediated lung disease. Semin Resp Med 12:143–245, 1991.

Rosenow EC, Myers JL, Swensen SJ, Pisani RJ: Drug-induced pulmonary disease. An update. Chest 102:239–250, 1992.

Gregory Tino   Michael Beers

DEFINITION

Primary pulmonary histiocytosis X (PPHX), also known as eosino-philic granuloma, is an uncommon interstitial lung disease characterized by accumulation of atypical histiocytes referred to as Langerhans or histiocytosis X cells in nodular granulomatouslike lesions. PPHX is often grouped under the general heading of *histiocytosis X* along with Letterer-Siwe disease and Hand-Schüller-Christian disease. These three disorders share a common histopathology. However, in contrast to these other disorders which are multisystemic in nature, PPHX is a disease which predominantly, and in most instances, exclusively involves the lungs.

EPIDEMIOLOGY

PPHX is a disease of young adults with peak incidence in the third and fourth decades of life. PPHX occurs almost exclusively in caucasians. Neither gender predominates. Although no occupational or geographic predisposition has been identified, the association with cigarette smoking is striking. In fact, more than 95 percent of patients are active or former smokers.

ETIOLOGY AND PATHOGENESIS

The etiology of PPHX is unknown; it is neither hereditary nor infectious. The possibility of a hypersensitivity or immune etiology has been raised by the finding of circulating immune complexes, diminished suppressor T lymphocyte (CD8) activity, increased lymphocyte cytotoxic activity, and granular IgG and complement deposition within alveolar and vascular walls. Additional support for this possibility is provided by the demonstration that histiocytosis X cells have phagocytic properties, release interleukin 1, and express cell surface HLA class II markers, suggesting their involvement in antigen presentation. This evidence has prompted the hypothesis that PPHX results from immune responses mediated by the histiocytosis X cell to an as yet unidentified inciting antigen. The role of cigarette smoking in pathogenesis is not understood.

PATHOLOGY

The pathologic features of PPHX are distinctive but vary depending on the stage and severity of disease. Early on, gross examination reveals multiple grayish nodules of varied size scattered throughout the lung parenchyma. Under light microscopy, nodules are highly cellular stellate lesions composed predominantly of large mononuclear cells which contain lobular nuclei and pale, eosinophilic cytoplasm. These so-called *histiocytosis X cells* are interspersed with fibrous tissue, eosinophils, and occasional multinucleated giant cells; true granulomas are not found. The nodular lesions are peribronchial in distribution, but may extend into alveoli, bronchial walls, or pulmonary vessels. Sometimes the nodules cavitate. As the disorder progresses, the cellularity of the nodules diminishes and the content of connective tissue increases. This process causes nodule retraction and distortion of normal lung architecture; at end stage, cyst formation and honeycombing ensue.

The histiocytosis X cell is a bone marrow-derived mononuclear phagocyte, related to, if not identical with, the Langerhans cells of skin. Several features distinguish these cells from resident alveolar macrophages: (1) the histiocytosis X cell stains for S-100 cytoplasmic protein and expresses CD1A cell surface antigen; and (2) electron microscopically, these cells contain characteristic tennis-racket or rod-shaped pentalaminar intracytoplasmic granules of unknown function known as X bodies or Birbeck granules. These cells, which are rarely, if ever, found in the respiratory tract of normal nonsmoking individuals, are occasionally found in small numbers in smokers without underlying lung pathology and in other interstitial lung diseases, e.g., sarcoidosis, hypersensitivity pneumonitis, and idiopathic pulmonary fibrosis. Therefore, the presence of these cells in histologic sections or bronchoalveolar lavage fluid is highly suggestive, but not pathognomonic, of PPHX.

CLINICAL MANIFESTATIONS

History As many as one quarter of patients are asymptomatic; the work-up is usually intiated after an abnormal chest radiograph is incidentally discovered. Two thirds of patients present with respiratory complaints, most commonly nonproductive cough and dyspnea; these are usually present for several months before diagnosis. Spontaneous pneumothorax, often recurrent, occurs in up to 20 percent of patients and is attributable to rupture of subpleural blebs. Up to one third of patients have constitutional complaints, including fever, fatigue, and weight loss.

Although PPHX is principally a disease of the lungs, in some patients extrapulmonary sites are involved. Osteolytic bone lesions involving the skull, ribs, or pelvis are found in up to 20 percent of patients; although often heralded by focal bone pain and tenderness, they may be clinically silent. An uncommon but distinctive feature of PPHX is diabetes insipidus, manifested by polyuria and polydypsia.

Physical examination The physical examination is usually unremarkable. When abnormalities are present, they are nonspecific: rales, rhonchi, and diminished breath sounds. Clubbing is rare.

Hepatosplenomegaly or peripheral lymphadenopathy are uncommon and should raise suspicion of other diagnoses. Affected bones may be tender to palpation. When pulmonary involvement is extensive and severe, signs of pulmonary hypertension and cor pulmonale are present.

USUAL DIAGNOSTIC TESTS

Chest radiograph The chest radiograph is consistently abnormal in individuals with PPHX. Typically, bilateral nodular densities are seen; these range in size from 1 mm to > 1 cm and are located primarily in the mid and upper lung fields, virtually sparing the costophrenic angles. Hilar and mediastinal lymphadenopathy, pleural effusions, alveolar opacities, and cavitation of preexisting nodules are uncommon. As previously mentioned, spontaneous pneumothorax may be a presenting feature or complication.

With progressive disease, the chest radiographic features typically evolve from a micronodular pattern to one of reticulonodular infiltrates and, ultimately, to honeycombing and cyst formation. Despite widespread interstitial infiltrates, lung volumes are typically preserved, in contrast to the diminished lung volumes associated with other fibrotic disorders. The preservation of lung volumes along with the mid and upper lung field predilection of disease provide valuable radiographic clues to the presence of PPHX.

Chest computed tomography usually adds little to the diagnosis. Both the plain and high-resolution techniques reveal multiple nodules and small thin-walled cysts, usually confirming the findings of plain films.

Pulmonary function studies Spirometry and lung volume measurements are normal in about 15 percent of individuals even in the presence of radiologic findings. In some instances, a decrease in diffusing capacity (DLco) may be the only abnormality. Features of airflow obstruction, including small airways disease, are found in as many as one fifth of patients, probably reflecting the peribronchial distribution of the pathologic process. Air trapping, as a consequence of the development of a cyst or bleb, may be manifested by a disproportionately low ratio of vital capacity (VC) to total lung capacity (TLC) or an increase in the residual volume (RV) to TLC ratio. The extent to which cigarette smoking contributes to the development of obstructive defects in PPHX has not been independently assessed. Although lung volumes are usually preserved, in rare instances of end-stage fibrotic disease, lung volumes decrease. Early in the course of the disease, arterial blood-gas levels are normal; as the disease progresses, the A-a gradient widens and arterial hypoxemia occurs during exercise, largely due to ventilation-perfusion mismatching.

Routine laboratory studies Routine laboratory tests are usually normal. In those patients with the syndrome of diabetes insipidus, urinary and serum electrolyte disturbances characteristic of this disorder are found.

Tissue biopsy A tissue diagnosis is indispensable and best obtained in early stages before fibrosis obscures the characteristic histopathology. Open lung biopsy remains the "gold standard" for diagnosis. However, in some clinics, fiberoptic bronchoscopy with bronchoalveolar lavage (BAL) and transbronchial biopsy has sufficed. In contrast to the finding of predominantly alveolar macrophages in normal individuals, lavage fluid in PPHX reveals increased numbers and percentages of lymphocytes and neutrophils. Identification of the histiocytosis X cell in lavage fluid or in transbronchial biopsy specimens provides strong but not definitive evidence in support of the diagnosis. Identification of these cells can be facilitated by immunohistochemical staining for S-100 protein and CD1A surface antigen, as well as by electron microscopic demonstration of Birbeck granules. When uncertainty remains concerning the diagnostic significance of histiocytosis X cells, open lung biopsy should be done. In patients with suspected PPHX and bony involvement, bone biopsy may be helpful in establishing the diagnosis.

DIFFERENTIAL DIAGNOSIS

The differential diagnosis of PPHX includes sarcoidosis, lymphangiomyomatosis, inorganic pneumoconiosis, desquamative interstitial pneumonitis (DIP), vasculitis, lymphangitic spread of tumor, and granulomatous diseases of infectious origin including miliary tuberculosis.

PROGNOSIS AND TREATMENT

The natural history of PPHX is variable and the prognosis generally favorable. In a recent clinical series in which follow-up was available for 60 patients, 25 percent of patients remained asymptomatic throughout their course, and another 25 percent had complete remission either spontaneously or with therapy; mortality was only 1 percent. This stands in marked contrast to the systemic histiocytic disorders, for which mortality rates may reach 40 percent. Uninvolved costophrenic angles on the chest radiograph are said to be associated with a more favorable prognosis in PPHX, whereas honeycombing portends a chronic course.

Investigations regarding therapy have been hampered by a variety of problems including small study groups, heterogeneous patient populations, and the high rate of spontaneous remission. These facts, coupled with the overall favorable natural history of PPHX, make decisions about instituting treatment difficult. Systemic corticosteroids are the most widely recommended form of therapy. However, their efficacy has not been established in placebo-controlled trials; indeed, in some studies, the rate of improvement mirrors the rate of spontaneous remission. A number of other agents, such as methotrexate, cyclophosphamide, vincristine, and 6-mercaptopurine, used either alone or in combination, have been tried in small clinical trials but, once again, their clinical efficacy is uncertain.

Therefore, decisions about treatment have to be individualized. In the asymptomatic or minimally symptomatic patient, a period of close observation with monitoring of the chest radiograph, pulmonary function tests, and arterial blood-gas values, is a reasonable approach. In patients in whom symptoms limit activity or in whom clinical deterioration is evident, prednisone therapy (1 mg/kg daily) should be initiated and maintained for several months. If the disease is progressive, alternative therapy with other immunosuppressive agents, such as alkylating agents or vinca alkaloids, should be considered.

Adjunctive therapeutic measures include (1) smoking cessation; (2) oxygen supplementation for resting or exercise-induced hypoxemia; (3) pleurodesis for recurrent episodes of spontaneous pneumothorax; (4) bronchodilator regimens for symptoms of obstructive lung disease; (5) management of diabetes insipidus by vasopressin replacement along with fluids and electrolytes; and (6) supportive measures for cor pulmonale, including diuresis, oxygen therapy, and inotropic agents for heart failure. Radiation of bony lesions usually alleviates bone pain.

BIBLIOGRAPHY

For a more detailed discussion, see Rosenow EC III: Primary pulmonary histiocytosis X, in Fishman AP (ed), *Pulmonary Diseases and Disorders,* 2d ed. New York, McGraw-Hill, 1988, pp 813–818.

Brambilla E, Fontaine E, Pison CM, Coulomb M, Paramelle B, Brambilla C: Pulmonary histiocytosis X with mediastinal lymph node involvement. Am Rev Respir Dis 142:1216–1218, 1990.

Fukuda Y, Basset F, Soler P, Ferrans VJ, Masugi Y, Crystal RG: Intraluminal fibrosis and elastic fiber degradation lead to lung remodeling in pulmonary Langerhans' cell granulomatosis (histiocytosis X). Am J Pathol 137:415–424, 1990.

Ha SY, Helms P, Fletcher M, Broadbent V, Pritchard J: Lung involvement in Langerhans' cell histiocytosis: Prevalence, clinical features, and outcome. Pediatrics 89:466–469, 1992.

Kulwiec EL, Lynch DA, Aguayo SM, Schwarz MI, King TE Jr: Imaging of pulmonary histiocytosis X. Radiographics 12:515–526, 1992.

Soler P, Kambouchner M, Valeyre D, Hance AJ: Pulmonary Langerhans' cell granulomatosis (histiocytosis X). Annu Rev Med 43:105–115, 1992.

David Murphy

Asbestos-related lung disease is subdivided into three categories: parenchymal, pleural, and associated conditions (Table 14-1). The designation *asbestosis* is reserved for parenchymal disease, in particular for interstitial fibrosis in which asbestos bodies or fibers can be demonstrated.

Although most exposure to asbestos occurs in occupational, paraoccupational, or environmental situations, asbestos is ubiquitous. Routine autopsy studies in large urban communities have revealed asbestos bodies in the lungs of about 30 percent of the general population. Workers most frequently exposed to asbestos are those engaged in the manufacture of asbestos cement products, floor tiling, insulation, fireproofing material, textiles, asbestos paper products, friction material, and the reinforcement of plastics. Asbestos was used in the filtration of alcoholic beverages and drugs, in gas masks during World War II, and as filter tips for some cigarettes in the United States. Exposure also occurs from mining the mineral.

ASBESTOS FIBERS

Asbestos is a collective term for fibrous mineral silicates which contain magnesium. Asbestos fibers are classified into two broad groups: amphibole and serpentine (Table 14-2). Serpentine fibers are curly, whereas amphibole fibers are needlelike. Commercial forms of asbestos—crocidolite, amosite, and chrysotile—have all been associated with asbestos-related disorders. Crocidolite has a greater carcinogenic effect than either amosite or chrysotile.

Most of the asbestos fibers in the lungs are < 5 μm long. Only a small proportion of all the asbestos fibers in the lungs are identifiable as "asbestos bodies." These appear under the microscope as brown or orange fibers, beaded or match stick in appearance, and about 50 to 100 μm in length. In general, a correlation exists between the concentration of asbestos fibers in the lung and the severity of the pulmonary fibrosis.

PARENCHYMAL DISEASE: ASBESTOSIS

Definition, Etiology, and Pathology

The term *asbestosis* should be reserved for interstitial fibrosis of the pulmonary parenchyma in which asbestos bodies or fibers are demonstrable. Pleural abnormalities are not part of this catagory.

TABLE 14-1 Asbestos-Related Conditions

Parenchymal	Pleural	Associated
Asbestosis	Benign pleural effusion	Bronchogenic carcinoma
Rounded	Pleural plaques	Peritoneal mesothelioma
atelectasis	Diffuse pleural thickening	
	Diffuse malignant	Associated malignant
	mesothelioma	conditions

TABLE 14-2 Asbestos Fibers

Amphibole group	Serpentine group
Crocidolite (blue)	Chrysotile (white)
Amosite (brown)	
Tremolite	
Anthophyllite	
Actinolite	

A latent period of 15 years or longer usually precedes clinical manifestations. There is no evidence that causal exposure to asbestos, as occurs in the general population, causes asbestosis.

Macroscopically, lungs that are the seat of asbestosis are smaller than normal. A gray opaque fibrosis extends from the subpleural regions into the parenchyma; the lobar and lobular septae are also thickened. Histologically, the initial reaction to the presence of asbestos fibers in the lung is an accumulation of macrophages and neutrophils in the alveolar spaces; release of their lysosomal enzymes leads to inflammation and later to fibrosis.

Early in the disease, the lower lobes are affected in a peribronchial distribution; this stage is succeeded by diffuse interstitial fibrosis. The more advanced stage is characterized by honeycombing with thick-walled air spaces from 1 to 15 mm in diameter. The visceral pleura is invariably involved in this fibrotic process.

Clinical

As with other occupational lung diseases, the diagnosis rests on an adequate history of exposure and a characteristic chest radiograph (Table 14-3). Biopsies of lung parenchyma are required only if the diagnosis is in doubt or for compensation purposes. Clinical findings include (1) dyspnea, initially present on exertion; (2) basilar rales, an early finding and usually first heard in the midaxillary line; and (3) clubbing of the fingers. Advanced stages of the disease may be associated with hypoxemic respiratory failure and cor pulmonale.

TABLE 14-3 Diagnostic Criteria for Asbestosis

Major Criteria
1. Reliable history of exposure
2. Appropriate interval between exposure and detection

Minor Criteria
1. Chest radiographic evidence of bilateral small irregular opacities
2. Restrictive pattern on pulmonary function testing
3. Diffusing capacity below the lower limits of normal
4. Bilateral late or paninspiratory rales at the posterior lung bases not cleared by cough

SOURCE: Am Rev Respir Dis 134:363, 1986.

Radiography

Typically, a reticular pattern is seen bilaterally in the lower lobes. Sometimes, the interstitial disease is accompanied by pleural plaques or diffuse pleural thickening. A diffuse nodular pattern also may occur.

Pulmonary Function

The effects of asbestos on pulmonary function are dose related, and pulmonary function abnormalities may occur without definite radiologic changes. For example, reduced expiratory airflow at low lung volumes occurs in asbestos-exposed individuals even when no abnormalities can be identified on the chest radiograph.

However, the usual pattern of abnormality in pulmonary function is a reduction in lung volumes: initially, inspiratory capacity and vital capacity are decreased while the functional residual capacity and residual volume reduction are preserved; the latter also decrease as the disease progresses. The forced expiratory volume in 1s/forced vital capacity (FEV_1/FVC) ratio is generally preserved. The diffusing capacity (DL_{CO}) is reduced in accord with the extent of the disease; the decrease correlates with the severity of histologic evidence of interstitial fibrosis. Lung compliance is decreased. Arterial hypoxemia occurs first during exercise and later at rest. In those who smoke cigarettes, a combined obstructive and restrictive pattern may be found.

Differential Diagnosis

The differential diagnosis includes usual interstitial pneumonitis; connective tissue disorders involving the lungs, such as rheumatoid arthritis, scleroderma, or systemic lupus erythematosis; sarcoidosis, lymphangitic carcinomatous; and radiation pneumonitis.

Treatment

No treatment is currently available to either prevent or retard the process of the asbestosis. Nor is there evidence that removal from the source of exposure affects the outcome of the disease.

Treatment of infections may be important because nonspecific inflammation may contribute to progression of the fibrosis. Corticosteroid therapy is not advocated. Supplemental oxygen therapy may be required to treat moderate-to-severe arterial hypoxemia.

Rounded Atelectasis or Pseudotumor

This is a localized fibrous folding of the parietal and visceral pleura causing a characteristic "comet sign" on the chest radiograph. The condition occurs in both upper and lower lobes and can mimic a tumor. The pathology is a nonspecific fibrous pleurisy with atelectasis of the underlying lung. Computed tomography (CT) scanning is helpful in identifying the nature of the lesion. However, if the diagnosis is in doubt, the lesion should be investigated as if it were a possible malignancy.

PLEURAL DISEASE

Asbestos-related pleural disease occurs in a variety of forms: benign pleural effusion, pleural plaques, diffuse pleural thickening, and diffuse malignant mesothelioma.

BENIGN PLEURAL EFFUSION

Definition, Etiology, and Pathology

Small exudative pleural effusions are one of the earliest consequences of asbestos exposure. They occur in about 7 percent of exposed workers, the incidence varying with the intensity of the exposure. The onset may be as early as 14 years after the start of the exposure. Many resolve within a year, but some recur years after the exposure, on the same or on the opposite side. The fluid is usually bloody and sterile and contains variable numbers of mesothelial cells along with lymphocytes, macrophages, and erythrocytes. Diagnostic criteria are shown in Table 14-3. In some long-term follow-up, 30 to 50 percent have proved to be associated with malignant mesothelioma.

Clinical and Radiographic Signs

The clinical and radiographic signs are those of a pleural effusion. The chest radiograph typically shows the meniscus sign. The presence of a subpulmonic effusion may be suggested by a shoulder on the normal diaphragmatic contour. Decubitus films are useful in confirming the presence of free-flowing fluid.

Differential Diagnosis

The major diagnosis to be excluded is diffuse malignant mesothelioma of the pleura. Other possible causes of pleural effusion also have to be discounted (see Part IX).

Treatment

A large pleural effusion may need to be drained to relieve dyspnea. More moderate effusions require no intervention.

PLEURAL PLAQUES

Definition, Etiology, and Pathology

Pleural plaques are discrete, elevated lesions of variable size and shape which occur most frequently on the posterolateral parietal pleura or on the diaphragmatic pleura, but not on the visceral pleura. Their surface may be shiny and smooth, bosselated, or nodular. Microscopically, the plaques consist of collagenous laminated connective tissue which is acellular except for a thin cover of mesothelial cells. Calcification is common. Asbestos fibers are present in the plaque and are uncoated. How the asbestos fibers reach the parietal pleura, and how they cause plaque formation, remains uncertain. In the general population, a prevalence of up to 3 percent has been reported. In contrast, in occupationally exposed, a prevalence of up to 85 percent has been found in individuals with 30 or more years of exposure.

Clinical

Pleural plaques, which serve as markers of exposure to asbestos, cause neither signs nor symptoms and produce no clinically significant reduction in pulmonary function.

Radiography

Chest radiographs identify only about 12 to 15 percent of the plaques found at autopsy. Most plaques produce smooth circumscribed elevations of the parietal pleura either on the posterolateral chest wall (between the seventh and tenth ribs), or on the diaphragm, or on the mediastinal pleura. Oblique views increase the diagnostic yield. Calcification in a plaque increases the chance of identification, especially when seen en face on the posteroanterior chest radiograph.

CT scanning is useful in identifying plaques not seen on conventional radiographs and in distinguishing pleural from parenchymal disease. Although plaques may occur in association with asbestosis, they are usually unaccompanied by interstitial fibrosis. There is no evidence that plaques precede the development of diffuse malignant mesothelioma of the pleura.

Differential Diagnosis

Bilateral plaques always suggest asbestos exposure (Table 14-4).

DIFFUSE PLEURAL THICKENING

Definition, Etiology, and Pathology

Diffuse pleural thickening is identified on the posteroanterior film as thickening of pleura (> 1 mm), below the fourth intercostal space (see Radiography below). In contrast to plaques which form on the parietal pleura, diffuse pleural thickening affects the visceral pleura. In one series of workers with 30 or more years of exposure, 20 percent had some pleural thickening, and 16 percent had pleural plaques. However, severe diffuse pleural thickening is uncommon. The pathogenesis of diffuse pleural thickening is uncertain, but it may be a sequel to a benign, asbestos-related, pleural effusion (Table 14-5).

Clinical

Complaints include dyspnea, chest tightness, or difficulty in completing an inspiration. Physical examination often reveals no

TABLE 14-4 Differential Diagnosis of a Unilateral Pleural Plaque

Uncalcified	Calcified
Metastatic disease	Trauma sequelae
Benign fibrous mesothelioma	Hemorrhage sequelae
Diffuse malignant mesothelioma	Infection sequelae
Lymphoma	Healed rib fractures
Myeloma	Radiation
Infection sequelae	Scleroderma
Trauma sequelae	Chronic mineral oil aspiration

SOURCE: Rosenstock L, Hudson LD: Occup Med 22:383, 1987.

TABLE 14-5 Benign Asbestos-Related Effusion: Diagnostic Criteria

- Exposure to asbestos
- Confirmation by chest radiography or thoracentesis
- No other disease-related pleural effusion
- No malignant tumor within 3 years

SOURCE: Epler GR: JAMA 247:617, 1982.

abnormalities except in severe cases, in which lung expansion may be diminished or a pleural rub heard.

Pulmonary Function

Extensive pleural involvement may result in a restrictive pattern of pulmonary function, with or without a reduction in DL_{CO}. The ratio of the DL_{CO} to alveolar ventilation (VA) can be helpful in distinguishing between asbestosis and an encased lung: a low DL_{CO}/VA ratio suggests asbestosis, whereas a high DL_{CO}/VA ratio suggests an encased lung. Pleural thickening in association with asbestosis exaggerates the abnormalities in pulmonary function tests. Extensive, severe bilateral pleural thickening can lead to respiratory failure or cor pulmonale.

Radiography

Diffuse pleural thickening due to asbestos exposure is often bilateral, involves the costophrenic angle(s), and rarely calcifies. It must be distinguished, especially in the obese, from extrapleural fat particularly in the region of the fourth to eighth ribs posterolaterally. CT is helpful in making this distinction. Visceral pleural changes, manifested by thickening of the interlobar fissures, may be the only radiographic signs of asbestos exposure.

Differential Diagnosis

Diffuse bilateral pleural thickening may occur with bilateral empyema, tuberculosis, scleroderma, rheumatoid arthritis, and systemic lupus erythematosis. Drugs such as methysergide and practolol may also cause bilateral pleural disease.

Treatment

Occasionally, decortication may be necessary if dyspnea is prominent. However, it should be considered only in the absence of parenchymal disease.

DIFFUSE MALIGNANT MESOTHELIOMA OF THE PLEURA

This topic is covered in Part IX.

SURVEILLANCE

A Canadian task force on occupational respiratory disease has recommended that occupationally exposed workers with normal chest radiographs should undergo chest radiography and spirometry every 2 years. If small irregular opacities or suspicious signs or symptoms are found, chest radiographs and spirometry should be performed yearly; complete pulmonary function and exercise testing should then be done every 2 years. Individuals with benign pleural abnormalities are monitored no more often than those with normal chest radiographs.

ASSOCIATED CONDITIONS

Bronchogenic Carcinoma

Lung carcinomas are uncommon in asbestos workers who do not smoke. Nonetheless, an association has been found between exposure to asbestos and bronchogenic carcinoma (see Part VII). The average latency period between first exposure and the detection of a carcinoma has ranged from 20 to 30 years. It is debatable whether asbestos itself causes lung cancer in nonsmokers. However, 40 percent of patients with asbestosis die from lung cancer.

CANCERS OF THE GASTROINTESTINAL TRACT AND LARYNX

Certain groups of asbestos workers have been reported to have increased risk of cancers of the gastrointestinal tract, larynx, kidney, pancreas, ovary, and eye. An increased risk of lymphoma has also been suggested. These findings remain unconfirmed.

BIBLIOGRAPHY

For a more detailed discussion, see Weill H, Jones RN: Occupational pulmonary diseases, in Fishman AP (ed), *Pulmonary Diseases and Disorders,* 2d ed. New York, McGraw-Hill, 1988, pp. 837–844.

Aberle DR: High-resolution computed tomography of asbestos-related diseases. Semin Roentgenol 26:118–131, 1991.

Kleinerman JI: Neoplasms of the pleura, chest wall and diaphragm, in Fishman AP (ed), *Pulmonary Diseases and Disorders,* 2d ed. New York, McGraw-Hill, 1988, pp 2033–2038.

Miller WT Jr, Gefter WB, Miller WT Sr: Asbestos-related chest diseases: Plain radiographic findings. Semin Roentgenol 27:102–120, 1992.

Raffn E, Lynge E, Korsgaard B: Incidence of lung cancer by histological type among asbestos cement workers in Denmark. Br J Ind Med 50:85–89, 1993.

Tuomi T, Huuskonen MS, Virtamo M, Tossavainen A, Tammilehto L, Mattson K, et al: Relative risk of mesothelioma associated with different levels of exposure to asbestos. Scan J Work Environ Health 17:404–408, 1991.

Tuberous Sclerosis and Lymphangiomyomatosis

Michael Beers   Gregory Tino

Because the *pulmonary* abnormalities (pathology, physiology, and clinical presentation) seen in both of these rare diseases are similar, they are presented together.

TUBEROUS SCLEROSIS

Definition

Tuberous sclerosis (Bourneville's disease) is an inherited disorder of unknown etiology involving a defect in connective tissue development. The full syndrome is characterized by the classic triad of epilepsy, mental retardation, and adenoma sebaceum (dermal angiofibroma). However, incomplete forms of the disease are common and organ systems other than the skin and brain are commonly involved. These include the eyes, thyroid, bones, kidneys, lymph nodes, heart, and *lungs.*

Etiology and Epidemiology

The disease is rare. Clinically recognized disease has been noted in about 1/150,000. Pulmonary involvement is even rarer; lung disease is estimated to occur in about 0.1 to 1.0 percent of all patients with tuberous sclerosis. In about 50 percent of the patients with tuberous sclerosis, the disease is sporadic; the others represent a hereditary autosomal dominant disorder. Men and women are equally affected.

Clinical Features

Skin lesions feature prominently in the diagnosis of tuberous sclerosis. The skin lesions are varied. Most distinctive is adenoma sebaceum which usually appears in early adolescence in the form of wartlike lesions on the face. Other lesions include hypopigmented spots on the trunk (hypomelanotic nodules) which often appear in childhood and sometimes precede adenoma sebaceum; discoloration and thickening of the skin (Shagren patches) in the lumbar region; and periungual fibromas.

Epilepsy and mental retardation comprise the rest of the triad. However, the occurrence of seizures and the degree of mental retardation are highly variable. Cerebral and paraventricular hamartomas are common.

In addition to the abnormalities of the skin and brain, other clinical and pathologic findings are common. These include pulmonary leiomyomatosis, cardiac rhabdomyoma, sclerotic bone lesions, renal angiolipoma, and renal cystic disease. Pneumothorax is a common complication of advanced pulmonary disease.

Pathology

The pathologic changes in the lung vary with the phase of the disease. The primary abnormality is a form of pulmonary leiomyomatosis characterized by proliferation and hypertrophy of smooth muscle in the walls of blood vessels, bronchioles, and lymphatics. In addition, adenomatoid nodules (alveolar hamartomas) are scattered throughout the lungs.

In the later stages of the lung disease, tuberous sclerosis can cause honeycombing and cyst formation. The cyst walls contain hypertrophied and hyperplastic smooth muscle. Subpleural blebs are common and predispose to pneumothorax.

Clinical Features of Pulmonary Involvement

Patients with pulmonary involvement from tuberous sclerosis generally present in one of four ways:

1. Spontaneous pneumothorax—in about one third of patients
2. Dyspnea—the most common initial pulmonary complaint
3. Chest pain—due to pneumothorax or associated with subpleural blebs
4. Hemoptysis—rare

Cyanosis and cor pulmonale are relatively late signs. Clubbing or pulmonary osteoarthropathy is rare.

As noted above, incomplete presentations of the disease are common. In contrast to the patients with neurologic abnormalities (generally < 20 years old), patients with pulmonary manifestations tend to be older (generally 30 to 35 years old) and predominantly female (80 percent are women). Not only do patients with pulmonary involvement manifest fewer signs of brain involvement (only 20 percent have seizures and 60 percent possess normal intelligence), but they also have more skin involvement.

In addition to parenchymal pulmonary disease, tuberous sclerosis can also involve the chest wall and pleura. Sclerotic bone lesions and cystic changes in the ribs do occur but are uncommon. Exudative (nonchylous) pleural effusions are rare.

Diagnostic Evaluation

Chest radiography   Early in the course of pulmonary disease, the chest radiograph shows diffuse interstitial lung disease predominantly at the bases. At first, the lesions assume a fine reticular or reticulonodular pattern. As the disease progresses, cysts and honeycombing supervene. Pneumothorax may ensue.

Pulmonary function tests These tests show a restrictive pattern and an abnormally low diffusing capacity.

Differential diagnosis Although exceedingly rare, pulmonary tuberous sclerosis should be considered in the differential diagnosis of interstitial lung disease in women of childbearing age (even in the absence of accompanying cutaneous or neurologic abnormalities). More common entities to be excluded include sarcoidosis, unusual interstitial pneumonitis (UIP), scleroderma, rheumatoid lung, histiocytosis X, lymphangitic tumor, and lymphangiomyomatosis.

Course and Prognosis

Most patients with pulmonary disease as part of tuberous sclerosis die of respiratory failure within 5 years of the onset of symptoms. The most frequent causes of death are cor pulmonale and recurrent spontaneous pneumothoraces. No effective treatment is known; corticosteroids have been tried without success.

LYMPHANGIOMYOMATOSIS

Definition

Lymphangiomyomatosis is a rare disorder of unknown etiology characterized by widespread proliferation of atypical smooth muscle in pulmonary lymphatics, venules, and small airways. The dominant clinical features of the disease are interstitial lung disease, chylous pleural effusions, and recurrent pneumothoraces.

Epidemiology

Lymphangiomyomatosis occurs exclusively in women, usually of childbearing age. Fewer than 150 cases have been reported. A genetic link is suspected but not proved.

Pathology and Pathophysiology

The fundamental pathologic abnormality in the lungs is widespread and uneven proliferation of atypical smooth muscle. Involvement of the parenchyma of the lungs by the proliferating venules, bronchioles, and lymphatics obstructs and distorts air spaces.

Chylous pleural effusions are common. They are attributed to obstruction and obliteration of lymphatics in the pleura or mediastinum which causes them to rupture. Obstruction of small airways leads to obstructive airways disease and hyperinflation. The interstitial disease is characterized by nodularity which is due to widespread but irregular muscular proliferation. Distended peribronchial lymphatics and interstitial edema are interspersed with the interstitial disease.

Clinical Features

In a woman of childbearing age, the diagnosis is suggested by the occurrence of progressive dyspnea, chylous effusions, repeated pneumothoraces, and hemoptysis, with or without evidence of interstitial lung disease. Dyspnea is the presenting symptom in > 50 percent of patients. It is insidious in onset and may be due to the presence of airflow obstruction, interstitial disease, or pleural effusion. Spontaneous pneumothorax is an initiating manifestation in about 25 percent of patients. Hemoptysis as a presenting sign occurs in < 10 percent of patients.

Diagnostic Evaluation

Chest radiography The three radiographic features of lymphangiomyomatosis are (1) widespread interstitial disease, usually reticular or reticulonodular in type; (2) pleural effusion, usually chylous, which occurs in more than two thirds of the patients in the course of the disease; and (3) pneumothorax, which occurs at some time in > 50 percent of the patients. As the disease progresses, the interstitial disease leads to widespread cyst formation, honeycombing, or hyperinflation.

Pulmonary function tests These reflect a combination of interstitial and obstructive lung disease, in varying combinations, and often disproportionately abnormal with respect to the radiographic changes. Spirometry reveals evidence of airways obstruction with a decrease in the forced expiratory volume in 1s/forced vital capacity (FEV_1/FVC) ratio and forced expiratory flow ($FEF_{25-75\%}$) and an increase in airway resistance. Static lung volumes often show increases in residual volume (RV) and functional residual capacity (FRC), suggesting air trapping. In contrast to other interstitial lung diseases, total lung capacity (TLC) is often preserved because of the combination of restrictive and obstructive disease. The diffusing capacity (DL_{CO}) is markedly reduced. Arterial hypoxemia, due to ventilation-perfusion mismatch, is common.

Biopsy Although the diagnosis of lymphangiomyomatosis may be suspected on clinical, radiographic, and physiologic manifestations, a positive diagnosis requires histologic examination of lung tissue. Transbronchial biopsies often provide sufficient material to establish the diagnosis but are often misinterpreted by inexperienced pathologists. When transbronchial biopsies are considered to be nondiagnostic by the experienced pathologist, open lung biopsy should be performed.

Differential diagnosis Lymphangiomyomatosis must be distinguished from conditions known to cause spontaneous pneumothoraces, interstitial lung disease, or chylous pleural effusions. Diseases which share one or several of these features include catamenial pneumothorax, cystic fibrosis, Marfan's syndrome, congenital cystic lung disease, sarcoidosis, lymphoma, eosinophilic granuloma, and idiopathic pulmonary fibrosis.

Prognosis and Treatment

The disease usually progresses insidiously, often leading to death from pulmonary insufficiency within 10 years of diagnosis. Therapeutic intervention is designed to inhibit or eliminate endogenous estrogen activity. This approach is based on evidence that proliferation of smooth muscle in the lungs is under estrogenic hormonal regulation.

1. Lymphangiomyomatosis often becomes worse either during pregnancy or after estrogen therapy; it sometimes undergoes remission after the menopause.
2. Both estrogen and progesterone receptors have been found in the lungs of the patients with this disease.

Hormonal manipulation has been attempted surgically by means of oophorectomy and medically by administering tamoxifen or progesterone. However, because of the rarity of this disorder, it has been difficult to prove that any of these modalities exerts a beneficial effect on the natural history of the disease. Currently, the favored therapy is progesterone, reserving oophorectomy as a second line intervention. Because of the detrimental effects of estrogen on the natural history of the disease, both pregnancy and the use of oral contraceptives must be avoided. Women of childbearing age must be counseled on alternative methods of birth control.

Recurrent pneumothoraces and symptomatic chylous effusions that do not respond to hormonal therapy should be treated by chemical pleurodesis. Prolonged drainage of chylous effusions by chest tube should be avoided because the loss of protein and of lymphocyte-rich pleural fluid will cause profound malnutrition and impair immune function. Several patients with far-advanced lung disease have had successful lung transplantation.

BIBLIOGRAPHY

For a more detailed discussion, see Fishman AP: Tuberous sclerosis and lymphangiomyomatosis, in Fishman AP (ed), *Pulmonary Diseases and Disorders,* 2d ed. New York, McGraw-Hill, 1988, pp 965–972.

Hauck RW, Konig G, Permanetter W, Weiss M, Wockel W, Fruhmann G: Tuberous sclerosis with pulmonary involvement. Respiration 57:289–292, 1990.

Lenoir S, Grenier P, Brauner MW, Frija J, Remy-Jardin M, Revel D, Cordier JF: Pulmonary lymphangiomyomatosis and tuberous sclerosis: Comparison of radiographic and thin-section CT findings. Radiology 175:329–334, 1990.

Sampson JR, Janssen LA, Sandkuijl LA: Linkage investigation of three putative tuberous sclerosis determining loci on chromosomes 9q, 11q, and 12q. The Tuberous Sclerosis Collaborative Group. J Med Genet 29:861–866, 1992.

Taylor JR, Ryu J, Colby TV, Raffin TA: Lymphangiomyomatosis: Clinical course in 32 patients. N Engl J Med 323:1254–1260, 1990.

Urban T, Kuttenn F, Gompel A, Marsac J, Lacronique J: Pulmonary lymphangiomyomatosis. Follow-up and long-term outcome with antiestrogen therapy; a report of eight cases. Chest 102:472–476, 1992.

III | MISCELLANEOUS DISORDERS

Paul E. Epstein

DEFINITION

The phrase *aspiration pneumonia* has been used to denote at least three separate syndromes: aspiration of gastric acid, aspiration of particulate matter, and pulmonary infection resulting from aspiration of any nongaseous material. Each of these syndromes is characterized by a distinct series of clinical findings, a distinct clinical course, and a distinct method of management. The apparent reason for the common practice of grouping them into a single clinical entity is that they all occur in similar clinical circumstances, frequently as a single event during gastrointestinal reflux or regurgitation.

NORMAL PROTECTIVE MECHANISMS

Normally, the respiratory tract is protected from liquid or solid soiling by a highly coordinated sequence of neuromuscular events involving the pharyngeal palate, epiglottis, vocal cords, pharyngeal constrictor muscles, and cervical esophagus. Once the glottis has been safely bypassed, the upper esophageal sphincter and esophageal peristaltic waves ordinarily ensure the normal unidirectional flow of swallowed material. Furthermore, the lower esophageal sphincter maintains a high resting tone, preventing reflux of gastric contents into the upper gastrointestinal tract. Even if the normal individual should experience regurgitation or vomiting, the coordinated, centrally mediated neuromuscular protection of the glottic opening is an effective mechanical barrier to aspiration of liquid or solid materials into the lungs. However, a variety of pathologic and iatrogenic circumstances can interfere with the coordination of neuromuscular events and predispose to aspiration.

PREDISPOSING FACTORS

Depression of consciousness automatically blunts the reflex response to aspiration. Surgical anesthesia, alcohol intoxication, narcotic overdose, and cerebrovascular accidents are common causes of depressed states of consciousness which frequently result in aspiration, particularly because these circumstances are associated with a propensity for vomiting. Operative procedures performed under general anesthesia are especially likely to be complicated by aspiration if the surgery involves the upper abdomen or insufficient time has elapsed after a meal for the stomach to empty. These circumstances are common in emergency abdominal surgery and in the course of obstetric anesthesia. Insertion of a cuffed endotracheal tube during surgery is helpful, but not infallible, in preventing aspiration of gastric contents.

Anatomic or functional alterations of the larynx or esophagus also predispose to aspiration of foreign materials. Bulbar palsy or vocal cord paralysis impair the coordinated protective movements of the larynx that commonly allow aspiration to take place. Achalasia or the presence of a Zenker's diverticulum produce a reservoir of particulate material that commonly washes back into the pharynx while the patient is asleep in a recumbent position. Tracheoesophageal fistulas, usually the result of carcinoma of the esophagus, allow free access of swallowed material into the tracheobronchial tree even though the pharynx and larynx function normally.

Among the iatrogenic factors involved in episodes of aspiration, two warrant special mention.

1. The presence of a nasogastric tube that disturbs laryngeal function and interferes with the function of the lower esophageal sphincter
2. Overfilling of the stomach by enteral nutrition through nasogastric or gastrostomy tube feedings which, in the critically ill patient, enhances the possibility of regurgitation and aspiration

PATHOPHYSIOLOGY AND CLINICAL CHARACTERISTICS

Aspiration of Gastric Acid

The syndrome produced by aspiration of gastric acid was first described by Mendelson in 1946. It should be distinguished from the effects of particulate or infective materials. The pH and the volume of aspirated liquid are the two most important factors determining the extent of damage produced by this event. If the pH of the gastric contents is 2.5 or higher, the adverse effects are dominated by the volume of aspirated liquid. When the pH of the aspirated liquid is 2.4 or lower, damage to the respiratory epithelium is a constant finding. Although other nonparticulate constituents of the gastric contents play a role in transient inflammation of the tracheobronchial tree, the physiologic effects usually disappear within 48 h.

Aspiration of small volumes of low pH fluid is common, occurring even in normal individuals during sleep. Although this is generally well tolerated, damage to the ciliated respiratory epithelial cells in the trachea and large bronchi potentially impair the normal defense mechanisms of the lung. Large aspirates of low pH liquid spread rapidly through the tracheobronchial tree to the alveoli, reaching the pleura within 12 to 18 s of aspiration. As the acid washes into the lung, ciliated cells in the bronchi are destroyed, surfactant is instantaneously inactivated, and cellular contents of the alveoli are lost due to chemical damage. In addition to the damage to type I and type II pneumocytes caused by acid aspiration, all structures of the alveolar capillary membrane are damaged, including the subepithelial basement membrane and the capillary endothelial cells. The resulting increase in alveolar-capillary permeability results in a massive shift of plasma and formed elements of the blood into the alveoli. Contact of gastric acid with proteins of the tracheobronchial mucus and with buffers in the bloody alveolar exudate leads to a rapid rise in the pH of aspirated fluid to nondamaging levels, but not before widespread destruction of pulmonary parenchyma has occurred.

Widespread damage to the alveolar capillary membrane also produces a sudden and dramatic rise in pulmonary arterial pressure, probably as a result of a variety of factors, including hypoxia, interstitial edema, local atelectasis, congestion and thromboses in the pulmonary microvessels, as well as release of vasoactive substances by damaged tissues. The coexistence of increased pulmonary vascular permeability and increased pulmonary pressure promotes the massive shifts of fluid out of the intravascular space and into the pulmonary interstitium and alveoli. Since ventilation to these alveoli virtually ceases as the pulmonary edema fluid fills the alveolar lumens, hypoxia worsens as blood flows through the unventilated areas. Meanwhile, the sudden decrease in intravascular volume often leads to tachycardia and systemic hypotension. The overall clinical picture is that of the adult respiratory distress syndrome, i.e., the sudden onset of tachypnea, refractory hypoxemia, and noncardiogenic pulmonary edema with systemic hypotension.

Aspiration of Solid Material

Large chunks of food are occasionally aspirated during a meal. The size of the bolus is usually large enough to be caught at the entrance of the glottis, causing blockage of air entry into the lungs. Since swallowing usually takes place closer to end-expiration than it does to end-inspiration, clearance of the upper airway by cough is usually unsuccessful. The natural tendency to attempt to fill the lungs is counterproductive in that the bolus is sucked further into the glottic chink. Asphyxia progresses rapidly and the individual is helpless as he becomes cyanotic and disoriented. The clinical appearance of the aspiration of a large chunk of food is that of an individual who has been eating calmly, but suddenly stands, unable to speak, begins to drool, and becomes progressively cyanotic. This is a true medical emergency that requires the Heimlich maneuver in which someone stands behind the affected individual, wraps the arms around the costal margin and locks hands in the epigastrium, and then applies a sharp, compressive motion to force air out of the chest and expel the food bolus from the glottis.

The aspiration of smaller particles of food can produce a different syndrome than that described above. They are generally aspirated during vomiting along with other gastric contents. Chewed or partially digested food particles are generally soft and small enough to enter the tracheobronchial tree. The entry of these food particles into the lower respiratory tract along with liquid gastric contents may block lobar, segmental, or subsegmental bronchial orifices and produce atelectasis. In addition, the foreign organic materials can cause an inflammatory response within the bronchial wall and lead to further impaction of the food particle. Certain vegetable products, such as nuts, are hydrophilic and tend to swell when trapped in the moist environment of the bronchial lumen. The clinical consequences of retained food particles include hypoxia, due to the flow of blood through atelectatic areas of lung, and the radiographic appearance of volume loss caused by atelectasis. In addition, persistently blocked bronchi are highly susceptible to infection.

Aspiration of Infective Agents

The excellent defense mechanisms of the lung usually render the lower respiratory tract sterile despite constant challenge by inhaled microorganisms. In addition, gastric contents are usually sterile as a result of the low pH of the stomach. Nonetheless, when gastric contents are aspirated into the lung, the material traversing the oropharynx frequently picks up microorganisms from the mouth. Damage to the mucociliary escalator, pooling of proteinaceous material in the alveoli, and altered access of white blood cells to the affected area contribute to the enhanced susceptibility of the lung to infection.

Despite these predisposing influences, infection is not a primary or early event after aspiration. Pulmonary infiltrates, fever, and hypoxia during the first few days following aspiration are due to chemical pneumonitis produced by the aspiration itself. Infection is heralded by cough with the production of purulent sputum and recrudescence of fever and leukocytosis at least three days after the aspiration. Infection takes the form of bronchopneumonia, lung abscess, necrotizing pneumonia, or empyema depending on the specific organisms involved and the mechanical factors enhancing the infection.

DIAGNOSTIC EVALUATION

As soon as aspiration is suspected, the oropharynx should be inspected for the presence and character (liquid or particulate) of vomitus. Auscultation of the chest often reveals rhonchi and wheezes in the affected areas. The chest radiograph may show focal abnormality in the dependent segments of lung, reflecting the position of the patient at the time that aspiration took place. Alternatively, a diffuse alveolar infiltrate of adult respiratory distress syndrome may also be seen.

Measurement of arterial blood oxygenation is the most effective means of assessing the severity of the aspiration event. Because hypoxia may develop gradually over the first several hours due to progressive congestion and atelectasis, serial sampling of arterial blood gases should start when the aspiration is first diagnosed and should be followed at intervals of 1 to 2 h until the patient is clinically stable. Because major fluid shifts occur in the course of serious aspiration and fluid replacement may be required, insertion of a Swan-Ganz catheter is appropriate to ensure optimal fluid balance.

TREATMENT

Oxygenation Supplemental oxygen administered by nasal cannula or face mask usually will maintain adequate oxygenation. However, when it becomes impossible to maintain oxyhemoglobin saturation of 90 percent or better while using a nonrebreathing oxygen mask, an endotracheal tube should be inserted and positive-pressure ventilation should be initiated.

Fluid management Hypotension in the course of aspiration is usually the result of loss of intravascular volume resulting from increased permeability of the pulmonary capillaries and flooding of the pulmonary parenchyma (noncardiogenic pulmonary edema). Intravascular volume must be replaced to maintain a tolerable blood pressure. However, pulmonary capillary wedge pressure should be kept as low as possible during the infusion of fluid to minimize the hydrostatic component of intrapulmonary capillary leakage. Crystalloids should be used for fluid replacement because colloids are likely to leak into the extravascular space and may retard fluid resorption as the lung begins to heal.

Corticosteroids Although attractive in theory because of their anti-inflammatory effects, there is little convincing evidence that administration of corticosteroids improves the outcome after an episode of aspiration. The use of steroids in this setting has therefore been abandoned.

Bronchoscopy Bronchoscopy should be performed only if bronchial obstruction by particulate matter is suspected. A rigid bronchoscope is more effective than a fiberoptic instrument for removing large particles. In the absence of atelectasis, bronchoscopy and bronchial lavage should be avoided because these can worsen the patient's clinical condition.

Treatment of infection Appropriate treatment of the infection depends on the evidence confirming its presence and the setting in which aspiration takes place. Antibiotic therapy is unnecessary at the time aspiration is first recognized, particularly if the patient has not been hospitalized for a prolonged period. When clear-cut pneumonia occurs, penicillin or clindamycin may be used. If the patient has been hospitalized for a long period and nosocomial infection is suspected, clindamycin should be combined with an aminoglycoside or third-generation cephalosporin to deal with gram-negative pathogens, including *Pseudomonas.* Before starting antibiotics, attempts should be made to obtain sputum for direct microscopic examination and for culture.

PREVENTION

The primary goal of the physician should be prevention of aspiration rather than treatment. Strict attention to predisposing causes and minimization of aggravating factors will decrease the incidence of aspiration dramatically. In addition, several studies have demonstrated the efficacy of decreasing stomach pH and promoting gastric emptying in obstetric and emergency surgical patients. The preoperative use of cimetidine and metoclopramide appears to achieve these goals in a clinically useful way.

BIBLIOGRAPHY

For a more detailed discussion, see Epstein PE: Aspiration diseases of the lungs, in Fishman AP (ed), *Pulmonary Diseases and Disorders,* 2d ed. New York, McGraw-Hill, 1988, pp 877–892.

Mullan H, Roubenoff RA, Roubenoff R: Risk of pulmonary aspiration among patients receiving enteral nutrition support. J Parenter Enteral Nutr 16:160–164, 1992.

Torres A, Serra-Batlles J, Ros E, Piera C, Puig de la Bellacasa J, Cobos A, et al: Pulmonary aspiration of gastric contents in patients receiving mechanical ventilation: The effect of body position. Ann Intern Med 116:540–543, 1992.

Michael Beers   Gregory Tino

DEFINITION

Primary or *classic pulmonary alveolar proteinosis* (PAP) is a clinical syndrome of unknown etiology characterized by excessive accumulation of surfactant phospholipids and apoproteins within the alveolar spaces. *Secondary PAP* or *pseudoproteinosis* occurs in association with certain environmental exposures, drugs, hematologic malignancies, and infections (Table 17-1), and shares many of the clinical, radiographic, and histologic features of the primary form.

PATHOGENESIS

The epithelium of the normal alveolar space is lined with lung surfactant, a phospholipid-rich, lipoprotein-like substance, that lowers alveolar surface tension and prevents atelectasis at end-expiration. Alveolar type II cells (granular pneumocytes) play a key role in normal surfactant metabolism, synthesizing, secreting, storing, and recycling both lipid and protein components of surfactant in a continuous and dynamic fashion. Alveolar macrophages, pulmonary lymphatics, and the mucociliary escalator contribute to the removal of surfactant from the alveolar space, but their role is thought to be minor.

Most evidence to date suggests that primary PAP results from decreased removal of surfactant by alveolar type II cells rather than to an increase in surfactant production. The mechanisms by which the diverse stimuli associated with the secondary form of alveolar proteinosis interfere with surfactant synthesis and uptake remain unknown.

PATHOLOGY

Primary PAP is a diffuse process characterized pathologically by the dense accumulation of periodic acid-Schiff (PAS)-positive phospholipid material in the alveoli, with preservation of the normal, delicate septal architecture. The phospholipid composition of the PAP material is similar biochemically to that of normal surfactant, whereas the total protein content of the material is abnormally high, due to increased amounts of surfactant-specific proteins, serum proteins (albumin), and immunoglobulins.

The biochemical and histologic characteristics of secondary PAP differ somewhat from those of primary PAP. Although accumula-

TABLE 17-1 Etiologic Classification of Alveolar Proteinosis

Primary (Pulmonary Alveolar Proteinosis)
1. Idiopathic
Secondary (Pseudoproteinosis)
1. Environmental exposure
a. Silica (silicoproteinosis)
b. Aluminum dust
c. Fiberglass
d. Volcanic ash
2. Drugs
a. Amphophilic cationic drugs—chlorphentermine
b. Amiodarone
c. Busulfan
3. Hematologic malignancy
a. Leukemia
b. Lymphoma
4. Infection
a. *Pneumocystis carinii*
b. *Mycobacterium tuberculosis*

tion of phospholipids is excessive in secondary PAP, limited data suggest that surfactant-specific apoproteins are present in normal amounts. Additionally, the distribution of both PAS-positive material and surfactant-specific apoproteins is less homogeneous. In contrast to the normal interstitium encountered in primary PAP, secondary PAP may be associated with interstitial inflammation or fibrosis.

EPIDEMIOLOGY

The disease is uncommon; fewer than 350 cases have been reported worldwide. Most patients with PAP are between 30 and 50 years of age. The incidence in men is two to four times that in women.

CLINICAL FEATURES

History The presenting symptoms of PAP are characteristically insidious in onset and nonspecific in nature. Typically, the patient presents with a nonproductive cough and progressive dyspnea on exertion. Pleuritic chest pain, hemoptysis, and weight loss are less frequently encountered. The abrupt onset of symptoms or the presence of fever should alert the physician to the likelihood of a superimposed opportunistic infection (see below).

Physical examination The most common finding on physical examination is the presence of widespread rales. Digital clubbing or cyanosis are seen in one third of patients. Physical findings suggestive of pulmonary hypertension and cor pulmonale are present in far-advanced cases.

USUAL DIAGNOSTIC TESTS

Chest radiograph Over half of patients with PAP will have the classic radiographic findings of bilaterally symmetric alveolar filling defects ("acinar pattern") which are predominantly perihilar ("bat-wing") in distribution and which spare the costophrenic angles. Although this pattern may mimic the radiographic findings of congestive heart failure, the heart size is normal, the pulmonary vasculature is not cephalized, and pleural effusions and Kerley B lines are notably absent. Less commonly, PAP may present radiographically as diffuse interstitial infiltrates or as multiple nodular densities. Intrathoracic adenopathy is not associated with primary PAP; its presence should suggest the possibility of concurrent lymphoma or infection.

Laboratory studies Arterial hypoxemia while breathing room air is common; in one study the mean P_{O_2} at presentation was 63 mmHg. An increase in the serum lactate dehydrogenase level (LDH) is characteristic. The LDH level has been shown in some studies to correlate with the activity and severity of the disease and may thus be a useful index to follow.

Pulmonary function testing The typical pattern seen in most patients with PAP is that of restrictive disease: static lung volumes (TLC, RV, and FRC) are reduced while airflow remains normal (normal FEV_1/FVC). In addition, the diffusing capacity is considerably decreased and the arterial O_2 saturation often falls during exercise. An appreciable right-to-left shunt, due to continued perfusion of fluid-filled, nonventilated alveoli, is almost universally present and is demonstrable by failure to achieve a normal level of arterial P_{O_2} during 100% O_2 breathing. Routine pulmonary function tests, as well as determination of the magnitude of the shunt fraction, are extremely useful in following the course of the disease and the response to therapy.

DIFFERENTIAL DIAGNOSIS

The diagnosis of PAP should be considered in any patient presenting with a history of chronic, insidious dyspnea in whom the chest radiograph shows bilateral alveolar or nodular infiltrates without evidence of mediastinal disease or interstitial edema. The differential diagnosis of such diffuse air space disease is broad and includes both cardiogenic and noncardiogenic pulmonary edema, bronchoalveolar cell carcinoma, lymphoma, alveolar hemorrhage, sarcoidosis, talc lung (secondary to illicit intravenous drug administration), and hypersensitivity pneumonitis.

SPECIAL DIAGNOSTIC EVALUATION

Fiberoptic bronchoscopy Two complementary techniques performed through a fiberoptic bronchoscope, bronchoalveolar lavage (BAL) and transbronchial lung biopsy, often provide sufficient material on which to base a diagnosis of PAP in the presence of compatible clinical and radiographic features. Fluid obtained by BAL in patients with PAP is characteristically turbulent or flocculent. Cytologic examination reveals lipid-laden macrophages. The proteinaceous material recovered by BAL is strongly PAS-positive but does not stain with alcian blue, a feature which differentiates this material from respiratory tract mucus. Electron-microscopic examination of the washings may demonstrate the presence of lamellar bodies, tightly coiled, concentrically arranged membranes identical to structures found in the cytoplasm of type II cells. Because the findings on BAL can be mimicked by unrelated disease processes or by secondary PAP, histologic examination of lung tissue is generally required to confirm the diagnosis. Tissue obtained by transbronchial biopsy and stained with PAS usually suffices to establish the diagnosis.

Open lung biopsy In situations where the diagnosis remains in doubt after bronchoscopy, open lung biopsy is indicated. The larger tissue samples provided by this procedure may be useful in identifying secondary causes of PAP, e.g., silicoproteinosis, lymphoma.

TREATMENT

Treatment is reserved for patients who are clearly symptomatic or in whom the disease is progressive. The preferred treatment for PAP is therapeutic whole lung lavage. The procedure is performed under general anesthesia, using a double-lumen endotracheal tube, which enables lavage of one lung while ventilating the other. Warm sterile saline is instilled into the lung and subsequently drained. The procedure is continued until the fluid drained from the lung is clear, which usually occurs after instillation of a total of 10 to 20 L saline, though up to 70 L has been required in some patients. After an interval of 3 to 7 days, the procedure is repeated on the other lung.

NATURAL HISTORY AND PROGNOSIS

The natural history of PAP is highly variable. The disease will remit spontaneously in approximately 25 percent of patients, but it is not possible to distinguish these patients a priori. Those who do undergo whole lung lavage usually respond dramatically, but the subsequent course of these patients is similarly unpredictable. Some will go into complete and sustained remission after only one lavage; others will relapse and require repeat lavage on one or numerous occasions. The need for repeat lavage is dictated by the patient's symptoms, pulmonary function abnormalities, and shunt fraction. Rarely, patients develop interstitial fibrosis and permanent respiratory disability.

Early clinical series suggested that patients with PAP were predisposed to the development of opportunistic pulmonary infections, particularly with *Nocardia* organisms. More recent studies, coming after the introduction of whole lung lavage, suggest that opportunistic infection is now an infrequent complication.

BIBLIOGRAPHY

For a more detailed discussion, see Claypool WD: Pulmonary alveolar proteinosis, in Fishman AP (ed), *Pulmonary Diseases and Disorders,* 2d ed. New York, McGraw-Hill, 1988, pp. 893–900.

Hoffman RM, Rogers RM: Serum and lavage lactate dehydrogenase isoenzymes in pulmonary alveolar proteinosis. Am Rev Respir Dis 143:42–46, 1991.

Honda Y, Takahashi H, Shijubo N, Kuroki Y, Akino T: Surfactant protein-A concentration in bronchoalveolar lavage fluids of patients with pulmonary alveolar proteinosis. Chest 103:496–499, 1993.

Hook GER: Alveolar proteinosis and phospholipoidosis of the lungs. Toxicol Pathol 19:482–513, 1991.

Tate K, Zoellner P, Bode ET: Bronchopulmonary lavage for pulmonary alveolar proteinosis. Mo Med 89:27–30, 1992.

IV | PULMONARY CIRCULATORY DISORDERS

Pulmonary Hypertension and Cor Pulmonale

Harold I. Palevsky   Alfred P. Fishman

The description *cor pulmonale* denotes enlargement of the right ventricle by either hypertrophy, or dilation, or both. Instead of intrinsic cardiac disease, the cause of cor pulmonale is disease in the respiratory apparatus: the airways, pulmonary parenchyma, respiratory control mechanism, chest bellows, or pulmonary vascular bed. Invariably, pulmonary hypertension precedes cor pulmonale. As in the case of systemic hypertensive cardiac disease, hypertrophy and dilation are involved in the ventricular enlargement; in acute conditions, right ventricular dilation predominates, whereas in chronic cor pulmonale, right ventricular hypertrophy is a prominent feature. As a rule, if the pulmonary hypertension is not relieved, right ventricular failure will ultimately ensue.

THE NORMAL PULMONARY CIRCULATION

The normal pulmonary blood flow is accomplished with an average drop in mean pressure of only 5 to 10 mmHg between the pulmonary artery and the left atrium (Table 18-1). In individuals at sea level, the upper normal limit of *mean* pulmonary artery pressure is of the order of 30 mmHg. The presence of pulmonary hypertension is often not recognized until an explanation is sought for right ventricular hypertrophy or right heart failure. The cause of the pulmonary hypertension is an increase in pulmonary vascular resistance defined by analogy with Ohm's Law of electrical resistance as follows:

$$\text{Pulmonary vascular resistance} = \frac{\substack{\text{Mean pulmonary} \\ \text{arterial pressure}} - \substack{\text{Pulmonary arterial} \\ \text{wedge pressure}}}{\text{Pulmonary blood flow (L/min)}}$$

Using the units indicated above, the normal pulmonary vascular resistance is approximately 1.0 unit. Resistance may also be expressed in dyne • sec • cm^{-5} by multiplying the numerator of the above equation by 80; expressed in this way, normal pulmonary vascular resistance is approximately 50 to 100 dyne • sec • cm^{-5}.

In practice, this resistance equation is more applicable to the abnormal than to the normal pulmonary circulation, because the abnormal vessel walls correspond more closely to the hemodynamic conditions on which the formulation is based.

Changes in the calculated pulmonary vascular resistance can have

TABLE 18-1 Normal Hemodynamic Values at Sea Level

	While at rest	During moderate exercise
Cardiac output (L/min)	6	16
Heart rate (beats/min)	80	130
Right atrial pressure (mmHg)	4–6	6–8
Pulmonary artery pressures (mmHg)		
Systolic	20–25	30–35
Diastolic	10–12	11–14
Mean	14–18	20–25
Pulmonary wedge pressure (mmHg)	6–10	10–14
Systemic arterial pressure (mmHg)	120/80	150/95
Mean	90–100	110–120
Pulmonary vascular resistance (units)	0.70–1.00	0.60–0.90

different clinical implications. For example, a decrease in calculated pulmonary vascular resistance due to an increased cardiac output accompanied by a decrease in pulmonary arterial pressure and an unchanged heart rate is more desirable clinically than is the same decrease in pulmonary vascular resistance caused by a greater increase in cardiac output in association with an unchanged pulmonary arterial pressure and tachycardia.

PATHOGENESIS OF PULMONARY HYPERTENSION

The major factor responsible for pulmonary hypertension is an increase in the pulmonary vascular resistance. This increase is localized primarily in the precapillary arteries and arterioles. This increase in vascular resistance may be anatomic or vasoconstrictive in origin; often both mechanisms are involved. Early in the evolution of pulmonary hypertension, as the extent or the distensibility of the pulmonary resistance vessels decrease, modest increments in cardiac output cause appreciable pulmonary hypertension. In time, as the pulmonary vascular tree is progressively curtailed and becomes less distensible, lesser and lesser increments in pulmonary blood flow (cardiac output) suffice to cause large increments in pulmonary arterial pressures. Eventually, even the resting cardiac output is enough to sustain high pulmonary arterial pressures.

Oxygen Tensions

The most potent stimulus for pulmonary vasoconstriction is alveolar hypoxia, acting on the small pulmonary arteries and arterioles. Systemic arterial hypoxemia augments the local effects of alveolar hypoxia. In chronic hypoxic states, the effects of these pulmonary vasoconstrictive stimuli are often augmented by increased blood viscosity due to secondary polycythemia.

Acid-Base Status

Acidosis (pH < 7.2) also elicits pulmonary vasoconstriction. In human beings, acidosis acts synergistically with hypoxia, whereas alkalosis diminishes the vasoconstrictive response to hypoxia.

Carbon Dioxide

Unlike hypoxia, carbon dioxide (CO_2) appears to contribute directly to pulmonary hypertension by way of the acidosis that it generates rather than by direct effect on the vessel walls. In addition, chronic hypercapnia, no matter how produced, e.g., metabolic alkalosis due to diuretics, depresses ventilation, thereby augmenting alveolar hypoxia and evoking hypoxic pulmonary vasoconstriction.

ETIOLOGIES OF PULMONARY HYPERTENSION AND COR PULMONALE

Pulmonary hypertension is usually secondary to an identifiable disease process rather than primary ("unexplained" or "idiopathic"). The mechanisms by which these underlying conditions cause pulmonary hypertension vary considerably (Table 18-2): heart diseases cause increased pulmonary venous pressure or increased pulmonary blood flow; in contrast, parenchymal lung diseases and thromboembolic disease obliterate or obstruct segments of the pulmonary vascular bed.

DIAGNOSIS OF PULMONARY VASCULAR DISEASE

Due to the large reserve capacity of the normal pulmonary circulation which allows it to accept large increases in pulmonary blood flow without substantial elevations in pulmonary arterial pressures, extensive pulmonary vascular changes must be present before pulmonary hypertension develops. When symptoms do develop, they occur first during exertion, presenting as easy fatigability, dyspnea, chest pain, or presyncope or syncope. Right heart failure occurs subsequently and manifests itself as peripheral edema, early satiety, or right upper quadrant pain.

Physical examination at rest, particularly before the pulmonary vascular changes have become extensive, is often normal. Unfortunately, early diagnosis is handicapped by the lack of noninvasive techniques for screening for pulmonary hypertension. Consequently, the prospect of pulmonary hypertension is often delayed

TABLE 18-2 Etiologies of Pulmonary Hypertension

Hyperkinetic
Intracardiac shunt lesions
  Atrial septal defect, ventricular septal defect, anomalous
  venous return (total and partial)
Pulmonary arteriovenous fistulas

Passive
Elevated left ventricular end-diastolic pressure
  Coronary heart disease, cardiomyopathy, aortic valve disease,
  constrictive pericarditis
Mitral valve stenosis or obstruction
Left atrial obstruction
  Myxoma, neoplasm, thrombus
Pulmonary venous obstruction
  Neoplasm, adenopathy, fibrosing mediastinitis

Obliterative
Pulmonary parenchymal disease
  Obstructive (bronchitis, emphysema, bronchiectasis)
  Restrictive physiology (fibrosis of any etiology, thoracic cage
  abnormalities)
Pulmonary arteritis
  Scleroderma, systemic lupus erythematosus, other collagen vascular
  disease and vasculitis, schistosomiasis

Obstructive
Pulmonary embolism—acute and chronic
  Venous thromboemboli, tumor emboli
Pulmonary arterial thrombosis
  Sickle cell disease, Eisenmenger syndrome, e.g., tetralogy of Fallot

Vasoconstrictive
Hypoxemia
  Sleep apnea syndromes, neuromuscular disorders, high altitude
  disease

Idiopathic
Primary pulmonary hypertension
  Including pulmonary veno-occlusive disease (small intrapulmonary
  veins)
Dietary-related pulmonary hypertension, e.g., aminorex, toxic oil
syndrome
Coexistent portal and pulmonary hypertension
Persistent fetal circulation

until severe symptoms or abnormalities in the chest radiograph or
electrocardiogram are present.

Symptoms

No symptom is specific for pulmonary hypertension. The most
frequent initial symptom of pulmonary hypertension is exertional
dyspnea. This dyspnea, as is the case with easy fatigability, is often
blamed on anxiety or being "out of shape." Various explanations

for this dyspnea have been proposed, including hypoxic stimulation of peripheral chemoreceptors, stimulation of interstitial irritant receptors, stimulation of stretch receptors in the pulmonary arteries, or inability of cardiac output to match metabolic need. It is likely that each explanation does play a role in some patients, although none has proved to be universal.

Syncope or presyncope (lightheadedness during exertion) is another symptom commonly seen in pulmonary hypertension. Most frequently, this occurs later in the course of the disease in patients with high resting pulmonary arterial pressures. This symptom is usually attributed to either an inability to adequately increase cardiac output during exertion (in association with exercise-induced systemic vasodilation) or to a bradyarrhythmia. It is generally considered to indicate a poor prognosis.

Chest pains occur in up to 50 percent of patients with severe pulmonary hypertension; these often resemble typical angina and are thought to be a consequence of right ventricular ischemia.

Hemoptysis occurs in pulmonary hypertension regardless of etiology: in postcapillary pulmonary vascular disorders, the bleeding may be from dilated submucosal veins in the airways; in precapillary pulmonary hypertension, aneurysms of alveolar capillaries may be responsible. In some instances, the underlying pulmonary inflammation causes bleeding by involving the pulmonary microvasculature.

Hoarseness occurs in long-standing, severe pulmonary hypertension. It is due to paralysis of the left vocal cord as the left recurrent laryngeal nerve is compressed between the aorta and the left pulmonary artery (Ortner's syndrome).

The advent of right heart failure and elevation of systemic venous pressure leads to early satiety or right upper quadrant epigastric pain due to hepatic congestion and distention of Glisson's capsule.

Signs

The physical signs of pulmonary hypertension are similar regardless of the underlying etiology or pathogenetic mechanism. Early on, the jugular venous pulse configuration is dominated by the a wave. As the pulmonary hypertension progresses and right heart failure with tricuspid insufficiency develop, the a wave becomes less prominent, and the v wave becomes proportionally larger. A right ventricular S_4 may be present with the prominent a wave. The right ventricle becomes palpable at the lower left sternal border or in the subxiphoid region, and pulmonary arterial valve closure becomes palpable in the second left intercostal space.

On auscultation, P_2 is accentuated and S_2 is initially narrowly split. Often a sharp systolic ejection click is heard over the pulmonary artery in the second left intercostal space. A right atrial S_3 gallop is often present. A tricuspid insufficiency murmur is frequently heard at the left sternal border. Due to the relatively large pressure gradient present across the tricuspid valve in pulmonary hypertension, the murmur present is high-pitched and quite different from the low-pitched, blowing insufficiency murmur associated with organic tricuspid disease. This murmur may not evidence significant respiratory variation. A pulmonic insufficiency murmur may also be appreciated.

In addition to presenting with the signs and symptoms of right ventricular hypertrophy or right heart failure, attention to the possibility of pulmonary hypertension may be drawn by unexplained arterial hypoxemia. Frequently, the hypoxemia responds poorly to the administration of supplemental oxygen, i.e., it suggests a shunting mechanism in the lungs. This shunt may reflect either increased flow through vessels in parts of the lungs that are poorly ventilated, or within the heart, i.e., via a reopened foramen ovale. An intravenous injection of $Tc^{99}MAA$ may be useful for distinguishing between these mechanisms: a patent foramen ovale shunts particles to the systemic circulation where they will be trapped in the brain, liver, and kidneys; imaging with a gamma camera will reveal these radioactive particles in these organs. Shunts at the pulmonary microvascular level will trap the imaging agent within the lungs so that imaging studies over systemic organs will be negative.

Diagnostic Studies

The unexpected finding of right ventricular hypertrophy on either an electrocardiogram or an echocardiogram, or of right heart enlargement or enlargement of the pulmonary arteries on a chest radiograph, should raise concern as to the presence of pulmonary hypertension and trigger further investigation. Except for cardiac catheterization (that includes measurements during exercise), currently available diagnostic techniques are more useful in following the course of documented pulmonary hypertension than for detecting early pulmonary hypertension.

Conventional laboratory tests sometimes shed light on the etiology of an unexplained pulmonary vascular disorder (Table 18-3). For example, polycythemia raises the possibility of chronic hypoxia or hemoglobinopathy; hypercoagulable states suggest thrombosis; abnormal liver function studies raise the possibility of concurrent pulmonary hypertension and portal hypertension; positive serologies can suggest the presence of a systemic connective tissue disorder.

Chest radiographs and pulmonary function tests (spirometry, lung volumes, and diffusing capacity) are useful in suggesting

TABLE 18-3 Evaluation of Suspected Pulmonary Hypertension

Laboratory studies—Complete blood count, coagulation profile, liver function tests, collagen vascular screen
Chest radiograph
Electrocardiogram
Pulmonary function tests—Spirometry, lung volumes, diffusing capacity, arterial blood gas
Ventilation-perfusion lung scan—Pulmonary angiogram (if lung scan or clinical history suggests proximal pulmonary embolism)
Echocardiogram
Exercise test
Right heart catheterization

disorders of the airways, intrinsic pulmonary parenchymal disease, or abnormalities of the mediastinum. A ventilation-perfusion lung scan is necessary in distinguishing between unresolved clot obstructing large vessels (surgically treatable) and other causes of unexplained pulmonary hypertension. Pulmonary angiography is generally reserved for patients with either a clinical history or a lung scan, suggestive of large obstructing pulmonary emboli in the major pulmonary arteries. An echocardiogram can demonstrate structural cardiac abnormalities such as valvular disease, septal defects, or myxomas. Right heart catheterization remains necessary for determining the degree of the pulmonary hypertension, for excluding certain cardiac lesions, and for testing the effectiveness of vasodilator agents.

Treatment of Pulmonary Hypertension

The treatment of pulmonary hypertension is directed toward reversing the underlying pathogenetic process while relieving hypoxemia, hypercapnia, or acidosis which might be contributing to right heart strain. In addition to specific measures, several categories of treatment may be helpful in patients with pulmonary hypertension regardless of etiology.

Oxygen Supplementation

In patients demonstrating either resting, exertion, or nocturnal arterial hypoxemia, careful oxygen supplementation is directed at treating the hypoxic vasoconstriction, thereby reducing the afterload on the right ventricle while decreasing the prospect of hypoxemic arrhythmogenesis. The performance of a sleep study looking for nocturnal arterial desaturation should be considered in all patients with unexplained pulmonary hypertension. Exertional arterial desaturation should be considered in all patients with a low diffusing capacity, e.g., < 60 percent of predicted; these patients should be exercised to tolerance while monitoring arterial O_2 saturation using pulse oximetry. Although oxygen administration entails some risk in patients with obstructive lung disease by potentially decreasing respiratory drive and alveolar ventilation and thereby worsening respiratory acidosis, the use of supplemental oxygen to maintain an arterial oxygen tension of > 60 mmHg, or an arterial oxygen saturation of $> 90\%$, reduces the mortality from cor pulmonale and improves cognitive function and quality of life.

A new therapy also directed toward improving arterial oxygenation in chronic obstructive pulmonary disease (COPD) involves the use of almitrine bismesylate, a carotid body stimulant which may also augment hypoxic vasoconstriction and improve ventilation-perfusion matching within the lungs without affecting minute ventilation. In a long-term, randomized, double-blind trial of this agent in hypoxemic, hypercapnic COPD patients, the study group had fewer hospitalizations and episodes of right heart failure than did the control group. However, these results await more extensive trials before this investigational drug can be used as a substitute for long-term oxygen supplementation.

Treatment of Heart Failure

Right heart failure in pulmonary hypertension and cor pulmonale may be transient if the exacerbating factors can be controlled. The usual therapies for heart failure are used: low-salt regimen, digitalis, and diuretics. Phlebotomy to decrease the circulating blood volume (and hematocrit) may be needed to maintain the benefit. Diuretics should be given with care, particularly in patients with abnormalities of ventilatory control, because metabolic alkalosis may complicate their use. Alkalosis, in turn, contributes to ventilatory insufficiency by depressing the ventilatory response to CO_2. Moreover, diuresis may increase blood viscosity by increasing the hematocrit. In critically ill patients, overdiuresis can result in inadequate filling of the right heart and may compromise cardiac output and arterial oxygenation.

Anticoagulation

Both acute and chronic pulmonary thromboembolism may result in pulmonary hypertension and right heart failure, and pulmonary hypertension of any etiology seems to have the potential to initiate in situ thrombosis in the pulmonary microvascular beds. Moreover, once the patient is in right heart failure, venous thrombosis and pulmonary embolism are frequent complications of the resultant venous stasis and decreased physical activity. Because of these observations, it is suggested that anticoagulation (or treatment with antiplatelet agents) be considered for any patient with pulmonary hypertension before the onset of overt right heart failure. Routine prophylaxis for venous thrombosis, usually with subcutaneous heparin, is advisable during periods of hospitalization or prolonged immobility. This is particularly important in critically ill patients who often have many factors predisposing to thrombosis and in whom symptoms relating to recent thrombosis may be difficult to discern.

Vasodilator Therapy

For more than 30 years, vasodilator therapy has been used to try to dilate the pulmonary resistance vessels and to decrease the right ventricular afterload. A major focus of these trials has been primary pulmonary hypertension. The current consensus is that vasodilator therapy has little role in secondary pulmonary hypertension, and is apt to be effective in only one third of patients with primary pulmonary hypertension. Moreover, vasodilator administration is potentially hazardous, necessitating that therapy be initiated in an intensive-care unit setting. The use of vasodilator therapy has been complicated by uncertainty as to the long-term significance of a favorable *acute* vasodilator response. Conversely, it is not known if the failure to elicit an acute response during a vasodilator trial indicates that there will be no benefit from long-term administration of vasodilators.

Among those who prove to be responders to acute vasodilator testing, calcium channel blockers, notably nifedipine or diltiazem, are most commonly administered orally for maintenance therapy. In patients with primary pulmonary hypertension, the maximum daily dose is determined in the course of cardiac catheterization by titrating the patient using successive hourly increments until the maximum tolerable level is reached. On rare occasion, other vasodilators, used singly or in combination, have proved effective. It must be stressed that most of these attempts at medical management are doomed to failure. Prolonged intravenous infusions of prostacyclin, or its analogues, are currently being used in some patients with primary pulmonary hypertension to stabilize those who have failed to respond to oral vasodilators and to sustain them for lung or heart-lung transplantation.

Transplantation

Despite the therapies above, the pulmonary hypertension and right heart failure often pursue a progressive course. For selected patients, transplantation of either a single lung or of two lungs, or of a lung-heart block, may provide dramatic relief of cardiorespiratory failure. Although these types of surgical interventions are still under development and are limited in availability, they can be lifesaving after the medical therapies have been exhausted. Recent reports have expanded the indications for lung transplantation and have documented improved patient survival with both lung and lung-heart transplantation.

BIBLIOGRAPHY

For a more detailed discussion, see Fishman AP: Pulmonary hypertension and cor pulmonale, in Fishman AP (ed.), *Pulmonary Diseases and Disorders,* 2d ed. New York, McGraw-Hill, 1988, pp. 999–1048.

Fishman AP (ed): *The Pulmonary Circulation: Normal and Abnormal.* Philadelphia, University of Pennsylvania Press, 1990.

Palevsky HI, Fishman AP: Diagnosis and treatment of pulmonary embolism and deep venous thrombosis, in Fishman AP (ed), *Update: Pulmonary Diseases and Disorders.* New York, McGraw-Hill, 1992, pp 451–464.

Palevsky HI, Fishman AP: Chronic cor pulmonale: Etiology and management. JAMA 263:2347–2353, 1990.

Rich S, Kaufmann E, Levy PS: The effect of high-dose calcium channel blockers on survival in primary pulmonary hypertension. N Engl J Med 327:76–81, 1992.

Rosenow EC III, Lie JT: The pulmonary vasculitides, in Fishman AP (ed), *Update: Pulmonary Diseases and Disorders.* New York, McGraw-Hill, 1992, pp 465–474.

Harold I. Palevsky

DEFINITION

Pulmonary thromboembolism refers to the lodging in the lungs of one or more venous thrombi from systemic veins. Materials other than bland blood clots also embolize to the lungs, e.g., talc injected by intravenous drug users, amniotic fluid during pregnancy, air, and infected thrombi. However, venous clots (thromboemboli) are, by far, the most common.

ETIOLOGY

Pulmonary embolism (PE) is so closely linked to deep venous thrombosis (DVT) that it can be considered as a clinical complication of DVT rather than as a separate disease. As defined above, PE does not occur without a systemic site of clot formation and propagation. Also, the risk of recurrence of PE depends directly on the clot that remains behind or propagates in the systemic vein after the original clot has broken off and moved to the lungs.

More than 90 percent of all clinically manifest PE originate in the proximal deep veins of the lower extremities, i.e., involving, or proximal to, the popliteal vein. The great majority of emboli to the lungs are asymptomatic. This is true not only for emboli that originate in the proximal deep veins of the lower extremities but also from the smaller and more distal veins of the calf.

Virchow's triad of stasis, hypercoagulability, and injury to the vessel wall identifies the factors that predispose to the development of venous thrombosis (Table 19-1). *Stasis,* most often a consequence of prolonged immobility or bed rest, is a major factor in the development of venous thrombosis in patients with concurrent medical conditions and after surgery. *Hypercoagulability* may be manifested either as a predisposition to venous thrombosis or as a failure of the mechanisms that normally inhibit propagation of thrombus. *Vascular injury,* particularly if it entails endothelial injury that exposes underlying basement membrane (collagen), causes platelet activation, the release of chemotactic substances and initiation of the clotting cascades. These factors are particularly important with respect to thrombi that form after trauma and surgery.

CLINICAL MANIFESTATIONS

The clinical consequences of PE range from asymptomatic (identified in the course of screening high-risk patients) to cardiorespiratory collapse and sudden death. The frequency with which the signs

TABLE 19-1 Virchow's Triad: Clinical States Predisposing to Venous Thrombosis

Stasis	Immobility
	Bed rest
	Anesthesia
	Congestive heart failure/cor pulmonale
	Prior venous thrombosis
Hypercoagulability	Malignancy
	Anticardiolipin antibody
	Nephrotic syndrome
	Essential thrombocytosis
	Estrogen therapy
	Heparin-induced thrombocytopenia
	Inflammatory bowel disease
	Paroxysmal nocturnal hemoglobinuria
	Disseminated intravascular coagulation
	Protein C and S deficiencies
	Antithrombin III deficiency
Vessel wall injury	Trauma
	Surgery

and symptoms of PE occur varies with patient population (Table 19-2). The so-called classic manifestations of PE, such as dyspnea, pleuritic chest pain, and hemoptysis, have proved to be the exception rather than the rule. These and other clinical indices have a specificity of only 37 percent for the diagnosis of PE.

After pulmonary embolization, the clinical state of the patient depends on three major influences, including (1) preexisting cardiac and pulmonary function; (2) the size of the embolus and the extent of the pulmonary vascular bed that has been obstructed; and (3) humoral mediators. Three separate lines of evidence suggest that humoral mediators play an important role in determining the clinical consequences. The changes in hemodynamics and gas exchange elicited by PE are often greatly excessive for the extent of the pulmonary vascular bed that has been obstructed. For example, in contrast to lobectomy or a pneumonectomy, which are generally well tolerated, a PE that obstructs a lobar or major pulmonary artery can be life threatening. In experimental models, cyproheptadine (a *nonselective* serotonin antagonist) and ketanserin (a *selective* serotonin antagonist) can block many of the hemodynamic and airway responses to PE. Bronchoconstriction, occasionally manifested by localized wheezing, sometimes occurs after PE.

Powerful pulmonary vasoactive substances, other than serotonin, are also released from both the formed elements of the blood and from the pulmonary vascular endothelium after PE. These include vasodilators as well as pulmonary vasoconstrictors. Moreover, neurohumoral reflexes have also been implicated in the pulmonary vasomotor response to embolization.

TABLE 19-2 Incidence of Signs and Symptoms of Pulmonary Embolism

	Massive PE* %	Submassive PE* %	PE without preexisting cardiac or pulmonary disease† %
Dyspnea	85	82	73
Pleuritic chest pain	64	85	66
Cough	53	52	37
Hemoptysis	23	40	13
Tachypnea	95 (>16 breaths/ min)	87 (>16 breaths/ min)	70 (>20 breaths/ min)
Tachycardia (>100 beats/min)	48	38	30
Increased pulmonic component of second heart sound	58	45	23
Rales	57	60	51
Phlebitis	36	26	11

*SOURCE: Data from NIH-sponsored urokinase and streptokinase clinical trials (Am J Med 62:355–360, 1977).
†SOURCE: Data from NIH-sponsored PIOPED study (Chest 100:598–603, 1991).

DIAGNOSTIC TESTS

Chest Radiography

The major diagnostic role of chest radiography is in excluding other entities that can mimic the clinical manifestations of an acute PE, e.g., pneumothorax. As a rule, the chest radiographs of the patient with a PE show some combination of a parenchymal infiltrate, atelectasis, and a pleural effusion. All of these manifestations are nonspecific. Although the parenchymal infiltrates are generally ascribed to pulmonary infarction, their pattern of rapid resolution is more suggestive of hemorrhagic edema than of tissue necrosis. Two other radiographic findings may be helpful in suggesting PE—the hypovascularity of a lung zone, especially when the oligemia is associated with an enlarged pulmonary artery, and one or more wedge-shaped, pleural-based densities (Hampton's hump) consistent with pulmonary infarction(s) secondary to PE.

Another important role for the chest radiograph is in evaluating ventilation-perfusion lung scans (see below).

Electrocardiogram

In the patient suspected of acute PE, the electrocardiogram (ECG) can be helpful in disclosing other clinical conditions, e.g., pericarditis or acute myocardial infarction. In most instances of PE, the ECG is nonspecific, manifesting only a sinus tachycardia or nonspecific changes in the ST-T segments.

Acute cor pulmonale can occur as a consequence of PE. The ECG may then show a p-pulmonale pattern, right axis deviation, right bundle branch block, or the classic $S_1Q_3T_3$ pattern. However, these findings are not only infrequent but they also occur in conditions other than acute PE. In large clinical trials (the urokinase and streptokinase pulmonary embolism trials), ECG evidence of acute cor pulmonale was found in only 32 percent of the patients with *massive* PE and in 26 percent of those with *submassive* PE. In contrast, the ECG was normal in 23 percent of the patients with submassive PE. Therefore, although the ECG can be helpful in suggesting an alternative diagnosis, it can, per se, neither make the diagnosis nor rule out PE.

Arterial Blood Gases

The distinctive abnormalities in the arterial blood gases are respiratory alkalosis and hypoxemia accompanied by a widened alveolar-arterial difference in Po_2 (A-a gradient). However, arterial pH, Po_2, and the A-a gradient are often either normal or only minimally perturbed. Variations in the degree of hypoxemia depend, in part, on the intensity of the humoral response. This variability has two important clinical implications. A normal arterial Po_2 or A-a gradient does not exclude the diagnosis of PE and in a patient who is a candidate for PE, the presence of hypoxemia without obvious cause should heighten suspicion of PE and encourage further evaluation.

Ventilation-Perfusion Lung Scans

In most pulmonary diseases or disorders other than PE, a perfusion defect is accompanied by a ventilation defect. In contrast, PE usually elicits perfusion defects that are unaccompanied by ventilation defects. Interpretation of ventilation-perfusion scans is based on the presence, size, and correspondence of ventilation and perfusion defects. Accordingly, scans for PE are classified into four categories, i.e., one *normal* and three abnormal: *high probability, intermediate (or indeterminate) probability,* or *low probability.*

A normal perfusion scan excludes clinically significant PE. If the perfusion scan is abnormal, a variety of etiologies, as well as PE, have to be considered. Correlation of the abnormal perfusion scan with the ventilation scan and with the chest radiograph greatly improves the accuracy of lung perfusion scans in detecting PE.

High probability lung scans Large perfusion defects, particularly when multiple and unmatched by ventilation defects, are most apt to represent substantial embolic events. Scans of this type are highly specific, i.e., they predict the presence of PE with a high degree of accuracy. In a recent multicenter trial (PIOPED), 88 percent of patients with high probability scans had angiographically documented PE. However, the predictive value of the high probability lung scans fell to 74 percent in patients with a prior history of PE, presumably because of residual perfusion defects due to the previous PE. In the patient who is a candidate for recurrent PE, follow-up lung scans, after the course of anticoagulation has been completed, may be helpful in setting a new baseline for detecting future emboli.

Although highly specific, the high probability scan is relatively insensitive in detecting PE. Thus, in the PIOPED study, scans were interpreted as high probability in only 41 percent of patients in whom PE was documented by angiography.

Non-high probability lung scans Intermediate and low probability lung scans are often considered together in dealing with patients suspected of PE because perfusion defects in both of these categories are smaller or fewer in number than in high probability scans and the management of the intermediate and low probability patient is similar. In patients suspected of having PE, intermediate and low probability scans are not diagnostic.

Correlating lung scans with clinical assessment When the interpretation of the lung scans and the clinical assessment are concordant in indicating either high or low probability of PE, the diagnostic accuracy is greater than that of the lung scan, per se (Table 19-3). In contrast, the accuracy of the lung scan decreases when the lung scan interpretation and the clinical assessment are discordant. The

TABLE 19-3 Prevalence of Pulmonary Embolism in PIOPED: Value of Correlating Lung Scan Interpretation with Clinical Assessment

		Clinical Assessment		
		High clinical suspicion for PE	Intermediate clinical suspicion for PE	Low clinical suspicion for PE
Lung scan interpretation	High probability of PE	96%	88%	56%
	Intermediate probability of PE	66%	28%	16%
	Low probability of PE	40%	16%	4%

SOURCE: Data modified after JAMA 263:2753–2759, 1990.

combination of lung scan and clinical assessment can fail to diagnose or exclude PE in up to two thirds of patients suspected of PE. In this circumstance, the next recourse is either pulmonary angiography or a diagnostic measure that can suggest PE by demonstrating a potential source of emboli in the lower extremities, e.g., impedance plethysmography, B-mode ultrasonography, or venography.

Noninvasive Diagnosis of Deep Vein Thrombosis

Although the "gold standard" for the diagnosis of venous thrombosis in the lower extremities continues to be contrast venography, this is an invasive procedure that has several serious drawbacks. It exposes the patient to radiation and to the risks of complications from the injection of large amounts of contrast media. In up to 10 to 20 percent of patients, the results do not suffice for interpretation. Accordingly, clinicians have come to rely increasingly on noninvasive techniques such as impedance plethysmography (IPG) and real-time (B-mode) ultrasonography. Under investigation are radiolabeled antibody imaging and several magnetic resonance imaging techniques.

Impedance plethysmography Of the noninvasive modalities available for the diagnosis of DVT in the lower extremity, IPG is the oldest and best validated. Although the technique is excellent for detecting DVT in the popliteal, femoral, and iliac veins (proximal DVT), it is not useful for the detection of thrombus in calf veins. For the detection of proximal DVT, the sensitivity of IPG is of the order of 95 percent and its specificity of the order of 96 percent. Serial IPG is useful in detecting *proximal propagation* of thrombi that begin in the calf veins even though it is not useful in diagnosing thrombosis in the calf veins, per se.

Real time (B-mode) ultrasonography B-mode imaging ultrasound is used to evaluate the deep venous system of the leg for patency, intraluminal thrombi, vein compressibility, evidence of blood flow, and response to hemodynamic maneuvers. This technique seems to be most useful for the diagnosis of femoral or popliteal DVT; it is neither accurate nor reliable for thrombi in the calf or iliac veins. Unfortunately, the diagnostic yield from this method is operator dependent. Therefore, it is unclear whether the favorable sensitivities and specificities reported from some medical centers are achievable in conventional practice. Real-time ultrasonography has the potential of being able to identify nonthrombotic causes of leg swelling, e.g., Baker's cyst. Although real-time (B-mode) ultrasonography does appear promising for the noninvasive diagnosis of proximal lower extremity DVT, it cannot be recommended as yet as the sole study on which to base therapeutic decisions.

TREATMENT OF THROMBOEMBOLIC DISEASE

Heparin The standard treatment for venous thromboembolic disease involves anticoagulation using heparin given intravenously followed by oral anticoagulation therapy using warfarin. The therapeutic guide for continuous, stable, and safe administration of heparin intravenously is an activated partial thromboplastin time maintained at between 1.5 and 2 times control values. When adequate anticoagulation is achieved with warfarin (as evidenced by increase in the prothrombin time to the therapeutic range), then heparin is discontinued.

Despite the apparent simplicity of this approach, several issues merit special consideration—the duration of heparin therapy before warfarin is started, how long to continue heparin, and how long to continue warfarin.

Despite the theoretical risk of generating a hypercoagulable state when warfarin therapy is begun in a heparinized patient, this risk has not materialized in practice. Therefore, warfarin can be started concurrently with, or soon after the start of, heparin therapy. The heparin infusion should be continued until the prothrombin time is in the therapeutic range (1.25 to 1.5 times control) for 3 days.

The duration of the heparin infusion is about 1 week, varying somewhat with when warfarin therapy was started and how long it takes to achieve therapeutic anticoagulation with warfarin. In some instances, long-term therapy using heparin administered subcutaneously may be preferable to warfarin therapy. In that event, the continuous infusion of heparin intravenously should be maintained for 1 week before switching to an adjusted-dose regimen of heparin administered subcutaneously.

Warfarin For long-term anticoagulation, the use of warfarin-type agents taken by mouth affords the simplest and least expensive means. As noted above in those patients who will need long-term anticoagulation, oral anticoagulant therapy with warfarin can be begun once continuous intravenous therapy with heparin has begun. The therapeutic goal for oral anticoagulation is to maintain the prothrombin time at a value of 1.25 to 1.5 times the control value. This level of anticoagulation should be maintained until the risk of recurrent thromboembolic events is low. In practice, our usual recommendation is to maintain anticoagulation with warfarin for approximately 4 months, reserving longer periods of time for those who have either had extensive DVT or large PE at the time of the initiation of therapy or who are at increased risk for recurrent thrombosis, e.g., prolonged inactivity or a hypercoagulable state.

Vena caval filters For patients with venous thromboembolism in whom anticoagulation is contraindicated, or for patients who are unlikely to survive a recurrent embolic event, percutaneous placement of a filtering device into the inferior vena cava has become standard practice. The incidence of clogging in the current generation of filters is low and the filters are safe, even when used in conjunction with anticoagulation or thrombolytic therapy.

Thrombolytic therapy Perhaps the most controversial aspect of managing venous thromboembolic disease is the role of thrombolytic therapy. Currently, three FDA-approved thrombolytic agents are available for the treatment of PE—streptokinase, urokinase, and recombinant tissue type plasminogen activator (Table 19-4). It is generally agreed that these agents should be used in treating PE that cause hemodynamic instability or significant respiratory compromise.

Less certain is the role of thrombolytic therapy in dealing with either *submassive* PE or a large proximal DVT. The major reason for thrombolytic therapy is to promote the rapid clearance of clot from pulmonary arteries. The diffusing capacity (DL_{CO}) in patients has been reported to improve more in patients treated with thrombolytic agents than in those treated with heparin. Also, in long-term follow-up, patients treated with thrombolytic agents had somewhat lower mean pulmonary arterial pressures and pulmonary vascular resistance at rest and during exercise than did patients treated with heparin. However, the hemodynamic differences were modest and their practical implications uncertain.

With respect to the treatment of proximal thrombi in the deep veins of the legs, thrombolytic therapy results in more rapid and complete clearance of clot, better preservation of venous valves, and seems to evoke fewer long-term complications (venous stasis and ulceration) than does heparin therapy.

However, enthusiasm for the use of thrombolytic therapy in venous thromboembolic disease is tempered by several practical considerations. (1) Thrombolytic therapy carries a greater risk of bleeding than does heparin therapy. (2) The optimal dosages and regimens for thrombolytic therapy, both in PE and in DVT, have

TABLE 19-4 Thrombolytic Therapy for Venous Thromboembolism

Agent	Loading Dose	Hourly Dose	Recommended Duration
Streptokinase	250,000 IU over 30 min	100,000 IU/h	PE: 24 h DVT: 48–72 h
Urokinase	4400 IU/kg over 10 min	4400 IU/kg/h	PE: 12 h DVT: not approved
Tissue-type plasminogen activator	none	50 mg/h	PE: 2 h DVT: not approved

not yet been identified. (3) Only a few long-term outcome trials are available in which thrombolytic therapy and conventional treatment with heparin are compared. After a course of thrombolytic therapy, standard anticoagulation is still necessary to prevent recurrent thromboemboli.

APPROACH TO MANAGEMENT

Our approach to treating venous thromboembolism emphasizes the role played by venous thrombosis in PE, and the noninvasive assessment of the amount of clot, both in the legs and in the lungs (Fig. 19-1). This approach presupposes hemodynamic and respiratory stability. It should be underscored that this approach applies to conventional anticoagulation; if thrombolytic therapy is being considered, the desirability of using invasive diagnostic tests has to be considered more seriously than usual since the greater risks of thrombolytic therapy usually require that the diagnosis of thromboembolic disease be unequivocal.

Certain key observations underlie this approach to management.

1. The vast majority (> 90 percent) of PE originate as DVT of the lower extremities.
2. Recurrent PE are associated with proximal DVT, whereas recurrent PE are rare if there is no proximal DVT.
3. High probability lung scans, especially when clinical suspicion of thromboembolism is high and the patient has no prior history of thromboembolic disease, are reliable tests for establishing the presence of PE.
4. A normal perfusion scan or a low probability ventilation-perfusion scan in conjunction with a low index of clinical suspicion is a reliable means of excluding PE.
5. Noninvasive evaluation of the lower extremities (particularly IPG), especially when repeated, can reliably establish or exclude the diagnosis of proximal DVT.
6. The outcome of patients in whom lung scans are not of high probability and in whom noninvasive evaluations (IPG) of the lower extremities for DVT are negative, especially on successive testing, are likely to be favorable, even if they are not anticoagulated.

Practical Aspects to this Approach

The patient suspected of having experienced pulmonary emboli and who is clinically stable is screened using ventilation-perfusion lung scans and IPG as shown in Figure 19-1. If both studies are negative, then other etiologies for the patient's symptoms are likely. If the lung scan is interpreted as high probability, and this interpretation

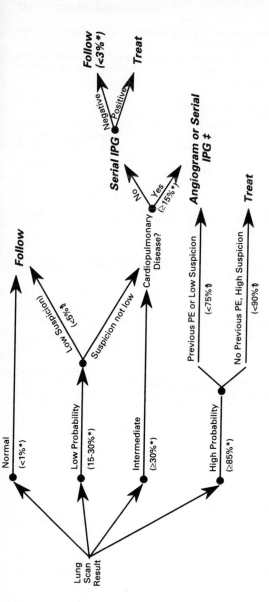

FIG. 19-1 Approach to management of pulmonary thromboembolism. The likelihood of pulmonary embolism is indicated in parentheses.
* Strongly supported by clinical studies.
† Suggested by clinical studies, needs confirmation.
‡ A serially negative impedance plethysmography result may not be sufficient to rule out thromboembolism.
(Reproduced with permission from Kelley MA et al: Diagnosing pulmonary embolism: New facts and strategies. Ann Int Med 114:300-306, 1991.)

is in keeping with the clinical impression, or if the IPG is positive, then the patient should be treated for venous thromboembolic disease. If the lung scan is non-high probability (but not normal) and the patient is clinically stable, then the decision to treat is often based on the results of IPG. If the IPG is negative, particularly if negative on repeated testing, then the risk of recurrent thromboembolism is small and treatment for thrombotic disease need not be instituted. Thus, most clinically stable patients can be evaluated noninvasively for the presence of thromboembolic disease.

Pulmonary angiography and venography are reserved for unstable patients or patients in whom the risks of anticoagulation or thrombolytic therapy are so high that an unequivocal diagnosis is necessary. Whether newer less invasive diagnostic modalities, e.g., real-time ultrasonography, monoclonal antibody imaging, or magnetic resonance imaging, can be substituted for invasive procedures, or used in an approach such as is outlined above, has not yet been established.

BIBLIOGRAPHY

For a more detailed discussion, see Kelley MA, Fishman AP: Pulmonary thromboembolic disease, in Fishman AP (ed), *Pulmonary Diseases and Disorders*. New York, McGraw-Hill, 1988, pp. 1059–1086.

Carson JL, Kelly MA, Duff A, Weg JG, Fulkerson WJ, Palevsky HI, Thompson BT, Popovich J Jr, Schwartz JS, Hobbins TE, Spera MA, Alavi A, Terrin ML: The clinical course of pulmonary embolism. N Engl J Med 326:1240–1245, 1992.

Goldhaber SZ, Morpurgo M for the WHO/ISFC Task Force on Pulmonary Embolism: Diagnosis, treatment and prevention of pulmonary embolism. JAMA 268:1727–1733, 1992.

Kelley MA, Carson JL, Palevsky HI, Schwartz JS: Diagnosing pulmonary embolism: New facts and strategies. Ann Intern Med 114:300–306, 1991.

Palevsky HI, Fishman AP: Diagnosis and treatment of pulmonary embolism and deep venous thrombosis, in Fishman AP (ed), *Update: Pulmonary Diseases and Disorders,* 2d ed. New York, McGraw-Hill, 1992, pp 451–464.

Deborah DeMarco

HYPERSENSITIVITY VASCULITIS

Definition

Also known as leukocytoclastic vasculitis or small vessel vasculitis, hypersensitivity vasculitis includes a variety of conditions in which inflammation of postcapillary venules and small arteries is the predominant feature. Although skin involvement predominates, any organ may be involved, especially the heart, lungs, and kidneys.

Etiology

Hypersensitivity vasculitis is designated as *primary* when no identifiable antigens or associated diseases are found. It is often caused by drugs, particularly sulfonamides, but may also result from infection, e.g., hepatitis B, streptococcus, or exposure to environmental agents such as insecticides.

Pathology

Characteristically, the precapillary and postcapillary vessels, especially the pulmonary venules, are the seat of neutrophilic infiltration, accompanied by leukocytoclasis and nuclear fragmentation. The capillaries may also be involved. All lesions are in the same stage of evolution. Immune complex deposition is believed to play a role in the pathogenesis of the lesions.

Clinical Features

The hallmark of hypersensitivity vasculitis is the abrupt development of skin lesions. The most common cutaneous expression of the syndrome is palpable purpura. But papular, petechial, and small ulcerative lesions are seen in 30 percent of patients. Bullous or vesicular lesions are seen in 20 percent of patients.

Constitutional symptoms, including fever and arthralgias, are common. Renal involvement is manifest by proteinuria and hematuria. Gastrointestinal bleeding may occur.

Pulmonary infiltrates, either nodular or diffuse, may be seen on chest radiograph, and pleural effusions have been described.

Diagnostic Tests

Laboratory indicators are not diagnostically useful. Diagnosis is based on the presence of a compatible clinical picture and characteristic histopathologic changes.

Treatment

Removal of the inciting antigen or successful treatment of the underlying disorder usually results in resolution of symptoms. If systemic symptoms or internal organ involvement is present, the use of oral glucocorticoids may be required. The initial dose depends on severity of symptoms and ranges from 20 to 60 mg prednisone per day.

CHURG-STRAUSS SYNDROME (ALLERGIC GRANULOMATOSIS AND ANGIITIS)

Definition

Churg-Strauss syndrome is a systemic disorder characterized pathologically by widespread necrotizing vasculitis and extravascular granulomas. As in Wegener's granulomatosis, the upper and lower respiratory tracts are predominantly affected. In contrast to Wegener's granulomatosis, it is almost invariably preceded by allergic manifestations, i.e., asthma, allergic rhinitis, or rarely, by a drug reaction.

Etiology

The cause is unknown. However, the strong association with allergic rhinitis and asthma, usually long-standing, suggests an antigen-antibody reaction. This suggestion is supported by increased levels of IgG and IgE in the blood in many patients. The immune reaction brings eosinophils to the site of injury setting into motion a cascade that aggravates the local damage, leading to necrosis, and prompts the formation of granulomas.

Pathology

The lungs show the usual features of asthma, generally in association with allergic rhinitis and sinusitis. In addition, foci of a distinctive pneumonia are widespread: the inflammatory cells in these lesions are predominantly eosinophils, often in association with multinucleated giant cells. Necrosis of the eosinophils is associated with granuloma formation. The lesions may resolve or result in scar. Vasculitis usually accompanies granulomas. Typically, the vasculitis affects small and medium-sized arteries and venules with eosinophilic granulomas in the adjacent lung. The necrotizing vasculitis often leads to thrombosis and aneurysms.

Systemic organs, such as brain, kidneys, and muscles, show similar lesions because of involvement of systemic vessels.

Epidemiology

This is a rare form of vasculitis. Usually it begins between 20 and 40 years of age. The ratio of men to women is about 1:1.

Clinical Features

Respiratory manifestations predominate and symptoms of asthma are usually the presenting complaint. Fever and weight loss are typical. A history of atopy is common. The mean duration of asthma before the onset of vasculitis is 8 years and often the asthma has become increasingly refractory to treatment.

Skin lesions are found in 60 percent of patients. Usually these are subcutaneous nodules, but petechiae or purpura also occur. About one third of patients develop congestive heart failure caused by infiltrative or pericardial disease. In 40 percent of patients, involvement of the gastrointestinal tract is manifested by bloody diarrhea or masses. Glomerulonephritis occurs in up to 40 percent of patients. Renal failure is uncommon. The peripheral nervous system is commonly involved, but central nervous system (CNS) disease is rare.

Diagnostic Tests

Peripheral blood eosinophilia is characteristic: eosinophils may account for 50 percent of the white blood cell count. When the disease is active, the sedimentation rate is high and anemia is present. Serum complement is normal. IgG and IgE levels have been increased in the few patients studied.

Abnormal chest radiographs occur in about 50 percent of patients. Findings include patchy, fleeting infiltrates; bilateral, diffuse nodular infiltrates without cavitation; or diffuse interstitial lung disease.

The diagnosis is made by biopsy of affected tissue in a patient with the typical clinical syndrome, i.e., middle-aged patient with history of asthma who develops characteristic skin lesions, pulmonary infiltrates and laboratory abnormalities.

Differential Diagnosis

The major diseases from which Churg-Strauss must be differentiated include Wegener's granulomatosis, lymphomatoid granulomatosis, sarcoidosis, eosinophilic pneumonia, and aspergillosis. These disorders can usually be differentiated by appropriate tests, i.e., culture, serologic studies, and histologic examination.

Treatment and Prognosis

The treatment of choice is glucocorticoids, e.g., prednisone 60 mg/day or its equivalent. Cytotoxic agents have been tried, but their effectiveness has not yet been established. Steroids are continued in high dosage until clinical improvement occurs. The dosage is then tapered. Most patients require a minimum of a year of therapy.

WEGENER'S GRANULOMATOSIS

Definition

As originally described, Wegener's granulomatous disease is a triad in which necrotizing, granulomatous vasculitis involves the upper and lower respiratory tracts and the kidney. In recent years, a limited form, without renal involvement, has also been described.

Etiology

Since respiratory manifestations usually predominate, an inhaled environmental antigen was originally believed to be responsible for the disease. Since then, a variety of immunologic mechanisms have gone in and out of favor. Most recently, a cell-mediated immune mechanism has been held responsible for the pathogenesis of the granulomatous vasculitis.

Pathology

The characteristic lesions are granulomatous lesions and vasculitis. The lesions can be found in almost any organ, but especially in the upper respiratory tract (nose, paranasal sinuses, nasopharynx, and adjacent regions), in the lower respiratory tract (airways, lungs), and kidneys. The lungs are almost always involved with typical lesions affecting both arteries and veins. The renal histology is more variable and may range from a nonspecific focal glomerulonephritis, to a diffuse glomerulonephritis and ultimately glomerulosclerosis. The lung is most apt to reveal distinctive changes on biopsy.

Epidemiology

Wegener's granulomatosis is a rare disease. Although it may affect any age group, it usually presents in the fourth and fifth decades. The incidence is slightly higher in men than in women.

Clinical Manifestations

Constitutional manifestations, consisting of malaise, anorexia weight loss, fever, and weakness, are virtually regular features often in association with arthralgias (particularly symmetrical involvement of small joints, but often polyarticular, also affecting large joints).

Respiratory involvement occurs in almost all patients, manifested by evidence of involvement of the lungs and nasal sinuses. Cough is common; less frequent are dyspnea and chest discomfort. Occasionally, spontaneous pneumothorax, pleural effusions, and atelectasis due to endobronchial lesions, are seen. Evidence of sinusitis, especially maxillary, can be striking or detectable only by radiography. It should be stressed that any organ, including skin, eyes, ears, brain, and heart, can contribute to the clinical manifestations because of the systemic nature of the disease.

Nasal involvement can range from rhinitis and epistaxis to destruction of the nasal septal cartilage, resulting in a "saddle nose" deformity.

In the "limited form," the patient is free of urinary abnormalities. In many instances, the "limited form" merely seems to mark one phase in the evolution of the systemic disease.

Diagnostic Tests

Chest radiography The usual presentation is that of solid nodules or cavitary infiltrates that may be single but more often are bilateral. An unusual presentation is atelectasis due to endobronchial obstruction. The onset with pleural manifestations (spontaneous pneumothorax, bronchopleural fistula, or pleural effusion) is rare.

Pulmonary function tests As a rule, the pattern is nondiagnostic. Pulmonary function tests may reveal the pattern of obstructive airway disease.

Laboratory tests The conventional laboratory tests, e.g., sedimentation rate and white blood cell count, are generally helpful only in indicating the activity of the process. Levels of circulating immunoglobulins are not diagnostic, but may be helpful in excluding Goodpasture's syndrome in which levels of circulating glomerular basement membrane (GBM) antibodies are high (and in which immunofluorescence reveals linear staining of the basement membranes in the lungs and kidneys).

Much more valuable is testing of the patient's serum for antineutrophil cytoplasmic antibodies (ANCA). ANCA is a class of autoantibodies that is demonstrated by indirect immunofluorescence of the patient's ethanol-fixed neutrophils and serum. Several different patterns of staining can occur. However, it is the cytoplasmic immunofluorescence that is highly specific for Wegener's granulomatosis (C-ANCA). A perinuclear pattern (P-ANCA) may also be encountered but is less specific for Wegener's granulomatosis, i.e., it may be seen in association with other vasculitides.

Although it is not yet clear whether these autoantibodies are pathogenic or simply an epiphenomenon, their clinical value in diagnosis has been shown convincingly. ANCA are also useful for following the activity of the disease and the response to therapy. Since the sensitivity of ANCA is only about 70 percent, a negative test does not rule out Wegener's granulomatosis.

Differential Diagnosis

As noted above, Goodpasture's syndrome, another pulmonary-renal syndrome, has to be ruled out by measurements of circulating anti-GBM antibodies and by immunofluorescent studies. Among the other possibilities that have to be considered are lymphomatoid granulomatosis, other vasculitic syndromes (systemic lupus erythematosus, Sjögren's syndrome, Henoch-Schönlein purpura, hypersensitivity vasculitis, and polyarteritis nodosa), allergic granulomatosis and angiitis (Churg-Strauss syndrome), and the granulomatous syndromes (sarcoidosis and midline granuloma).

Midline granuloma Similar in histologic appearance to that of either Wegener's granulomatosis or of lymphomatoid granulomatosis, sometimes midline granuloma is a prelude to full-blown Wegener's granulomatosis, but sometimes it persists as a locally destructive process. In contrast to full-blown or limited forms of Wegener's granulomatosis, midline granuloma usually responds poorly to cyclophosphamide-prednisone regimens. Instead, it responds to high doses of radiation (which have not been tested in Wegener's granulomatosis).

Treatment

Without treatment, the disease is reputed to have a high mortality rate within a few years after initial presentation. Cyclophosphamide (1 to 2 mg/kg/per day orally) in conjunction with oral corticosteroids (equivalent of 60 mg prednisone daily) is the standard initial therapy for Wegener's granulomatosis. After 2 to 4 weeks, decrease in the steroid dose is generally possible. Using this regimen, complete remission is usually achieved in more than 90 percent of patients. Treatment in modified dosage is continued for at least a year after complete remission.

Higher doses of cyclophosphamide (4 to 5 mg/kg daily), along with prednisone (2 mg/kg daily), may be needed in the severer forms of the disease. Depending on the severity and rate of progression, different clinics use variations in the dosages and routes of administration of both the cytotoxic agent and the corticosteroids. Daily plasma exchange for the first 7 days of treatment is used in some clinics. Recently, the antimicrobial agent trimethoprim-sulfamethoxasole has been advocated, either as an addition to cyclophosphamide and prednisone, or as a sole agent. However, this suggestion has not yet been subjected to extensive clinical trials.

LYMPHOMATOID GRANULOMATOSIS

Definition

Once confused with Wegener's granulomatosis because of similar clinical presentation, lymphomatoid granulomatosis is now felt to be a separate entity. Although it, too, is angiocentric and angiodestructive in nature, the lesions lack granuloma formation and fibrinoid necrosis. Almost 50 percent of patients who develop this disease eventually develop a malignant lymphoma which is refractory to chemotherapy.

Etiology

Lymphomatoid granulomatosis is believed to represent a post-thymic T-cell proliferative disorder.

Pathology

The histologic appearance can range from benign lymphocytic angiitis and granulomatosis to malignant lymphoma. Organ involvement is widespread. With the affected organ, the arteries and veins show destructive, inflammatory infiltrates composed of atypical lymphoreticular cells. Distinct granulomas are not found. Immunohistologic staining using monoclonal antibodies has shown that most of the lymphocytes are T cells. In addition to the lungs, other organs such as the kidney, liver, brain, spleen, adrenal glands, skin, and heart, are often involved.

Epidemiology

Lymphomatoid granulomatosis is a rare disease, with a slight male predominance, and the usual onset of disease is the fourth to fifth decades.

Clinical Manifestations

The disease usually presents with constitutional manifestations, i.e., weight loss, malaise, and fever. Cough, shortness of breath, and chest pain are also usually present at the onset. Also common are macular or nodular skin lesions, CNS abnormalities, which depend on the sites of the lesions, arthralgias, myalgias, and gastrointestinal complaints.

Diagnostic Tests

There are no specific diagnostic laboratory abnormalities. In some patients, leukopenia is present; in about 50 percent, the sedimentation rate is high. Definitive diagnosis is based on tissue biopsy and demonstration of the characteristic histologic features.

Chest radiography The chest radiograph usually shows bilateral nodular densities, some of which may be cavitary. Pleural effusions sometimes occur; hilar adenopathy is rare. Diffuse fluffy alveolar and reticulonodular infiltrates occur occasionally.

Treatment and Prognosis

Although corticosteroids and cyclophosphamide have occasionally been reported to be successful in the treatment of lymphomatoid granulomatosis, as a rule, the disorder progresses inexorably to death. In contrast, benign lymphocytic angiitis and granulomatosis usually responds favorably to cytotoxic agents and corticosteroids. Also in contrast to lymphomatoid granulomatosis, benign lymphocytic angiitis and granulomatosis has several distinctive features: (1) high concentrations of IgE in serum; (2) few, if any, extrathoracic manifestations; (3) responsiveness to a cytotoxic agent; (4) usual remission after treatment for about 6 months; and (5) no progression to malignancy.

RHEUMATOID ARTHRITIS

Pulmonary vasculitis is uncommon in rheumatoid arthritis. The clinical features are similar to those of primary pulmonary hypertension. The presumed antigen is an immunoglobulin and immune complex deposition seen in walls of small and medium-sized pulmonary arteries. The treatment therefore consists of high-dose corticosteroids combined with cytotoxic agents. No controlled trials have evaluated this therapeutic regimen.

SYSTEMIC LUPUS ERYTHEMATOSUS

Although pulmonary vascular pathology is common in lupus erythematosus, vasculitis of pulmonary vessels is uncommon. Although vasculitis may occur as extension of the parenchymal lung disease, most patients with lupus pneumonitis do not have vascular abnormalities.

Deposition of immune complexes in small and medium-sized arteries can cause massive hemorrhage by disrupting the vessel walls. This picture may also be seen with capillaritis and venulitis. Treatment includes high-dose corticosteroids and cytotoxic agents.

BIBLIOGRAPHY

For a more detailed discussion, see Strauss L, Lieberman KV, Churg J: Pulmonary vasculitis, in Fishman AP (ed), *Pulmonary Diseases and Disorders,* 2d ed. New York, McGraw-Hill, 1988, pp 1127–1156.

Fienberg R, Mark EJ, Goodman M, McCluskey RT, Niles JL: Correlation of antineutrophil cytoplasmic antibodies with the extrarenal histopathology of Wegener's (pathergic) granulomatosis and related forms of vasculitis. Hum Pathol 24:160–168, 1993.

Jennette JC: Antineutrophil cytoplasmic autoantibody-associated diseases: A pathologist's perspective. Am J Kidney Dis 18:164–170, 1991.

Michel BA: Classification of vasculitis. Curr Opin Rheumatol 4:3–8, 1992.

Rosenow EC III, Lie JT: The pulmonary vasculitides, in Fishman AP (ed), *Update: Pulmonary Diseases and Disorders.* New York, McGraw-Hill, 1992, pp 465–474.

Staples CA: Pulmonary angiitis and granulomatosis. Radiol Clin North Am 5:973–982, 1991.

V | DISEASES OF THE AIRWAYS

Robert L. Vender

ETIOLOGY

Mechanisms responsible for upper airway obstruction can be divided into two general categories.

1. Structural abnormalities that are grossly visible; these cause mechanical obstruction because of their size or destructive nature.
2. Factors or disease processes which cause neuromuscular dysfunction of the upper airway in the absence of grossly visible lesions.

Taken together, these processes encompass a wide range of pathologic entities ranging from immunologic and infectious to malignant (Table 21-1).

In some instances such as epiglottitis, upper airway obstruction may represent an isolated phenomenon. In others, upper airway obstruction may be part of a systemic disease, e.g., myasthenia gravis or relapsing polychondritis; frequently, symptoms related to the upper airways may be the initial manifestation of the systemic disorder.

At times, upper airway obstruction may be at its peak when first seen, e.g., aspiration of a foreign body. Alternatively, it may develop insidiously over months to years, e.g., postintubation tracheal stenosis, or progress very rapidly, e.g., anaphylaxis or thermal injury.

Sometimes, a pathologic process that obstructs the upper airway is accompanied by signs or symptoms remote from the site itself, e.g., fever and toxicity that accompany a retropharyngeal abscess.

ABNORMAL PHYSIOLOGY

Resistance to flow through the upper airways exhibits exponential characteristics (Fig. 21-1). The major reason for this pattern is that resistance varies inversely as the fourth power of the radius of the lumen. At normal flow rates, considerable luminal narrowing can occur without appreciable increase in resistance. However, once a critical level of airway occlusion is achieved, i.e., the break point in Figure 21-1, resistance begins to increase dramatically. Small decrements in the lumen of the airway below the critical value effect large increases in resistance, thereby reducing ventilatory capacity. Moreover, as inspiratory flow rates increase, e.g., during exercise, the break point develops at a relatively lesser degree of luminal narrowing.

TABLE 21-1 Common Etiologic Causes of Upper Airway Obstruction

Structural Lesions

Abscess	Macroglossia
Anaphylaxis/angioedema	Malignant tumors
Benign polyps	Postextubation edema/stenosis
Caustic injury	Relapsing polychondritis
Epiglottitis	Thermal injury
Foreign body	Thymoma-thyroid goiter
Granulomatous disorders	Trauma
Hematoma	Viral papillomatosis

Neurologically Mediated Obstruction

Dystonic spasm (Meige syndrome)
Guillain-Barré syndrome
Myasthenia gravis
Stroke-occlusive cerebral vascular disease
Postextubation laryngospasm
Bilateral vocal cord paralysis—postthyroid surgery
                                        Idiopathic
                                        Malignancy

Types of Upper Airway Obstruction

Based on the standard flow-volume loop, upper airway obstruction can be categorized physiologically as *fixed* or *variable*. Before considering the specific features of these different types of obstruc-

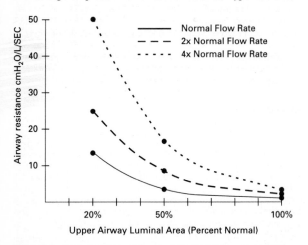

FIG. 21-1 The relationship between reduction in airway luminal dimensions and its effect on upper airway resistance measured at various flow rates compared to normal.

tion, it is worth emphasizing that in upper airway obstruction, the most marked flow limitation during expiration occurs at the start of the maneuver, i.e., at high lung volumes close to total lung capacity (TLC) where flow rates are *effort dependent*. In contrast, the most marked limitation to expiratory flow in diffuse disease of the peripheral airways occurs in the lower range of lung volumes nearer to the residual volume (RV), i.e., in the *effort-independent* portion of this maneuver (Fig. 21-2*A*).

Fixed Obstruction

Fixed obstruction is characterized by a reduction in cross-sectional area of the airway, which persists despite variations in the transmural pressure gradient (extraluminal-to-intraluminal pressure differences) that occur during either phase of the respiratory cycle; the resistance remains unchanged throughout the respiratory cycle. Lesions resulting in fixed obstruction are usually circumferential, e.g., postintubation tracheal stenosis. Flow is compromised during both inspiration and expiration and the characteristic plateau configuration is seen in both limbs of the flow-volume loop (Fig. 21-2*B*).

Variable Obstruction

Variable obstruction is characterized by dynamic changes in the degree of obstruction and, therefore, in resistance that depend on the phase of respiration. In contrast to the fixed obstruction, the physiologic behavior of a variable obstruction does depend on the differences between extraluminal and intraluminal pressures; these differences, in turn, are dictated by the anatomic site of obstruction and the phase of respiration. Two types of variable obstruction can be identified—extrathoracic and intrathoracic.

Variable extrathoracic obstruction The extrathoracic airways (above the sternal notch) are subjected to a constant extraluminal pressure that is equal to atmospheric pressure. In variable extrathoracic obstruction, the transmural pressure gradient favors luminal narrowing due to intraluminal pressure becoming inordinately subatmospheric during inspiration while extraluminal pressure remains atmospheric. This effect is exaggerated as the flow rate through the area of narrowing is increased by strenuous muscular efforts. Conversely, a forced expiratory maneuver tends to dilate the obstruction as intraluminal pressure becomes positive with respect to extraluminal pressure. Consequently, in variable extrathoracic obstruction, the inspiratory portion of the flow-volume loop shows an absolute reduction in the magnitude of flow rates, and a linear plateau in the curve over a considerable range of the vital capacity whereas expiratory characteristics remain normal (Fig. 21-2*D*).

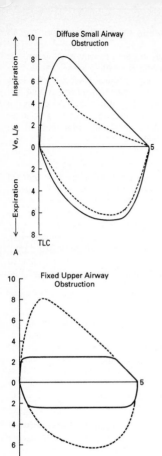

FIG. 21-2 Representative examples of normal and abnormal flow-volume tracings characteristic of the three classifications of upper airways obstruction. *A. Obstruction of small airways.* The solid line displays the normal pattern. The dashed line indicates the pattern of diffuse obstruction of small airways characteristic of disease processes like asthma, bronchitis, and emphysema where the greatest degree of reduction in flow occurs at the mid-low range of the forced vital capacity (FVC) maneuver. *B. Fixed upper airway obstruction.* The solid line depicts reduction in flow rates during both the inspiratory and expiratory phase of the flow-volume loop characteristic of fixed upper airway obstruction. The dashed line displays a near-normal pattern following correction of the pathologic process.

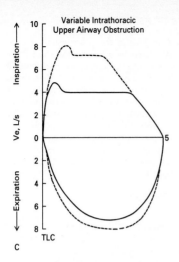

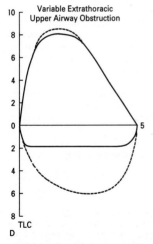

FIG 21-2 *C. Variable intrathoracic obstruction.* The solid line depicts flow limitation only during the expiratory portion of the FVC maneuver but with normal inspiratory flow characteristic of variable intrathoracic obstruction. The dashed line represents improvement but not total normalization after appropriate therapy. *D. Variable extrathoracic upper airway obstruction.* The solid line displays flow limitation only during inspiration characteristic of variable extrathoracic upper airway obstruction. The dashed line represents improvement after therapy. (Adapted from Miller RD.)

Variable intrathoracic obstruction This is the more usual type of variable obstruction, generally caused by a lesion that arises from one side of the trachea and extends into the lumen; the contralateral wall is spared and remains pliable and responsive to changes in transmural pressure. The pressure around the intrathoracic segment of the upper airway reflects pleural pressure, which is negative with respect to intraluminal pressure during inspiration and positive during forced expiration. Thus, with variable intrathoracic obstruction, transmural pressure differences favor airway dilatation and normal flow characteristics during inspiration, whereas a forced expiration elicits marked expiratory flow limitation because of dynamic compression (Fig. 21-2C).

CLINICAL-PHYSIOLOGIC CORRELATIONS

The presence and severity of respiratory symptoms and signs depends on the degree of reduction in airway luminal diameter (Table 21-2). The normal diameter of the laryngotracheal lumen is 15 to 25 mm. Patients with narrowing of either the vocal cords or the tracheal dimension are usually asymptomatic until this diameter is reduced to < 10 mm. Reduction to approximately 8 mm is frequently accompanied by exertional dyspnea; the values of arterial P_{O_2} and P_{CO_2} remain normal at rest. Critical narrowing to 5 mm or less is associated with dyspnea at rest and is accompanied by respiratory distress, substernal retractions, and cyanosis; arterial hypoxemia and hypercapnia are present. In the extreme, the combination of a severe reduction in airway lumen in association with strenuous muscular efforts to sustain high flow rates through the area of stricture can contribute to inspiratory muscle fatigue and predispose to respiratory failure. The converse is also true: a modest increase in airway caliber after successful therapy can cause

TABLE 21-2 Clinical-Pathophysiologic Correlates of Laryngotracheal Obstruction

Degree of narrowing	Approximate diameter	Symptoms and signs	Arterial blood-gas measurements
Normal	15–25 mm	None	Normal
Mild	10 mm	None or mild dyspnea on exertion	Normal
Moderate	8 mm	Dyspnea on exertion Exercise limitation Tachypnea	Normal
Severe	5 mm	Dyspnea at rest Obvious distress Substernal retractions Cyanosis Stridor	Elevated P_{CO_2} Decreased P_{O_2}

a significant decrease in airway resistance and a dramatic relief of respiratory complaints.

It should be stressed that the absence of respiratory symptoms does not eliminate the possibility of significant upper airway luminal narrowing. Conversely, the development of hypercapnia and dyspnea at rest, even in the absence of obvious respiratory distress, portends a very serious, life-threatening degree of airway obstruction that mandates immediate intervention.

Inspiratory stridor This is a valuable clinical sign of upper airway obstruction. However, the absence of inspiratory stridor does not exclude the possibility of upper airway disease when either the degree of luminal narrowing is only minor or the degree of obstruction is so severe that no appreciable airflow can be generated across the orifice.

Hoarseness This sign affords a valuable clue to the presence of lesions involving the larynx, particularly edema, epiglottitis, or tumor. An important exception is bilateral vocal cord paralysis, which generally causes the voice amplitude to decrease without hoarseness.

DIFFERENTIAL DIAGNOSIS

Clinically, upper airway obstruction often has to be distinguished from obstructive diseases of the more peripheral airways, notably asthma and chronic obstructive pulmonary disease.

DIAGNOSTIC EVALUATION

Pulmonary function testing As discussed above, the flow-volume loop is of vital importance in documenting the presence of upper airway obstruction and in distinguishing upper airway obstruction from the more common obstructive lung diseases involving the more distal airways. The pattern of upper airway obstruction on the flow-volume loop is useful in identifying the nature of the lesion. Whereas most fixed lesions and variable extrathoracic lesions are benign, neoplasms account for a large portion of variable intrathoracic obstruction.

Other information provided by routine pulmonary function testing in favor of the diagnosis of upper airway obstruction includes:

Test	Values
• FEV_1 (ml)/PEFR (L/min)	≥ 10 ml/L/min
• MVV (L)	$< 30 \times FEV_1$ (L)
• $FEV_1/FEV_{0.5}$	≥ 1.5
• FEF50%/FIF50%	≥ 1

Although these indices are nonspecific, abnormal values should prompt the examination of the flow-volume loop for more definitive evidence of upper airway obstruction.

Radiographic studies Narrowing of the tracheal air column can occasionally be seen on the posterior-anterior chest radiograph in patients with upper airway obstruction. However, this technique is insensitive. Lateral neck radiographs and computed tomographic examination of the upper airways are sometimes helpful.

Bronchoscopy/laryngoscopy Direct visualization of the upper airways is an essential component of the evaluation of upper airway obstruction. This procedure must be undertaken with caution because it runs the risk of precipitating respiratory failure in the patient in whom the airway is critically narrowed. To deal with this prospect, the operator must be prepared to establish an airway quickly, either by endotracheal intubation or tracheostomy. Therefore, inspection of the airway by either bronchoscopy or laryngoscopy should only be undertaken by physicians skilled in the emergency management of the compromised airway.

TREATMENT

Of primary importance is ensuring a secure and patent airway. If the obstruction is causing respiratory distress, endotracheal intubation or tracheostomy should be performed. Rigid bronchoscopy is preferable to flexible bronchoscopy if the site of obstruction is apt to bleed during manipulation or biopsy. Control of the airway to ensure patency is essential before definitive therapy is directed at the primary cause of the obstruction.

Two temporizing measures have been used in special circumstances to alleviate the obstruction in patients in whom the degree of airway narrowing is deemed not to be critical. In situations where laryngeal edema contributes to upper airway obstruction, e.g., anaphylaxis and postextubation laryngeal edema, the administration of racemic epinephrine by nebulizer may increase airway caliber sufficiently, albeit modestly, to obviate the need for intubation or tracheostomy. This form of therapy should be used with caution in the elderly or patients with underlying cardiac disease. The second measure consists of the inhalation of a mixture of 80% helium/20% oxygen (which has a lower density than ambient air); this therapy is sometimes effective in decreasing the resistance to flow through a narrowed upper airway. Neither of these measures should be used as the sole mode of therapy nor should they delay establishment of a secure airway in a patient with critical upper airway obstruction.

An uncommon complication of acute upper airway obstruction is the development of noncardiogenic pulmonary edema. This complication may accompany the obstruction or may develop shortly after the obstruction is relieved. In most instances, the pulmonary edema is self-limited and does not require intervention beyond the use of supplemental oxygen.

BIBLIOGRAPHY

For a more detailed discussion, see Miller RD: Obstructing lesions of the larynx and trachea: Clinical and pathophysiological aspects, in Fishman AP (ed), *Pulmonary Diseases and Disorders,* 2d ed. New York, McGraw-Hill, 1988, pp 1173–1186.

Horner RL, Guz A: Some factors affecting the maintenance of upper airway patency in man. Respir Med 85 (suppl A):27–30, 1991.

John SD, Swischuk LE: Stridor and upper airway obstruction in infants and children. Radiographics 12:625–643, 1992.

Kuna ST, Sant'Ambrogio G: Pathophysiology of upper airway closure during sleep. JAMA 266:1384–1389, 1991.

Pickering R, Martinez FJ: Helium flow-volume loop in an asthmatic patient. Respir Care 36:1157–1159, 1991.

Wilson RS: Upper airway problems. Respir Care 37:533–550, 1992.

Chronic Obstructive Pulmonary Disease (COPD)

Reynold A. Panettieri, Jr.   Richard K. Murray

DEFINITIONS

The term chronic obstructive pulmonary disease (COPD) may be used to describe a variety of pulmonary disorders including asthma, chronic bronchitis, emphysema, cystic fibrosis, and bronchiectasis. However, its use is generally restricted to chronic bronchitis and emphysema. Unlike asthma, COPD implies, in part, irreversible airway obstruction. The clinical manifestations of these diseases overlap considerably so that features of emphysema and chronic bronchitis may coexist in the same individual with airway obstruction.

Chronic bronchitis is a clinical diagnosis that stems from chronic excessive secretion of mucus associated with obstruction to airflow and mucous plugging; it is manifested by a chronic or a recurrent productive cough. These symptoms should recur most days for a minimum of 3 months per year, for no less than 2 consecutive years.

Emphysema is an anatomic alteration of the lungs characterized by abnormal enlargement of airspaces distal to the terminal, nonrespiratory bronchioles, accompanied by destructive changes in the alveolar walls.

PATHOLOGY AND PATHOGENESIS

Chronic Bronchitis

Pathologically, the bronchial mucous glands are enlarged and accompanied by an increase in the number (hyperplasia) of mucous-secreting cells. Although an increase in the ratio of the thickness of bronchial mucous glands to that of the bronchial wall (Reid index) has been advocated as a basis for the diagnosis of chronic bronchitis, this histologic index is not specific for chronic bronchitis since other obstructive airway diseases may also induce alterations in this ratio.

Emphysema

In contrast to chronic bronchitis, emphysema is an anatomic diagnosis. It is characterized by irreversible, abnormal increases in the size of airspaces distal to the terminal bronchiole (acinus). *Centrilobular emphysema,* which occurs most commonly as a result of, or in association with, cigarette smoking, affects the proximal segment of the respiratory bronchiole. *Panacinar emphysema,* which occurs in the elderly and in patients with α_1-antiprotease deficiency, uniformly affects the entire respiratory bronchiole. Panacinar and centrilobular emphysema often coexist in the same lung. It is the degree of functional impairment from emphysema, not the type, which determines the clinical significance of the disease.

Tobacco Smoking and COPD

In the United States, most patients with emphysema and chronic bronchitis are either current or former smokers. Curiously, however, only about 15 percent of smokers develop COPD. Although the pathogenesis of emphysema remains speculative, accumulating evidence suggests that cigarette smoke induces an imbalance between protease and antiprotease activity in the lung, resulting in an increase in elastase activity and destruction of the elastic fibers in the alveolar walls. According to this hypothesis, cigarette smoke induces a relative increase in elastase activity, both by increasing the elastase burden in the lung, i.e., by recruiting neutrophils to the lung, and by oxidizing and thereby inactivating endogenous antiproteases. Consistent with the protective role postulated for the endogenous antiproteases is the fact that patients with α_1-antitrypsin deficiency, a hereditary disease characterized by a lack of α_1-antitrypsin activity in homozygotic individuals, develop emphysema.

The mechanisms that induce the pathologic changes of chronic bronchitis are also speculative. However, cigarette smoking again appears to be causally related. In addition, acute or chronic exposure to dusts, fumes, air pollution, and respiratory viruses has been associated with the onset of chronic bronchitis.

PATHOPHYSIOLOGY

Pulmonary Mechanics

Chronic airflow limitation, a hallmark of emphysema and chronic bronchitis, may occur via several mechanisms: (1) airway lumens may be partially occluded by excessive and tenacious secretions, e.g., in patients with chronic bronchitis; (2) contraction of airway smooth muscle and bronchial wall edema and inflammation may also induce airway obstruction by decreasing the luminal diameters of the airways; and (3) destruction of lung parenchyma, e.g., in patients with emphysema, may diminish the tethering forces exerted on airway lumens; in emphysema, moderate-sized airways, which are not surrounded by cartilage, become "floppy" and limit airflow especially during forced expiratory maneuvers. Because all three mechanisms may occur concomitantly, therapeutic efforts should be directed at reversing airway smooth muscle contraction, decreasing airway inflammation, and augmenting sputum expectoration. Unfortunately, the loss of radial traction of the airways and the decrease in the elastic recoil of the lung, as seen in emphysema, is irreversible.

Despite the variety of mechanisms that can induce airway obstruction, pulmonary mechanics in chronic airway obstruction are altered in a predictable manner: expiratory flow rates and volumes are diminished throughout the expiratory cycle; because airflow limitation prolongs expiration time and prevents complete emptying of affected alveoli, lung volumes increase. The increases in lung volume alter the length-tension relationship of the diaphragm in such a way as to place it at a mechanical disadvantage.

Gas Exchange

In patients with COPD, ventilation-perfusion mismatch occurs commonly and induces alterations in both oxygenation and alveolar ventilation. Perfusion of poorly ventilated areas of lung (low ventilation-perfusion ratio) results in widening of the arterial-alveolar gradient for oxygen and, in more severe cases, in arterial hypoxemia. Similarly, some areas of lung may be relatively overventilated for the degree of perfusion, resulting in increased deadspace ventilation and impaired excretion of CO_2.

Control of Ventilation

Although patients with severe airflow limitation (< 0.8 L) are more likely to retain CO_2, there is considerable individual variation: some patients with COPD, particularly those with severe chronic bronchitis, develop CO_2 retention, whereas others with comparable airflow limitation do not.

In patients with COPD, the work of breathing is increased due, in part, to increased airway resistance and altered respiratory muscle mechanics. In addition, the ventilatory response to inhaled CO_2 may be subnormal. One popular hypothesis is that patients with COPD retain CO_2 to compensate for an increased work of breathing. However, the mechanism that induces CO_2 retention in these patients is unknown and is likely to be multifactorial.

CLINICAL MANIFESTATIONS

History The patient with COPD usually comes to the physician seeking relief from dyspnea or an upper respiratory tract illness. A pointed history reveals moderate shortness of breath with exertion that has been insidious in onset. The patients are usually in the sixth or seventh decade of life and usually give a history of cigarette smoking. Similar symptoms in the fourth or fifth decade of life should prompt the physician to consider alternative diagnoses such as asthma, α_1-antitrypsin deficiency, or congenital lung disease. Although cough is a common complaint, it is rarely debilitating. Patients in whom bronchitis is a predominant component of their disease will complain of marked and persistent sputum production. Although hemoptysis, weight loss, or a severe cough may occur in patients with chronic bronchitis or emphysema, these symptoms should raise the suspicion of lung cancer or tuberculosis.

Other manifestations that occur late in the course of the disease generally represent complications of COPD. For example, leg swelling suggests right-sided congestive heart failure. Morning headache, lethargy, and confusion are common symptoms of CO_2 retention. Although exertional dyspnea often occurs in patients with moderate-to-severe COPD, exertional dyspnea may also be a manifestation of ischemic heart disease, a common comorbid condition in patients with a significant smoking history.

The "pink puffer" (type A) and the "blue bloater" (type B) syndromes are historical descriptions of two subsets of patients with COPD. The "pink puffer" is tachypneic, with labored respirations and pursed-lip breathing, but arterial oxygenation is well preserved. In contrast, the term "blue bloater" refers to patients who present predominantly with cyanosis (due to arterial hypoxemia), hypercapnia, leg swelling, and right-sided congestive heart disease; as a rule, the patients tend to be obese and they produce copious amounts of sputum. The "pink puffers" were pictured as suffering predominantly from emphysema, whereas the "blue bloaters" were primarily patients with chronic bronchitis. Pathologic studies have since established that emphysema may be present in both groups. This classification of COPD patients is occasionally useful in defining the predominant underlying process; unfortunately, there is a significant degree of overlap, and few patients fall exclusively into either subset.

Physical examination On auscultation, examination of the chest often reveals distant breath sounds, expiratory wheeze, and a prolonged expiratory phase. If airway obstruction is moderately severe, then increased lung volumes are manifested by an increased anteroposterior diameter of the chest, large, hyperresonant lung fields, and limited respiratory excursion of the diaphragm. A palpable liver edge without evidence of hepatomegaly results from caudal displacement of the diaphragm. Hypertrophy of accessory muscles of respiration (sternocleidomastoid and trapezius) also suggests severe chronic airflow limitation. Cyanosis is uncommon in patients with stable COPD; however, during acute exacerbations, cyanosis indicates considerable arterial oxygen desaturation. Signs of pulmonary hypertension and right-sided congestive heart failure, i.e., neck vein distention, hepatomegaly, peripheral edema, usually occur in patients with long-standing arterial hypoxemia stemming from ventilation-perfusion abnormalities. Consequently, they are most apt to occur in the predominantly chronic bronchitic "blue bloater" than in the patient with predominantly emphysema, i.e., the "pink puffer."

USUAL DIAGNOSTIC STUDIES

Chest radiography The chest radiograph from patients with emphysema characteristically shows hyperinflation manifested by radiolucent lung fields, a flattened diaphragm, and a slender cardiac silhouette. Although the chest radiograph is useful in confirming a diagnosis of COPD, particularly emphysema, it is not specific since patients with acute exacerbations of asthma, cystic fibrosis, bronchiectasis, or chronic bronchitis may have identical chest radiographs. Also, the chest radiograph may not reflect the severity of COPD determined by pulmonary function testing.

Pulmonary function testing Pulmonary function testing in patients with COPD is valuable in assessing the severity of the disease, in confirming the diagnosis, in evaluating reversibility, and in determining prognosis. Spirometry reveals a decrease in both the forced expiratory volume in 1 s (FEV_1) and the forced vital capacity (FVC). The FEV_1/FVC ratio is also decreased and is diagnostic of obstructive airway disease. Although most patients with COPD do not manifest an increase in FEV_1 in response to aerosolized bronchodilators, approximately 20 percent are bronchodilator responsive, i.e., the FEV_1 increases by 20 percent after administration of an aerosolized β-agonist. Lung volumes, determined by body plethysmography, are increased in emphysema but may be normal in chronic bronchitis. The increase in total lung volume, a consequence of airflow limitation and air-trapping, includes an increase in the functional residual volume and the residual volume (Fig. 22-1).

In COPD, lung volumes measured by body plethysmography are often higher than those measured by single-breath helium dilution technique. In the face of significant airflow obstruction, helium is incompletely distributed throughout the lung after a single breath, thereby underestimating the true lung volume. In emphysema, the single-breath diffusing capacity (DL_{CO}) is decreased because of loss of alveolar-capillary units. In contrast, the DL_{CO} is well preserved in patients with chronic bronchitis or asthma. Consequently, this test is of value in distinguishing patients with predominantly emphysema from those with predominantly chronic bronchitis or asthma.

Arterial blood-gas values are relatively insensitive measures of

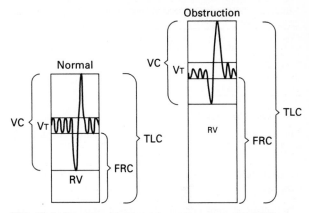

FIG. 22-1 Spirometry and lung volumes in patients with COPD. As a consequence of airflow limitation and loss of elastic recoil in the lung, expiratory time is prolonged and complete emptying of alveoli is prevented. The residual volume (RV) measures the volume of gas in the lungs at end expiration, then increases and induces a decrease in vital capacity (VC). In patients with COPD, the increase in functional residual capacity (FRC) and total lung capacity (TLC) results from an increase in residual volume. The tidal volume (VT) may be less than normal.

the severity of COPD. In early stages of emphysema, an increase in the arterial-alveolar oxygen difference is common. In later stages of the disease, hypoxemia or hypercapnia may occur at rest. Reactive erythrocytosis, manifested by increases in hematocrit, is a consequence of chronic hypoxemia that may be reinforced by high carboxyhemoglobin levels due to cigarette smoking.

NATURAL HISTORY AND PROGNOSIS

The natural history of COPD is highly variable. Although population studies have defined certain trends, the course in the individual patient is difficult to predict. Prognosis correlates best with measurements of FEV_1. In one large series, median survival was approximately 10 years when the FEV_1 was 1.4 L, 4 years with an FEV_1 of 1 L, and slightly over 2 years with an FEV_1 of 0.5 L. The onset of cor pulmonale and right heart failure portends a particularly poor prognosis. Respiratory failure is the most common cause of death in patients with COPD. The natural history of COPD is favorably altered by smoking cessation and by oxygen administration; the ability of other common interventions such as bronchodilators to influence outcome remains unproven.

TABLE 22-1   Differential Diagnosis of Obstructive
Airway Disease

Asthma
Chronic bronchitis
Emphysema
Bronchiectasis
Cystic fibrosis
Congenital bullous lung disease

DIFFERENTIAL DIAGNOSIS

Chronic airflow obstruction characterizes a number of disorders
listed in Table 22-1.

MANAGEMENT

Smoking Cessation

The benefits of smoking cessation are well established. In young
smokers (< 35 years old) who have mild obstructive airway disease
(80 percent predicted > FEV_1 > 60 percent predicted), the FEV_1 will
return to normal after the patient stops smoking. In older patients,
cessation of smoking will slow, but not eliminate, further decrements
in the FEV_1. The recently introduced transdermal nicotine patch,
intended to attenuate the physiologic effects of nicotine withdrawal,
provides an important, though imperfect, tool in assisting patients
with smoking cessation. In one large study involving approximately
290 smokers, use of the transdermal patch was associated with a
1-year abstinence rate of 17 percent, which compared favorably to
the placebo-associated rate of only 4 percent. Use of the nicotine
patch should be combined with counseling and psychological
support.

Bronchodilators

Ipratropium bromide, a quaternary anticholinergic agent which
blocks muscarinic receptors on airway smooth muscle, decreases
vagal tone, inhibits smooth muscle contraction, and decreases
mucous secretion. As a single agent, inhaled ipratropium bromide
is at least equal to and, in many studies, a better bronchodilator
than methylxanthines or inhaled β-agonists. Additionally, ipratropium is associated with fewer side effects than these other agents.
Moreover, the bronchodilator potency of the anticholingeric agents
is not attenuated by continued administration, whereas patients
treated with β-agonists for prolonged periods may experience
blunted bronchodilator responses to β-agonists. Beta-agonists also
may induce pulmonary vasodilation, which worsens ventilation-per-

fusion mismatching, occasionally resulting in a decrease in the arterial Po_2; ipratropium bromide does not have this effect.

Ipratropium is delivered by metered-dose inhaler (18 μg/puff) two puffs four times daily for a maximum of four puffs four times daily. Although effective as monotherapy, the addition of ipratropium to β-agonists therapy elicits an additive bronchodilator effect.

Theophylline

Despite the use of methylxanthines in the treatment of COPD for over 100 years, the mechanism by which this agent improves dyspnea or decreases airway obstruction remains unknown. Theophylline is a weak bronchodilator in comparison to β-agonists or ipratropium. Given the narrow therapeutic window, the use of theophylline should be tailored to the individual patient, and "optimal" bronchodilator effects may occur in the low therapeutic range (5–15 mg/dL; Table 22-2). Theophylline clearance may be affected by a variety of other medications, and dosing regimens should be individualized and serum levels checked regularly (Table 22-3).

In COPD patients, the therapeutic benefit of theophylline may be a consequence of effects other than bronchodilation. Apart from increasing cyclic adenosine monophosphate (cAMP) levels by inhibiting phosphodiesterase activity, methylxanthines have been reported to increase the contractility of "fatigued" diaphragms and increase mucociliary action in normal airways. Moreover, methylxanthines also increase hypoxic drive to ventilation in hypercapnic COPD patients and increase right and left ventricular ejection

TABLE 22-2 Theophylline Dosing* † in Adults with Acute Bronchospasm

Dosing	Intravenous aminophylline
Loading dose†	
History of theophylline use	
None	6 mg/kg over 20 min
Oral theophylline use	0–3 mg/kg over 20 min
Maintenance dose§	
Patient category	
Nonsmoker	0.5 mg/kg/h
Smoker	0.3 mg/kg/h
Critically ill	0.5 mg/kg/h
Congestive heart failure	0.2 mg/kg/h
Severe pneumonia	0.2 mg/kg/h

*Dosing expressed in aminophylline equivalents (theophylline dose = 0.8 × aminophylline dose).
†If possible, serum theophylline levels should be obtained prior to administration. Initial target serum concentration for theophylline is 10 mg/ml.
§Theophylline levels should be measured 12–24 h after loading and more frequently if symptoms or signs of theophylline toxicity are evident.

TABLE 22-3 Physiologic Factors and Drug Interactions
Altering Theophylline Metabolism

Increases serum levels	Decreases serum levels
Advanced age	Carbamazepine
Obesity	Dilantin
Erythromycin	Rifampin
Cimetidine	Cigarette smoking
Oral contraceptives	Phenobarbital
Propranolol	
Allopurinol	
Hepatic disease/congestion	
Congestive heart disease	
Quinolines (ciprofloxacin, etc.)	

fractions through vasodilation and through direct myocardial stimulation.

Steroids

Although the benefit of steroids is well established in the management of asthma, the efficacy of steroids in the management of COPD is less well established. Therapy with corticosteroids has been reported to provide both subjective and objective benefits in some patients with COPD. Unfortunately, few clinical predictors identify which patients will respond to steroids. Some COPD patients who do not respond to bronchodilators improve with steroid therapy. Therefore, a therapeutic trial of corticosteroids seems justified in any patient with COPD. For the therapeutic trial, the patient undergoes pretreatment pulmonary function testing and then receives a 2-week course of methylprednisolone or prednisone at a dose of 20 to 40 mg/day. Pulmonary function testing is then repeated. If the testing shows improvement, the dose of steroids is slowly tapered to a maintenance level; if no improvement, steroid therapy is discontinued. Patients with COPD do not benefit from inhaled or alternate-day steroid therapy.

High-dose intravenous corticosteroids are commonly used in the treatment of acute respiratory failure complicating COPD. Again, however, their efficacy in this setting is not firmly established.

Mucolytics

In some COPD patients who manifest excess production of mucus, adjunctive use of mucolytic expectorants appears to improve the quality of life, decreases cough, and decreases the duration of acute exacerbations of dyspnea. One to 8 weeks of iodinated glycerol therapy at a dose of 60 mg four times daily has been effective in reducing symptoms in such patients. However, mucolytic agents, such as acetylcysteine (inhaled or oral), glycerol guaiacolate (guaifenesin) and ambuxol, have not been as effective. If conventional therapy fails to relieve cough or chest tightness, an 8-week trial of iodinated glycerol taken by mouth may be beneficial.

Antibiotics and Vaccines

The administration of antibiotics, e.g., trimethoprim-sulfamethoxazole, amoxicillin, or doxycycline, to patients with COPD during an acute exacerbation decreases the duration of the episode and promotes rapid improvement in peak expiratory flow rates. However, no evidence supports the prophylactic use of antibiotics in COPD patients. Antibiotics are administered for 7 to 10 days during an acute exacerbation.

Although the pneumococcus is one of the two pathogens most often cultured from the sputum during an exacerbation, most exacerbations are not due to bacterial infections. No evidence indicates that pneumococcal bacteremia or sepsis is particularly common in COPD patients. Large scale trials examining the clinical efficacy of the pneumococcal vaccine in patients with COPD have failed to demonstrate a clear benefit. Nonetheless, because there is little downside to this intervention, most physicians advocate its use. Patients with COPD should receive the influenza vaccine annually.

Supplemental Oxygen

When administered for a minimum of at least 12 h/day, supplemental O_2 is the only drug that has reduced mortality in COPD. The current indications for home O_2 therapy include (1) resting $Pa_{O_2} <$ 55 mmHg or an arterial oxygen saturation $< 90\%$; (2) Pa_{O_2} of 55 to 59 mmHg with evidence of cor pulmonale or polycythemia; or (3) significant exercise- or sleep-induced hypoxemia that reverses with supplemental O_2 therapy. Supplemental O_2 should be titrated to maintain the Pa_{O_2} between 65 and 80 mmHg.

Pulmonary Rehabilitation

Exercise limitation in patients with COPD may be due to a variety of pathophysiologic mechanisms including abnormal pulmonary mechanics, impaired gas exchange, abnormal perceptions of dyspnea, impaired cardiac performance, and poor nutritional status. Pulmonary rehabilitation programs have been reported to decrease the need for hospitalization, improve quality of life, decrease respiratory symptoms (dyspnea), and improve endurance time and exercise tolerance in severe COPD patients. Unfortunately, because exercise is ventilation limited in these patients, classic training effects do not occur.

Lung Transplantation

Both unilateral and bilateral lung transplantation can be performed in patients with COPD. Some centers use unilateral procedures for patients over the age of 50 and bilateral procedures for those under the age of 50. The criteria for lung transplantation vary slightly among institutions; however, COPD patients are considered for transplant if they have severe and progressive obstructive disease that substantially limits daily activities. In addition, the patient must be ambulatory with rehabilitative potential, have adequate cardiac function without significant coronary heart disease, and have adequate nutritional and psychosocial profiles. Patients are excluded if they have significant nonpulmonary disease, coronary artery disease, or if they continue to smoke.

Investigational Therapy

Respiratory Muscle Training/Strengthening

Repetitive inspiration against resistive loads improves respiratory muscle strength and endurance in COPD patients. Although exercise tolerance improves in some patients after resistive load conditioning, it is generally unaccompanied by improvement in pulmonary function tests, maximal voluntary ventilation, or maximal sustainable ventilation. Advocates of this approach stress improved quality of life rather than improved physiologic measurements.

Antielastase Therapy

Since emphysema may be induced by an imbalance between neutrophil elastases and serum antiproteases, therapy directed toward increasing serum antiproteases or decreasing neutrophil elastases may prove beneficial in the management of patients with emphysema. In patients with α_1-antitrypsin deficiency, plasma α_1-antitrypsin may be given intravenously once weekly (60 mg/kg) or once monthly (250 mg/ml) to maintain serum α_1-antitrypsin levels above 11 μM. These doses increase lung α_1-antitrypsin levels and restore lung antineutrophil elastase defense mechanisms into the normal range. Although α_1-antitrypsin replacement therapy is efficacious in restoring serum levels of antiprotease activity in patients with α_1-antitrypsin deficiency, it is unclear that this approach will slow the decrease in lung function or improve survival. In any event, replacement therapy has no role in patients with COPD unless they are shown to have underlying α_1-antitrypsin deficiency.

BIBLIOGRAPHY

For a more detailed discussion, see Reid LM: Chronic obstructive pulmonary diseases, in Fishman AP (ed), *Pulmonary Diseases and Disorders,* 2d ed. New York, McGraw-Hill, 1988, pp 1247–1272.

Campbell EJ, Senior RM: Emphysema, in Fishman AP (ed), *Update: Pulmonary Diseases and Disorders.* New York, McGraw-Hill, 1992, pp 37–51.

Chapman KR: Therapeutic algorithm for chronic obstructive pulmonary disease. Am J Med 91:17S–23S, 1991.

Shapiro SH, Erst P, Gray-Donald K, Martin JG, Wood-Dauphinee S, Beaupre A, Spitzer WO, Macklem PT: Effect of negative pressure ventilation in severe chronic obstructive pulmonary disease. Lancet 12:1425–1429, 1992.

Turino GM: Natural history and clinical management of emphysema in patients with and without alpha-1-antitrypsin inhibitor deficiency. Ann NY Acad Sci 624:23–30, 1991.

Richard K. Murray   *Reynold A. Panettieri, Jr.*

DEFINITION AND ETIOLOGY

Asthma is a chronic disease characterized by reversible obstruction to airflow within the lungs. In contrast to emphysema or chronic bronchitis, patients with asthma may have essentially normal lung function between episodes. Although the etiology of asthma remains unknown, airway hyperreactivity in response to inhalational challenge using methacholine or aerosolized allergen is a hallmark of this disease. In some patients, narrowing of the airways may be part of an allergic reaction triggering the release of biologically active mediators. In other patients, specific stimuli trigger episodes and suggest an etiologic relationship (exercise, airway cooling, or stress). In the majority of patients, the cause of the airway hyperreactivity is unknown. Specific causes that have been proposed include imbalances within the nervous system, deficiency of β-receptors, excess contraction of airway smooth muscle, imbalances in mediator production, and immune regulatory defects.

EPIDEMIOLOGY

Asthma is a prevalent disease now affecting approximately 4 percent of the United States population. The prevalence of asthma has increased by 25 percent over the last decade independent of demographic factors. In addition, the mortality of asthma has increased by 31 percent during the past decade with a disproportionate rise in mortality in young African Americans, particularly from urban areas.

PATHOLOGY

The pathology of asthma includes narrowing of the airway lumen and thickening of the airway wall. Mucus and sloughed epithelial cells are seen within the airway lumen and an infiltrate of inflammatory cells, especially eosinophils, is seen within the airway wall. Edema within the airway wall is also a prominent finding. Recent studies of biopsies in asthmatic patients have shown increased numbers of T lymphocytes, mast cells, macrophages, and eosinophils compared to normal controls.

ABNORMAL PHYSIOLOGY

Increased resistance to airflow is the sine qua non of the asthmatic attack. In large part, the increase in airway resistance is due to contraction of airway smooth muscle cells, but other mechanisms contribute to the obstruction to airflow, notably thickening of the airways by edema and cellular infiltration as well as intraluminal collections of mucus, secretions, and cellular debris. Small changes in airway diameter have dramatic effects on airway resistance.

An increase in resistance to airflow causes a series of physiologic alterations including abnormalities of lung mechanics and gas exchange. Spirometry reveals an obstructive pattern manifested by a decrease in forced vital capacity (FVC) and forced expiratory volume at 1s (FEV_1) and a decrease in the FEV_1/FVC ratio. The functional residual capacity (FRC) is increased and the lungs appear hyperinflated on the chest radiograph. The work of breathing is increased and the efficiency of the respiratory pump is decreased because of altered compliance and a pressure-volume relationship that places the respiratory muscles at a suboptimal length-tension relationship. Thus, as airflow is restricted, the work of breathing is increased.

Regional inhomogeneity in the distribution of inspired air leads to ventilation-perfusion ($\dot{V}/\dot{Q}$) mismatch and impaired gas exchange. Areas of low $\dot{V}/\dot{Q}$ contribute to the development of hypoxemia. Dead-space ventilation is increased but adequate elimination of CO_2 is maintained in mild-to-moderate asthma by a compensatory increase in minute ventilation. In severe asthma, the combined effects of augmented CO_2 production, impaired CO_2 elimination, and respiratory muscle fatigue lead to the development of hypercapnia and respiratory acidosis, eventuating in respiratory failure if therapy is unsuccessful.

CLINICAL MANIFESTATIONS

History A detailed history is an essential part of formulating a diagnosis of asthma in a patient with unexplained dyspnea. Patients with asthma typically have a history of intermittent episodes of shortness of breath, wheezing, and chest tightness. In some patients, cough, unaccompanied by wheezing or breathlessness, may be the sole manifestation of their asthma.

A history should attempt to determine if any environmental factors or other exposures appear temporally or causally linked to the exacerbation of symptoms. For example, some patients will report exercise- or cold-induced symptoms. Other patients may report symptoms related to prior upper respiratory tract infections or exposure to specific irritants. Exacerbation of symptoms early in the week followed by improvement over the weekend suggests an occupationally induced cause for the asthma. A detailed history concerning pet exposures, travel history, how symptoms change seasonally, type of home heating and air conditioning systems, and effects of vacations may suggest other specific trigger factors that may be avoided by the patient.

If the patient already carries the diagnosis of asthma, the history should also focus on number of emergency room visits, pattern of exacerbations, admissions to the hospital, admissions to the intensive care unit, or prior need for intubation. These factors, along with a history of prior steroid requirements to control asthma, may help identify patients who are at increased risk for severe or fatal asthma.

Physical examination The physical examination of the asthmatic during an acute attack frequently reveals an uncomfortable and anxious patient obviously short of breath. Use of accessory muscles and nasal flaring suggest particularly severe obstruction. The chest is resonant to percussion, and the diaphragm may be low with reduced movement. Auscultation frequently reveals polyphonic wheezes radiating throughout the chest during expiration. Although such wheezing is usually described as diffuse in that it may be heard in many locations over the chest wall, acoustic analysis usually reveals only two or three discrete wheezes in a given patient. The finding of only a single localized wheeze favors a tracheal or endobronchial obstruction as may be seen with tumor or a foreign body. The expiratory phase is prolonged up to four or five times the inspiratory phase and thus inspiration is brief and forceful. Auscultation of the heart should be normal other than for tachycardia and distant heart sounds. The heart examination is important because an S_3 suggests an alternative diagnosis (congestive heart failure/cardiac asthma) for the patient's dyspnea and wheezing. Pulsus paradoxus may result from wide swings in intrapleural pressure. Cyanosis may be seen in severely ill patients; clubbing or edema should not be present. The presence of nasal polyps suggests triad asthma as a possible etiology (aspirin sensitivity, asthma, and nasal polyps). In patients with hysterical vocal cord dysfunction presenting as asthma, direct laryngoscopy examination may show inappropriate apposition of the vocal cords during both inspiration and expiration.

USUAL DIAGNOSTIC TESTS

It is important to remember that asthma is a clinical diagnosis. The diagnosis is suggested by the onset of wheezing, breathlessness, and cough in patients exposed to certain trigger factors. The "gold standard" for the diagnosis of asthma is the reversibility of symptoms either spontaneously or in response to therapy. Not all signs and symptoms or laboratory abnormalities need be present at one time in a particular patient.

Pulmonary function testing Since the symptoms and signs of asthma often do not correlate with the severity of the bronchoconstriction, objective measures of lung function are essential for the diagnosis and assessment of patients with asthma. Simple spirometry, which provides a measure of FEV_1 and the FVC, is the most useful way to diagnose increased resistance to airflow. Even when asymptomatic, the FEV_1 and the FVC are usually low in the patient with asthma. The reduction in peak expiratory flow rates (PEFR), which correlates well with a reduction in the FEV_1, may also be used to objectively assess airflow obstruction. Patients can measure their PEFR by using an inexpensive, hand-held flowmeter at home while documenting their symptoms in a diary. This approach allows correlation of the patient's symptoms with an objective measure of airflow. Other measurements of pulmonary function may be helpful in distinguishing asthma from other causes of increased resistance to airflow. For example, the single-breath diffusing capacity is normal in asthma but is low in emphysema. Flow-volume loops can be important in ruling out upper airway obstruction that can mimic asthma.

Bronchoprovocational testing of airway responsiveness to methacholine, histamine, or exercise is sometimes useful in supporting the diagnosis. As the patient inhales increasing doses of either histamine or methacholine, serial FEV_1 measurements are obtained. A 20 percent decrement in the FEV_1 (PD_{20}) at a dose of 8.0 mmol methacholine or 16 mg/ml histamine indicates airway hyperresponsiveness. To evaluate exercise-induced bronchospasm, serial measurements of FEV_1 are performed before, during, and after exercise to determine whether the patient experiences an exercise-induced increase in airflow resistance. A decrease in the FEV_1 by 20 percent with exercise is considered a positive test.

Chest radiography During the acute attack of asthma, the chest radiograph usually reveals hyperinflation of the lungs in association with a small elongated, cardiac silhouette. More importantly, the chest radiograph is helpful in evaluating suspected complications of acute asthma, such as rib fractures from protracted coughing, pneumomediastinum, atelectasis, or pneumonia. It can also be helpful in patients with upper airway obstruction rather than asthma in whom wheezing and dyspnea are due to foreign bodies or extrinsic compression of the trachea by tumor or goiter, or in making the diagnosis of congestive heart failure.

Other tests Differential white blood counts frequently reveal eosinophilia (5 to 15 percent) in patients with asthma. However, absolute eosinophilia (cell count > 300 per cubic millimeter) suggests alternative diagnoses, e.g., Loeffler's syndrome, idiopathic hypereosinophilia syndrome, allergic bronchopulmonary aspergillosis, drug reactions, chronic myelogenous leukemia, Churg-Strauss syndrome, or parasitic infections.

Total serum IgE levels are often high in allergic asthma and are not useful for characterizing the severity of the disease. Normal skin tests, as well as normal total serum IgE levels, suggest alternative diagnoses; however, nonatopic patients with asthma may also have negative tests.

DIFFERENTIAL DIAGNOSIS

Table 23-1 lists entities frequently confused with asthma.

NATURAL HISTORY AND OUTCOME

The natural history of asthma is not well characterized. Childhood asthma often persists into adulthood and the prognosis of children with asthma appears to be related to the age of onset of respiratory symptoms, history of exposure to cigarette smoke, the magnitude of the decrease in the FEV_1 while asymptomatic, airway hyperreactivity (as demonstrated by inhalational challenge), as well as the degree of atopy at presentation. Some patients who are severely hyperresponsive to methacholine as children develop irreversible airflow obstruction as adults despite "adequate" treatment of their asthma with corticosteroids. Further studies aimed at identifying risk factors for the development of irreversible bronchoconstriction in asthma are needed to better understand this progression.

Although asthma is generally regarded as a benign disease, and deaths due to asthma are uncommon, mortality due to asthma has been rising. Most of these deaths occur outside the hospital and the mortality for hospitalized asthmatics remains < 1 percent. Factors related to increased asthma mortality are shown in Table 23-2.

TABLE 23-1 Differential Diagnosis of Asthma

Mass Lesions
  Endobronchial or intratracheal tumor
  Extrinsic compression of the trachea, e.g., goiter
  Foreign body
Inflammatory or Immunologic
  Anaphylaxis or anaphylactoid reactions
  Laryngeal edema or laryngospasm
  Epiglottis
  Endobronchial sarcoidosis
  Amyloidosis
  Vasculitis, e.g., Wegener's granulomatosis
  Pulmonary embolus (mediator release)
Airway Edema
  Congestive heart failure
Psychological
  Hysterical vocal cord dysfunction

TABLE 23-2 Circumstances Associated with Fatal Asthma in the United States

Demographics
  Occurs more frequently in urban, African-Americans
History
  Prior history of intubation or admission to an intensive care unit for asthma
  Two or more hospitalizations for asthma in the past year
  Serious psychiatric disease or psychosocial problems
Other
  Patients with large diurnal variations in airflow are at greatest risk
  Usually associated with inadequate assessment and treatment

TREATMENT

Successful treatment of the patient with asthma requires the appropriate choice of medication as well as an emphasis on patient education. The goals of patient education include avoidance strategies for specific trigger events as well as treatment strategies for exacerbations. Studies have clearly shown that frequent contact between the physician and the asthmatic patient can play a major role in decreasing the severity of episodes.

The pharmacotherapy of asthma is focused mainly on bronchodilation and on reducing inflammation within the airways. Bronchodilators, acting primarily on smooth muscle to effect relaxation, include β-adrenergic agents, anticholinergic agents, and theophylline.

Anti-inflammatory agents include inhaled steroids and systemic steroids. Other agents such as cromolyn sodium are more difficult to classify.

While the use of inhaled β-agonists may cause a prompt increase in airway caliber and thus make the patient feel better, they do not treat the airway inflammation and hyperresponsiveness that characterize the late phase of asthma. For these reasons as well as recent studies demonstrating excess mortality in patients treated with long-acting or regularly scheduled β-agonists, combination therapy with β-agonists and anti-inflammatory drugs, e.g., inhaled steroids, is considered to be the most appropriate approach for most patients.

β-Adrenergic agents These agents act to increase cAMP within airway smooth muscle and cause a decrease in force production leading to a widening of the airway. They are available both as oral and inhalational agents (and intravenous in a few cases). Inhaled β-adrenergic agents have a wider therapeutic index than oral adrenergic agents. Table 23-3 summarizes the currently recommended use of inhaled bronchodilators in asthma.

Theophyllines Theophylline preparations are prescribed frequently for asthma although their role in therapy is declining. The mecha-

TABLE 23-3 Aerosolized, β-Adrenergic Agents

Drug	β₂-specific	Onset of action (min)	Peak effect (min)	Duration (h)	Aerosol dose by nebulizer*	Aerosol dose by metered-dose inhaler
Isoproterenol	no	5	15	1	2.5–5 mg	250 mg/2 puffs
Isoetharine	yes	10	30	2–3	5 mg	680 mg/2 puffs
Metaproterenol	yes	10	45	3–6	15 mg	1300 mg/2 puffs
Albuterol	yes	10	60	4–6	2.5–5 mg	180 mg/2 puffs
Terbutaline	yes	10	60	4–6		400 mg/2 puffs
Pirbuterol	yes	10	60	4–6		400 mg/2 puffs
Bitolterol†	yes	10	60	3–8		1050 mg/3 puffs
Fenoterol†	yes	10	60	4–8		400 mg/2 puffs
Salmeterol†	yes	10	60	8–10		50 mg/puff
Formoterol†	yes	10	60	8–10		12 mg/puff

*Aerosol dose by nebulizer diluted in 3 ml saline.
†Not available in the United States.

nism of action of theophylline is still unclear; the major therapeutic effect is relaxation of airway smooth muscle. The dosing of theophylline is confounded by erratic absorption, unpredictable excretion kinetics, and a narrow therapeutic range. Despite serum levels in the therapeutic range, many patients experience anxiety, tremor, palpitations, and gastrointestinal symptoms. In addition, aminophylline effects only a slightly greater increase in indices of airflow to that achieved by inhaled β-agonists. Currently, theophylline preparations are generally reserved for those patients who cannot be adequately treated with β-agonists. For those patients receiving theophylline, the target concentration in the blood is 10 to 20 mg/ml. A variety of drugs affect theophylline metabolism through interaction with the hepatic P450 enzyme system; concurrent use of these drugs necessitates that the dose of theophylline be adjusted according to measured blood levels.

Anticholinergics Ipratropium bromide blocks muscarinic receptors in the airways leading to a modest bronchodilation. Though inhaled anticholinergic therapy is as effective as β-agonist therapy in patients with chronic obstructive pulmonary disease, the same is not true in asthma. Thus, the role of ipratropium in asthma remains as a second line therapy to β-agonists.

Steroids Corticosteroids, unlike bronchodilators, treat the consequences of airway inflammation that include cellular infiltration, edema, and mediator release. Corticosteroids have no acute effects on airway caliber and exert their effects only after a delay of 3 to 6 h. The most significant recent advance in the use of steroids in asthma has been the introduction of inhaled corticosteroids that achieve an anti-inflammatory effect localized to the airways without significant systemic side effects. The three agents currently available in the United States are beclomethasone dipropionate, triamcinolone acetonide, and flunisolide. Inhaled steroids are given as a metered-dose inhaler (MDI) and, as with β-agonists, the patient must learn the effective use of an inhaler to ensure delivery of the drug to the airways. Although inhaled steroids at currently approved doses are free from systemic side effects, delivery of a significant amount of the steroid to the oropharynx may result in symptomatic oral *Candida* infections. Such infections may be prevented by proper MDI technique, the use of a spacer, or by gargling after each dose of the inhaled steroid.

Systemic steroids play an important role in the management of acute and chronic asthma because they represent the most effective anti-inflammatory therapy available. In acute exacerbations of asthma, short courses of prednisone or methylprednisolone (intravenous or oral) may be necessary in patients already taking inhaled steroids or too sick to use them. There is little evidence that doses higher than 40 to 60 mg prednisone or equivalent four times a day result in further improvement of airway obstruction. Despite the well-known complications of chronic steroid use, short courses of even high-dose corticosteroids are generally well tolerated. Hypokalemia, hyperglycemia, muscle weakness, and alterations in mental status can occur but usually resolve promptly. The optimum method to taper steroids is unclear. Patients are usually switched from parenteral methylprednisolone to either oral prednisone or methylprednisolone once symptoms and airflow are clearly improving. Dosing frequency is cut to either once or twice daily, and the dosage is tapered to a target of 20 mg/day over 10 to 14 days. In many patients, inhaled steroids can fully replace this dose of prednisone and the oral steroids can then be discontinued.

Cromolyn Cromolyn, which inhibits mast cell degranulation, can inhibit both the early and late phases of allergen-induced bronchoconstriction. It is most effective when used as prophylaxis in patients with exercise-induced asthma. Cromolyn is not a bronchodilator, and it is ineffective in treating acute asthma and in adults with chronic severe asthma.

Experimental agents A number of therapeutic agents useful in some patients with asthma are under various stages of investigation. Investigational bronchodilators include leukotriene receptor antagonists, calcium channel blockers, potassium channel agonists, intravenous magnesium, and inhaled diuretics.

The immune modulatory effects of low-dose methotrexate and cyclosporine are currently under investigation as steroid-sparing agents in patients requiring chronic high-dose systemic steroids. Although both agents appear to be able to decrease the required daily dose of steroids, their use is limited by substantial toxicity. Some agents, such as the macrolide antibiotics troleandomycin (TAO) and erythromycin, also appear to be "steroid-sparing" in some patients.

BIBLIOGRAPHY

For a more detailed discussion, see: McFadden ER Jr: Asthma: General features, pathogenesis, and pathophysiology, in Fishman AP (ed), *Pulmonary Diseases and Disorders,* 2d ed. New York, McGraw-Hill, 1988, pp 1295–1310.

Barnes PJ: A new approach to the treatment of asthma. N Engl J Med 321:1517–1527, 1989.

McFadden ER Jr: Asthma: Acute and chronic therapy, in Fishman AP (ed), *Pulmonary Diseases and Disorders,* 2d ed. New York, McGraw-Hill, 1988, pp 1311–1323.

McFadden ER, Gilbert IA: Asthma. N Engl J Med 327:1928–1937, 1992.

Murray RK, Panettieri RA: Management of asthma: The changing approach, in Fishman AP (ed), *Update: Pulmonary Diseases and Disorders.* New York, McGraw-Hill, 1992, pp 67–82.

Pueringer RJ, Hunninghake GW: Inflammation and airway reactivity in asthma. Am J Med 92:32S–38S, 1992.

Widdicombe JG: Airway hyperreactivity. Am Rev Respir Dis 143:S1–S82, 1991.

Stanley Fiel

DEFINITION

Cystic fibrosis (CF) is a fatal hereditary disorder of infants, children, and young adults in which there is widespread dysfunction of the exocrine glands, leading to chronic pulmonary disease, pancreatic insufficiency, and abnormally high levels of electrolytes in the sweat.

EPIDEMIOLOGY

The disease is transmitted as a simple autosomal recessive trait. CF is the most common lethal genetic disease in the caucasian population, occurring once in every 3500 live births. The disease is less frequently encountered in other racial and ethnic groups; for example, it occurs in only 1/14,000 live African-American births, and 1/25,500 live Asian births. At present, there are > 30,000 CF patients in the United States. Dramatic increases in longevity and survival have been achieved since World War II, primarily resulting from improvements in antibiotic therapy and more aggressive nutritional management. The median survival has increased from < 2 years in the 1940s to > 29 years today. One third of the present CF population consists of adolescents and adults.

PATHOGENESIS

Recent evidence indicates that the widespread exocrine gland dysfunction which characterizes CF stems from an underlying defect in epithelial cell chloride conductance. The genetic basis for this defect was defined in 1989 when the CF gene was identified. A three base pair deletion, resulting in loss of a phenylalanine residue at position 508, represents the most common defect identified. The protein product of this gene, termed the *cystic fibrosis transmembrane regulator* (CFTR), functions as a chloride channel and, when defective, leads to impaired chloride transport across cell membranes. Defective chloride conductance is reflected in an abnormal transepithelial potential difference. This increased potential difference has been shown to exist across CF nasal, respiratory, and sweat gland epithelium.

In the respiratory epithelium, trapping of chloride ions inside the cell and concomitant excessive reabsorption of sodium leads to desiccation of respiratory secretions. The thick, sticky, dehydrated mucus that forms in the airways results in mechanical obstruction and impaired mucociliary clearance, trapping bacteria in the airways and giving rise to chronic infection. Further contributing to the pathogenesis of lung disease in CF is the host inflammatory response; neutrophils recruited to the lung release a variety of proteolytic enzymes and inflammatory mediators. The end result of chronic infection and inflammation in the airways is irreversible damage to the bronchial walls producing widespread bronchiectasis.

CLINICAL MANIFESTATIONS

History The clinical manifestations of CF are protean, reflecting the multisystemic nature of the disease. However, pulmonary involvement tends to predominate and accounts for most of the morbidity and nearly all of the mortality associated with CF. Patients typically complain of chronic cough and sputum production. Commonly, the course of pulmonary involvement is marked by periods of exacerbation, presumably reflecting worsening airway infection. During periods of exacerbation, the cough becomes more intense, and sputum is increased in volume and purulence and may be blood streaked. Pulmonary exacerbations are often accompanied by anorexia, weight loss, and low-grade fevers. As pulmonary function deteriorates, dyspnea is noted. Ultimately, chronic respiratory insufficiency leads to the development of pulmonary hypertension and cor pulmonale. Respiratory failure and death follow.

A number of other respiratory problems may complicate the course of patients with CF. Pneumothorax, caused by rupture of subpleural blebs, occurs in 17 to 20 percent of adults with CF and is usually heralded by the sudden onset of chest pain and dyspnea. Minor hemoptysis occurs in > 50 percent of adults; massive and potentially life-threatening hemoptysis is seen in approximately 8 percent of adults. Allergic bronchopulmonary aspergillosis occurs with increased frequency in CF patients; persistent wheezing and evidence for reversible airflow obstruction on pulmonary function testing provide important clues to its presence. Upper respiratory tract complications include sinusitis and nasal polyps, present in approximately 90 percent and 40 percent of adult patients, respectively.

The most commonly encountered nonrespiratory manifestation of CF is malabsorption due to pancreatic exocrine insufficiency. Other nonrespiratory manifestations include diabetes mellitus, pancreatitis, intestinal obstruction, intussusception, cholelithiasis, bililary cirrhosis, and azoospermia.

Physical examination Patients typically appear underweight. The thorax is often expanded in the anteroposterior dimension ("barrel chest"), reflecting hyperinflation of the lungs. Auscultation of the lungs reveals course inspiratory crackles, typically more pronounced in the upper lung fields. Wheezing may be present, due either to mechanical obstruction of airways with mucus or to true bronchospasm. Use of accessory muscles of respiration, cyanosis, evidence of pulmonary hypertension (increased P_2, right ventricular heave) and signs of right heart failure (hepatomegaly, jugular venous distention, lower extremity edema) indicate advanced pulmonary disease. Clubbing, usually pronounced, is present in the vast majority of adults.

DIAGNOSIS

Sweat chloride test The diagnosis rests on the demonstration of an elevated sweat chloride concentration in association with either chronic pulmonary disease or pancreatic insufficiency. More than 98 percent of patients with CF have sweat chloride concentrations > 60 mEq/L. Use of the Gibson and Cook iontophoresis method allows separation of non-CF from CF patients with almost no overlap in the pediatric age group; in the adult population some overlap occurs. Despite the normal increase in values of sweat chloride and sodium with age, however, the sweat test remains an excellent diagnostic test in adults. In the future, use of DNA analysis will likely supplant the sweat chloride test.

Chest radiography The chest radiograph typically demonstrates hyperinflation, with flattening of the diaphragms and enhancement of the retrosternal air shadow. Thickening of the bronchial walls is manifest radiographically as an increase in interstitial markings. When viewed in cross section, the thickened and dilated bronchial walls appear as ring shadows; viewed longitudinally, they appear as parallel lines ("tram lines"). With more advanced disease, cystic changes occur and are often most pronounced in the upper lobes. When fully filled with pus, these cysts take on a nodular appearance. Hilar adenopathy is radiographically apparent in a minority of patients.

Pulmonary function tests An obstructive pattern is characteristically present. Commonly, the residual volume is increased, reflecting air trapping. The diffusing capacity usually remains normal until late in the disease course. Arterial blood gases are normal in mild disease, but manifest progressive hypoxemia as lung function deteriorates; hypercapnia is present with advanced disease.

DIFFERENTIAL DIAGNOSIS

Clinically, CF may be confused with a number of other chronic pulmonary disorders. Because of the presence of airflow obstruction, patients may be misdiagnosed as having asthma or chronic obstructive pulmonary disease. Bronchiectasis and recurrent pulmonary infections may also be seen in immunoglobulin deficiency states, e.g., common variable hypogammaglobulinemia, immotile cilia syndrome, and allergic bronchopulmonary aspergillosis. The radiographic appearance of CF may mimic fungal pulmonary disease, tuberculosis, sarcoidosis, eosinophilic granuloma, or lymphoma.

TREATMENT

Antibiotics Intravenous antibiotics are, at present, the treatment of choice for acute pulmonary exacerbations. Antibiotics are usually selected on the basis of the results of sputum cultures. Since *Pseudomonas aeruginosa* is the most frequent pathogen in the adult, the antibiotics selected are often a combination of a semisynthetic penicillin or a third-generation cephalosporin, i.e., ceftazidime, and an aminoglycoside, such as tobramycin, which have been shown to have synergistic effects against *Pseudomonas* in vitro. A 2- to 3-week course of therapy is usually administered. Conventionally, patients are hospitalized for the entire course of antibiotic therapy. However, home use of parenteral antibiotic therapy is rapidly becoming a widely accepted practice for the stable patient. For mild exacerbations, a 2-week course of oral ciprofloxacin is commonly used.

The precise role of antibiotics will not be known until the mechanism for pulmonary colonization with *Pseudomonas* is understood. Multicenter trials now under way are expected to provide information about the optimal timing and duration of antibiotic therapy and the most efficacious drug combinations. At the present time, it is generally agreed that intravenous antibiotics should be used for acute exacerbations. No such consensus exists with respect to the use of prophylactic and suppressive oral antibiotics to retard lung damage from chronic infection. The role of aerosolized antibiotics, e.g., tobramycin, is presently being evaluated in a randomized fashion.

Bronchodilators Aerosolized β-agonists and atropine derivatives appear to improve pulmonary function in some CF patients with documented airway hyperreactivity. These agents are also commonly used during periods of exacerbation as an adjunct to chest percussion and postural drainage. There are reports of paradoxical worsening of pulmonary function in response to bronchodilator therapy. In sum, the need for and response to bronchodilator therapy varies among CF patients and should be assessed on an individual basis.

Corticosteroids The host inflammatory response within the airways is thought to contribute to local destruction of the bronchial walls; anti-inflammatory agents may therefore be beneficial. A large multicenter trial of alternate-day prednisone therapy, sponsored by the Cystic Fibrosis Foundation, has been in progress for several years. Until the results of this study are reported, corticosteroid therapy should be limited to the segment of CF adults who develop allergic bronchopulmonary aspergillosis, to infants with severe bronchiolitis, and to patients with significant reversible airway obstruction unresponsive to bronchodilators alone. No evidence to date indicates that patients receiving steroid therapy in conjunction with antipseudomonal antibiotics undergo a worsening of bacterial infection.

Chest physical therapy and exercise Removal of mucous secretions from the lungs of CF patients has long been a staple of treatment. Postural drainage with percussion, breathing exercises, and exercise therapy are all used to effect mucous removal. There have been few controlled studies of the long-term benefits of these measures, although postural drainage has been shown to have short-term clinical utility. Because routine chest physical therapy is time consuming and compliance is poor, vigorous coughing is sometimes used as an alternative.

Many adult patients choose to substitute programs of exercise for conventional chest physical therapy. Supervised physical conditioning has been shown to significantly increase exercise tolerance, peak oxygen consumption, and cardiorespiratory fitness. Patients should, however, be alerted to the possibility of exercise-induced bronchospasm, and an exercise test to determine tolerance and detect potential oxygen desaturation should be performed before an exercise program is begun.

Oxygen therapy Oxygen therapy is indicated in patients with exercise-related or resting hypoxemia and in patients with cor pulmonale. Supplemental oxygen alleviates dyspnea associated with exercise-induced arterial desaturation and improves the patient's sense of well-being. Generally, a greater degree of hypoxemia is associated with a worsening of pulmonary hypertension and right-sided heart strain. There is evidence that pulmonary hypertension related to CF can be reduced with oxygen therapy, and that the development of cor pulmonale may be prevented through the early use of oxygen. Transtracheal oxygen delivery techniques are more acceptable cosmetically and may become the preferred mode of therapy for younger, more active patients.

Cardiopulmonary transplantation When heart-lung transplants were first performed in patients in the 1960s, it was generally believed that CF patients would not be suitable candidates because of the risk of chronic infection. By 1989, largely as a result of improved antibiotics and use of immunosuppressive agents, CF had become the leading indication for both heart-lung and double lung transplantation. In the United States, double lung transplantation has supplanted heart-lung transplantation as the procedure of choice for CF patients. Successful transplantation leads to marked improvement in pulmonary function, exercise tolerance, and quality of life; many patients are able to resume a normal activity level. There has been no documented recurrence of the underlying disease in the transplanted lungs. Indeed, studies of the luminal electrochemical gradient in heart-lung recipients 36 months after transplant have shown that these patients no longer show an abnormal mucosal potential difference below the tracheal anastomosis, whereas the upper trachea retains the high CF potential. The 3-year survival rate after lung transplantation approximates 60 percent; current data are insufficient to predict long-term survival rates.

Evolving therapies A number of therapeutic interventions are currently under investigation in the treatment of CF. Two new therapies, amiloride and UTP/ATP are intended to correct abnormal ion transport in the airways and thus prevent dehydration and thickening of respiratory secretions. The diuretic amiloride acts by inhibiting uptake of sodium by respiratory epithelium. The nucleotides ATP and UTP have been shown in vitro to stimulate uptake of chloride by CF respiratory epithelial cells, presumably by using a pathway for chloride uptake distinct from that mediated by CFTR. A preliminary trial of aerosolized amiloride demonstrated a decrease in the rate of decline of pulmonary function in treated patients; larger scale trials are planned as are clinical trials with aerosolized ATP/UTP.

The highly viscous quality of CF airway secretions is due, not only to desiccation, but also to an unusually large content of DNA released by white blood cells. The enzyme DNase is capable of degrading DNA and, when directly mixed with CF mucus, renders CF mucus thin and fluid. Early short-term clinical experience with aerosolized recombinant DNase in CF patients suggests that this therapy is well tolerated, facilitates clearance of secretions, and improves pulmonary function.

As previously discussed, neutrophil-mediated inflammation is believed to contribute to airway injury, in part, through the release of destructive proteases such as elastase. Trials are currently under way to evaluate the therapeutic efficacy of elastase inhibitors including the naturally occurring *secretory leucoprotease inhibitor* (SLPI). The use of the nonsteroidal anti-inflammatory agent ibuprofen is also being investigated.

Discoveries illuminating the process by which *P. aeruginosa* and other bacteria colonize the lungs have led to preliminary work on a vaccine.

Most exciting on the horizon of therapeutic interventions is the prospect of gene therapy. Successful transfer of the normal CFTR gene into defective cells, with resultant correction of abnormal chloride conductance, has been achieved in tissue culture, and gene transfer has also been successfully performed in animal models. Transfer of the CF gene may be accomplished either through use of viral vectors (adenovirus, retroviruses) or through nonvector systems such as liposomes or DNA-protein complexes. Currently, three centers in the United States are poised to begin clinical trials of gene therapy in CF patients.

PROGNOSIS

CF remains a progressive and ultimately lethal disease, with the vast majority of patients dying of respiratory failure or cor pulmonale. However, the prognosis for patients afflicted with this disease has improved dramatically over the past several decades, and the median survival has increased from < 1 year in the 1940s to > 29 years in 1991. Indeed, it is now estimated that individuals born with CF today can be expected to live well into their forties.

Because of marked variability in the course of disease, it has proven somewhat problematic to identify reliable and accurate prognostic factors which can be applied to the individual patient. In general, the prognosis is somewhat more favorable for males than females. Colonization of the airways with *Pseudomonas cepacia* may be associated with an accelerated decline. A recent study of > 600 patients suggests that patients with a $FEV_1 < 30$ percent predicted have a 2-year mortality rate exceeding 50 percent.

BIBLIOGRAPHY

For a more detailed discussion, see Scanlin TF: Cystic fibrosis, in Fishman AP (ed), *Pulmonary Diseases and Disorders,* 2d ed. New York, McGraw-Hill, 1988, pp 1273–1294.

Collins FS: Cystic fibrosis: Molecular biology and therapeutic implications. Science 256:774–779, 1992.

Fiel SB: Clinical management of pulmonary disease in cystic fibrosis. Lancet 341:1070–1074, 1993.

Fiel SB: Providing comprehensive care to adults with cystic fibrosis. J Respir Dis 12:669–682, 1991.

Iannuzzi MC, Collins FS: Genetic defect in cystic fibrosis, in Fishman AP (ed), *Update: Pulmonary Diseases and Disorders.* New York, McGraw-Hill, 1992, pp 83–92.

Koch C, Hoiby N: Pathogenesis of cystic fibrosis. Lancet 341:1065–1069, 1993.

Kubesch P, Dork T, Wulbrand U, Kalin N, Neumann T, Wulf B, et al: Genetic determinants of airways' colonisation with *Pseudomonas aeruginosa* in cystic fibrosis. Lancet 341:189–193, 1993.

Gerald Weinhouse

The term *bronchiectasis* refers to permanently dilated bronchi, usually proximal subsegmental airways. In *wet bronchiectasis,* the involved airways are inflamed and edematous and full of purulent, foul-smelling sputum. In contrast, in *dry bronchiectasis,* the involved airways are the seat of mucosal erosion and ulceration and may develop abscesses.

The dilation of the bronchi is caused by destruction of both the muscular and elastic components of the bronchial wall. Although bronchiectasis is generally confined to the airways, severe cases may cause recurrent pneumonias that may lead to permanent scarring. Although bronchiectasis may be the result of a process confined to the lungs, e.g., bronchial obstruction or recurrent infection, it is often apt to be a manifestation of a more generalized disorder (Table 25-1).

Bronchiectasis may be either focal or diffuse; the disease is bilateral in 30 percent of patients. The lower lobes are most often affected, probably due to anatomic features which affect drainage and patency of the airways.

Focal bronchiectasis may be a consequence of foreign body aspiration (especially in children), adenopathy, benign tumors, and mucous plugging; it is less likely to be caused by malignant tumors for two reasons: (1) the course of the disease may be too rapid for bronchiectasis to develop; or (2) the neoplasm is treated successfully.

Diffuse bronchiectasis may follow aspiration of gastric contents or inhalational injury, both of which cause widespread tracheobronchial inflammation. Intravenous drug abuse may also cause diffuse bronchiectasis, possibly due to lymphatic obstruction by injected particulate matter (see Table 25-1). Although the incidence of bronchiectasis has lessened in the United States due, in part, to the availability of antibiotics, it remains a significant health problem worldwide.

PATHOGENESIS

The fundamental abnormality that culminates in bronchiectasis is an inflammatory destruction of the components of the bronchial wall. The changes in tracheal pressure during respiration and coughing, in association with peribronchial fibrosis, lead to characteristic abnormalities of the airways, i.e., accompanied by impairment of mucociliary clearance and cellular defense mechanisms.

Although infectious, anatomic (obstructive), and congenital factors may predispose to bronchiectasis; a necrotizing infection is

TABLE 25-1 Predisposing Factors for Bronchiectasis

Categories	Specific entities
Bronchopulmonary Infections	
Childhood diseases	Pertussis; measles
Other bacterial infections	Infections due to *Staphylococcus aureus*, *Klebsiella*, *Mycobacterium tuberculosis*, *H. influenzae*
Other viral infections	Infections due to adenovirus (particularly types 7 and 21), influenza, herpes simplex; viral bronchiolitis
Miscellaneous infections	Mycotic infections (histoplasmosis); ? mycoplasmal infections
Bronchial Obstruction	
Foreign body aspiration	Peanut; chicken bone; grass inflorescence, etc.
Neoplasms	Laryngeal papillomatosis; adenomas; bronchogenic carcinoma
Hilar adenopathy	Tuberculosis; histoplasmosis; sarcoid
Mucoid impaction	Allergic bronchopulmonary aspergillosis; bronchocentric granulomatosis; postoperative mucoid impaction
Chronic obstructive pulmonary disease	Chronic bronchitis; bronchial asthma
Acquired tracheobronchial disease	Relapsing polychondritis; amyloidosis
Congenital Anatomic Defects	
Tracheobronchial	Bronchomalacia; bronchial cysts; cartilage deficiency (Williams-Campbell syndrome); tracheobronchomegaly (Mounier-Kuhn syndrome); ectopic bronchus; endobronchial teratoma; tracheoesophageal fistula
Vascular	Pulmonary (intralobar) sequestration; pulmonary artery aneurysm
Lymphatic	Yellow nail syndrome
Immunodeficiency States	
IgG deficiency	Congenital (Bruton's type) agammaglobulinemia; selective deficiencies of subclasses (IgG$_2$, IgG$_4$); acquired immune globulin deficiency
IgA deficiency	Selective IgA deficiency +/– ataxia-telangiectasia syndrome
Leukocyte dysfunction	Chronic granulomatous disease
Hereditary Abnormalities	
Ciliary defects of respiratory mucosa	Kartagener's syndrome; immotile cilia syndrome; ciliary dyskinesis
1-Antitrypsin deficiency	Production of abnormal antitrypsin molecules; failure of gene transcription
Cystic fibrosis (mucoviscidosis)	Typical early childhood syndrome; adolescent presentation with solely pulmonary symptoms

TABLE 25-1 Predisposing Factors for Bronchiectasis (*Continued*)

Categories	Specific entities
Miscellaneous Disorders	
Young's syndrome	Obstructive azoospermia with sinopulmonary infections
Recurrent aspiration pneumonias	Alcoholism; neurologic disorders; lipoid pneumonia
Inhalation of irritants	Ammonia, nitrogen dioxide, or other irritant gases; smoke; talc; silicates; detergents
Following combined heart-lung transplantation	Associated with obliterative bronchiolitis

SOURCE: From Swartz MN: Bronchiectasis, in Fishman AP (ed), *Pulmonary Diseases and Disorders*, 2d ed. New York, McGraw Hill, 1988, p 1559.

almost always involved. The dramatic decline in the incidence of bronchiectasis in the postantibiotic era testifies to the importance of infection in its pathogenesis. Congenital bronchiectasis, once thought to be common, is now recognized to be rare. When congenital defects do occur, e.g., abnormalities in tracheobronchial cartilage, cilial defections, abnormalities in respiratory mucus, they predispose to bronchiectasis but require infection to complete the picture.

PATHOPHYSIOLOGY

Pulmonary function test abnormalities in bronchiectasis are generally nonspecific and difficult to distinguish from the condition which predisposed the patient to bronchiectasis. In patients in whom bronchiectasis is localized and not associated with chronic bronchitis, pulmonary function tests are usually normal. In contrast, in patients with severe diffuse bronchiectasis, pulmonary function tests are often indistinguishable from those of chronic obstructive pulmonary disease (COPD).

Mucociliary transport is adversely affected in bronchiectasis for several reasons: (1) loss of normal ciliated epithelium; (2) hereditary ciliary defects that underlie some instances of bronchiectasis; and (3) abnormal composition of the respiratory mucus. The sputum in bronchiectasis is abnormally viscid because of its high DNA content and its high concentration of disulfide linkages; it is mucoid secondary to hyperactivity of the submucosal glands.

Bronchiectasis can have important hemodynamic consequences because of proliferation of the bronchial circulation in its vicinity. The major hemodynamic alteration is a left-to-right shunt at the precapillary level secondary to anastomoses between the bronchial and pulmonary arterial circulations. The shunt is usually quite modest, e.g., 3 to 12 percent of pulmonary flow, and of little hemodynamic consequence. However, in rare instances of widespread severe bronchiectasis, it may lead to left ventricular overload and failure.

CLINICAL MANIFESTATIONS

History A variety of clues to the presence of bronchiectasis may be gained from the history: (1) a history of a contagious disease (involving the lungs) in childhood; (2) purulent sputum, worse in the morning, large in quantity, and foul in odor; (3) a family history of cystic fibrosis or other inherited functional anatomic abnormality; (4) a history of pneumonia, especially if recurrent; (5) hemoptysis occurs in up to 50 percent of patients; (6) sinusitis, e.g., associated with cystic fibrosis or Kartagener's syndrome; (7) history of pleuritis; and (8) a history of difficult to manage asthma. Cough may be paroxysmal.

Physical examination The physical examination can arouse suspicion of the presence of bronchiectasis in several different ways: (1) clubbing of the digits in a patient with chronic cough or evidence of chronic bronchitis and/or emphysema (clubbing is exceedingly rare in COPD); (2) nasal polyps and increased nasal secretions; and (3) "moist" crackles over the involved lobe(s); typically these begin early in inspiration and fade out by end-expiration.

Frequently, other pulmonary abnormalities are found in patients with bronchiectasis, e.g., diffuse rhonchi and prolonged expiration, dullness to percussion and decreased breath sounds over the involved lobe(s), and bronchial breath sounds if pneumonia is present.

DIAGNOSTIC EVALUATION

As a rule, conventional laboratory tests are of little help in the diagnosis of bronchiectasis. For example, the sputum often shows a mixed flora on Gram stain and is often nondiagnostic on culture. Also, except for severe or widespread disease, the peripheral blood only occasionally shows a leukocytosis and the anemia of chronic disease.

Special tests, when indicated by the history and clinical findings, are apt to be more informative. For example, the sweat chloride test may be indicated in the young adult or adolescent who has a history of an antecedent pneumonia, obstruction, or other apparent cause of bronchiectasis. Serum immunoglobulins can be useful in young patients, especially males, who have a history of recurrent pneumonias. In patients with asthma who are difficult to manage medically, an antibody titer for *Aspergillus* species may be useful.

Other tests may be in order in accord with the possibilities listed in Table 25-1.

RADIOGRAPHY

The chest radiograph often raises the possibility of bronchiectasis and is useful in supporting the clinical suspicion. For example, it may show linear radiolucencies accompanied by parallel markings radiating from the hila ("tram lines"). Thick parallel lines ("toothpaste lines") or clustered cysts, sometimes with air-fluid levels, may also be seen. Nonspecific findings include peribronchial haziness, atelectasis, and consolidation.

Computed tomography (CT) can be invaluable; its sensitivity approaches that of bronchography. It also has the advantage of being easier to perform technically, better tolerated by patients, and safer. In addition, it allows both lungs to be visualized and the parenchyma to be assessed.

Bronchoscopy is indicated in the patient with localized disease to exclude an obstructing lesion. It may also be useful in localizing the site of bleeding especially if resection is under consideration.

Bronchography used to be the diagnostic "gold standard" but has been replaced by high-resolution CT. In those institutions where high-resolution CT is unavailable, bronchography may still be indicated in specific cases, i.e., if surgery is contemplated for local disease. However, it should not be done during an acute exacerbation. It may be useful with respect to surgical resection if (1) the patient has persistent hemoptysis and bronchoscopy fails to disclose the source or (2) the diagnosis is known but the site is believed to be in a single, poorly defined segment or lobe. Bronchography is sometimes helpful in guiding chest physical therapy.

PROGNOSIS AND COMPLICATIONS

Before the use of antibiotics became widespread, bronchiectasis had a grave prognosis. However, since the advent of antibiotics, most patients with bronchiectasis do well, undergoing little deterioration in lung function; only few patients manifest progression of disease. In these few, increasing disability may be a serious problem: progressive suppuration, hemoptysis and major pulmonary hemorrhage, obliteration of peripheral airways with associated bronchitis and emphysema. Chronic respiratory failure and cor pulmonale in some of these patients is attributable to underlying COPD and not to the bronchiectasis. Although recurrent pulmonary infections, often associated with antibiotic-resistant organisms, continue to occur in some patients, improved antimicrobial therapy has decreased the incidence of such ominous consequences as metastatic brain abscess and amyloidosis. The incidence of cancer of the lung is not increased in patients with bronchiectasis.

TREATMENT

Antibiotics are the mainstay of therapy. The choice of agents depends on the results of sputum culture for aerobes, anaerobes, and mycobacteria. The most common offending organisms in patients with bronchiectasis (except for those with cystic fibrosis) are *Haemophilus influenzae* and *Streptococcus pneumoniae.* Therefore, empirical coverage should include one of a variety of broad-spectrum agents, including the penicillins, cephalosporins, sulfonamides, tetracyclines, chloramphenicol, and trimethoprim. The penicillins (especially amoxicillin) and cephalosporins (cefaclor is the most effective oral cephalosporin against *H. influenzae*) are the most effective and should be used as the first line for empirical therapy.

There are no set guidelines for either dosage or duration of therapy. Some patients may require higher than conventional doses of amoxicillin possibly because of poor penetration into the abnormal airways or to the presence of β-lactamases. Patients with frankly purulent secretions are most apt to require the higher doses. Treatment is usually continued for 5 to 14 days. However, some patients benefit from the use of prophylactic antibiotics given continuously or for a set number of weeks per month. During an acute flare, success of therapy is reflected in the patient's symptomatic improvement; in those treated long-term prophylactically, successful treatment results in improvement in the sense of well being.

In addition to antibiotics, certain procedures may be helpful: (1) chest physical therapy, involving postural drainage, chest clapping, humidification, and mucolytics; (2) bronchodilators for patients with airway hyperreactivity; (3) management of the underlying disease, e.g., administration of intravenous immunoglobulins in those patients with immunodeficiency; (4) immunization against potential pulmonary pathogens, e.g., pneumococcal and influenza vaccines; and (5) surgery for one of three major reasons—massive hemoptysis complicating bronchiectasis when the site of bleeding is known, local disease refractory to medical management, or in patients unwilling or incapable of taking antibiotics. Alternatives to surgery for massive hemoptysis are either endobronchial balloon tamponade using a Fogarty balloon or selective embolization of the bronchial arteries that supply the bleeding site.

BIBLIOGRAPHY

For a more detailed discussion, see Swartz MN: Bronchiectasis, in Fishman AP (ed), *Pulmonary Diseases and Disorders,* 2d ed. New York, McGraw Hill, 1988, pp 1553–1581.

Barker AF, Bardana EJ Jr: Bronchiectasis: Update of an orphan disease. Am Rev Respir Dis 137:969–978, 1988.

Conway JH, Fleming JS, Perring S, Holgate ST: Humidification as an adjunct to chest physiotherapy in aiding tracheo-bronchial clearance in patients with bronchiectasis. Respir Med 86:109–114, 1992.

McGuinness G, Naidich DP, Leitman BS, McCauley DI: Bronchiectasis: CT evaluation. AJR Am J Roentgenol 160:253–259, 1993.

Murray JF: New presentations of bronchiectasis. Hosp Pract 26(3A):55–58, 61–64, 67–68, 1991.

...

William Sexauer

DEFINITION AND ETIOLOGY

For clinical purposes, *alveolar hypoventilation* is said to exist when the arterial P_{CO_2} exceeds 45 mmHg. Hypoventilation may occur both acutely, e.g., drug overdose, or chronically. This chapter addresses only the chronic forms of alveolar hypoventilation.

Alveolar hypoventilation can be categorized into two groups depending on whether the lungs are inherently normal, i.e., where intrinsic pulmonary disease is not the initiating mechanism, or abnormal due to intrinsic disease of the lung parenchyma or airways (Table 26-1). Alveolar hypoventilation in association with normal lungs can arise from inadequate drive from the central nervous system to the chest bellows or from mechanical derangement of the chest bellows. Although this classification is useful in conceptualizing the major syndromes responsible for hypoventilation, in many instances more than one abnormality is responsible for hypercapnia.

CLINICAL MANIFESTATIONS

Symptoms in patients with chronic alveolar hypoventilation may have two sources: (1) the underlying disorder responsible for the alveolar hypoventilation; and (2) alveolar hypoventilation, per se. An abnormally high P_{CO_2} causes cerebral vasodilation, which may produce headache particularly after sleep when alveolar hypoventilation is apt to become more severe. Thus, "morning headache" that resolves quickly on awakening is a common complaint in patients with chronic alveolar hypoventilation. An acute increase in alveolar and arterial P_{CO_2} can depress mental status and even cause coma (CO_2 narcosis). Alveolar hypoventilation is invariably accompanied by hypoxemia. Therefore, patients in whom chronic alveolar hypoventilation is severe or long-standing often manifest polycythemia, cyanosis, pulmonary hypertension, or cor pulmonale.

SPECIFIC ETIOLOGIES

The disorders that follow have in common chronic hypercapnia even though the routes to chronic CO_2 retention may be strikingly different in the various disorders.

Airway and Parenchymal Lung Disease

Chronic obstructive pulmonary disease (COPD), usually chronic bronchitis, is the most common cause of chronic hypercapnia. The mechanism is primarily that of ventilation-perfusion mismatch,

TABLE 26-1 Causes of Chronic Alveolar Hypoventilation

Normal Lungs*
I. Inadequate nervous system output/transmission
   1. Functional depression of ventilatory drive
      Drugs (narcotics, sedatives)
      Metabolic alkalosis
      Hypothyroidism
   2. Structural derangement of respiratory neurons
      a. Central:
         Encephalitis
         Poliomyelitis
         Brain-stem neoplasm or infarction
      b. Peripheral:
         Poliomyelitis
         Amyotrophic lateral sclerosis
         Cervical spinal cord injury
         Guillain-Barré syndrome
         Bilateral phrenic nerve injury
   3. Primary (idiopathic) alveolar hypoventilation
II. Mechanical impairment of the chest bellows
      Kyphoscoliosis
      Thoracoplasty
      Obesity hypoventilation syndrome
      Muscular dystrophies
      Myasthenia gravis
Abnormal Lungs or Airways
I. Chronic obstructive pulmonary disease
II. Upper airway obstruction (any cause)

*Free of intrinsic disease of the airways or pulmonary parenchyma or both.

which leads to increased dead-space ventilation and, therefore, to reduced effective alveolar ventilation. Other factors that may be involved in the pathogenesis of hypercapnia in COPD include abnormalities of ventilatory control, abnormalities in respiratory muscle function leading to fatigue, and altered patterns of breathing. Restrictive lung disease, which is generally associated with low alveolar P_{CO_2} during virtually all of its course, often progresses through a stage of normocapnia and then to hypercapnia as end-stage disease is approached.

Primary (Idiopathic) Alveolar Hypoventilation

Primary alveolar hypoventilation is a rare disease characterized by chronic hypercapnia (and hypoxia) in the absence of detectable lung, airway, musculoskeletal, or neurologic abnormalities. By definition, it is a diagnosis of exclusion. The underlying defect appears to be a failure of the central respiratory controller to respond appropriately to respiratory stimuli. Distinct anatomic lesions are not found in *primary* alveolar hypoventilation, thereby distinguishing this entity from *secondary* causes of central alveolar hypoventilation, e.g., encephalitis or brain-stem neoplasm.

Primary alveolar hypoventilation usually occurs between the ages of 20 and 50, although it has been reported in all age groups. The disease is usually recognized only when far advanced, i.e., to the stage of chronic hypercapnia, hypoxia, and cor pulmonale. Characteristically, dyspnea is minimal. In some instances, the onset may be precipitated by the administration of sedatives or anesthesia. Disturbances in mentation and sleep are common in advanced stages.

Laboratory evaluation reveals normal spirometry, lung volumes, respiratory system compliance, and respiratory muscle strength. The maximum voluntary ventilation is normal and the patients usually can hyperventilate voluntarily to normal, or even reduced, levels of arterial P_{CO_2}. The ventilatory response to breathing CO_2 enriched air is consistently reduced and is generally reduced to hypoxic inspired mixtures as well.

Obesity Hypoventilation Syndrome

A few markedly obese individuals develop chronic hypercapnia, i.e., the obesity hypoventilation syndrome (OHS). As a rule, the alveolar hypoventilation seems to result from a complex interplay of multiple factors. For example, massive obesity decreases the compliance of the respiratory system and increases the work of breathing. Additionally, a diminished respiratory responsiveness to CO_2 can be demonstrated, suggesting that respiratory drive is blunted. The existence of an abnormality in respiratory control is also suggested by the ability of respiratory stimulants, e.g., progesterone, to increase ventilation and decrease arterial P_{CO_2}.

Because of their frequent association, obstructive sleep apnea has been suggested as a cause of OHS. However, obstructive sleep apnea is unlikely to be the sole cause on two accounts: (1) only a minority of patients with obstructive sleep apnea have daytime hypercapnia; and (2) in only a few instances does successful therapy of obstructive apnea correct hypercapnia. In some patients with OHS, concomitant obstructive airways disease or respiratory muscle dysfunction contributes to the pathogenesis of the disorder.

Abnormalities of the Chest Bellows

These disorders may be grouped into two main categories: (1) severe deformity of the chest wall or pleura; and (2) respiratory muscle weakness. Abnormalities of the lung parenchyma may accompany the chest deformity or muscle weakness as a secondary event, e.g., atelectasis or retained secretions due to impaired cough. Disorders of the chest bellows leading to alveolar hypoventilation are characterized by a restrictive ventilatory defect on pulmonary function testing.

Severe deformity of the chest wall, e.g., in kyphoscoliosis or thoracoplasty, decreases respiratory system compliance and increases the work of breathing. In turn, these derangements in the mechanics of breathing cause a pattern of breathing characterized by small tidal volumes and a rapid respiratory rate. This pattern, while minimizing the work and oxygen cost of breathing as well as decreasing the patient's sense of effort in breathing, increases ventilation of the dead space at the expense of alveolar ventilation. Because of limitations imposed by the chest wall deformity, the patient is unable to increase alveolar ventilation appropriately in response to exercise or infection.

Respiratory muscle weakness or paralysis may result in alveolar hypoventilation. The respiratory muscle dysfunction may be generalized, e.g., muscular dystrophy or myasthenia gravis, or localized, e.g., bilateral diaphragmatic paralysis due to phrenic nerve injury. As a rule, as long as the lungs are free of disease, hypercapnia does not occur until respiratory muscle strength (as measured by maximal inspiratory and expiratory pressures) is < 50 percent of predicted.

In a patient with alveolar hypoventilation who has evidence of generalized skeletal muscle weakness, respiratory muscle weakness is an obvious possibility. However, suspicion is not as easily raised when diaphragmatic weakness or paralysis is the sole abnormality. Patients with diaphragmatic weakness or paralysis are characteristically asymptomatic in the upright position, but develop dyspnea when supine. In the supine position, paradoxical inward movement of the upper abdomen during inspiration can occur due to passive movement of the diaphragm into the thorax as a result of the negative inspiratory pressures generated by the intercostal and accessory muscles of the neck. Paradoxical movement is usually absent in the upright position due to the effect of gravity on the abdominal contents. Laboratory findings that support the diagnosis of severe diaphragmatic weakness or paralysis include a fall in vital capacity of > 30 percent on moving from the seated to the supine position, fluoroscopic demonstration of paradoxical upward movement of the diaphragm during a forceful sniff ("sniff test") in the supine position, and a transdiaphragmatic pressure < 25 cmH$_2$O.

Miscellaneous Causes

Sedative drugs may produce either acute or chronic hypercapnia. Metabolic alkalosis causes a functional depression of respiratory drive that may either produce hypercapnia itself or increase the degree of hypoventilation due to another etiology. Certain electrolyte disturbances such as hypophosphatemia, hypocalcemia, or hypokalemia may produce respiratory muscle weakness sufficient to produce hypercapnia. Severe hypothyroidism can cause alveolar hypoventilation in several ways: (1) depressed central respiratory drive; (2) generalized muscle weakness; or (3) upper airway obstruction due to macroglossia or myxedematous infiltration of pharyngeal structures.

DIAGNOSTIC EVALUATION

Analysis of arterial blood gases confirms the presence of a compensated respiratory acidosis (hypercapnia with a slightly subnormal pH), generally accompanied by arterial hypoxemia while breathing ambient air. The arterial-alveolar P_{O_2} gradient (A-a gradient) remains normal in pure hypoventilatory states but may widen if there is accompanying parenchymal or airways disease. In some instances, the history (drug ingestion, loud snoring with fragmented sleep, and daytime hyposomnolence) or physical examination (severe kyphoscoliosis, generalized muscle weakness, massive obesity) may suggest the underlying etiology.

All patients should have a chest radiograph and blood studies consisting of a complete blood count, serum electrolytes (including magnesium, calcium, and phosphate levels), and an assessment of thyroid function. An electrocardiogram and echocardiogram are helpful in evaluating the possibility of cor pulmonale.

Pulmonary function studies are also done routinely. Spirometry and lung volumes are useful in assessing the presence and severity of both obstructive and restrictive ventilatory defects. The flow-volume loop is useful in looking for upper airway obstruction. Maximal inspiratory and expiratory pressures are used to assess respiratory muscle strength. If diaphragmatic weakness is suspected, measurement of transdiaphragmatic pressures using a catheter equipped with esophageal and gastric balloons may be helpful.

Measurement of arterial blood gases after a period of maximal voluntary ventilation (MVV) may be helpful in distinguishing patients who "can't breathe," i.e., severe obstructive lung disease, from those who "won't breathe," i.e., primary alveolar hypoventilation. Patients with disturbances of ventilatory control will usually be able to lower their P_{CO_2} by > 10 mmHg after performing an MVV, whereas those with mechanical impairments usually show little or no change.

Because of the common occurrence of sleep-disordered breathing in hypoventilatory syndromes, polysomnography (a sleep study) is frequently indicated. All patients with OHS, symptoms of obstructive sleep apnea, or hypoventilation of uncertain etiology should have a sleep study.

If a disturbance of ventilatory control is suspected, measurement of the ventilatory response to CO_2 rebreathing or hypoxia is sometimes done. However, these tests can be difficult to interpret because chronic CO_2 retention itself can depress the central response to hypercapnia, chronic hypoxia can blunt peripheral chemoreceptor responsiveness, and because patients with advanced obstructive or restrictive ventilatory defects may be unable to increase ventilation due to mechanical impairment of the respiratory apparatus.

THERAPY

The initial approach should aim at the identification and correction of reversible causes of chronic hypoventilation. This includes the discontinuance of sedative or narcotic drugs, correction of electrolyte and mineral disorders, replacement therapy for hypothyroidism, optimization of bronchodilator therapy for COPD, and correction of metabolic alkalosis. Careful attention to factors that may worsen hypercapnia, e.g., diuretics that cause metabolic alkalosis, or precipitate respiratory failure, e.g., sedatives, should be stressed. Intermittent or continuous oxygen supplementation may be necessary if other measures do not correct significant oxygen desaturation.

Several respiratory stimulants have been used to treat disorders associated with depressed ventilatory drives. Progestational agents, e.g., medroxyprogesterone, have provided long-term benefits in some patients with primary alveolar hypoventilation and OHS. Acetazolamide may decrease P_{CO_2} in patients with a combined metabolic alkalosis and respiratory acidosis by producing a bicarbonate diuresis; however, this agent places the patient at risk of severe acidemia if dosage is excessive. Other agents that can stimulate ventilation, including tricyclic antidepressants and aminophylline, are not consistently effective.

If obstructive sleep apnea is associated with a hypoventilation syndrome, therapy is directed at relieving nocturnal apnea or hypopnea. Nasal continuous positive airway pressure (CPAP) is now the treatment of choice for the management of patients with these nocturnal events. However, even though the symptoms and quality of life are sometimes improved by successful management of sleep apnea, only a few patients normalize daytime blood gases in response to therapy directed solely at relieving sleep apnea.

Many patients with chronic alveolar hypoventilation require assisted ventilation. In recent years, there has been a resurgence of interest in negative pressure ventilation. These devices assist ventilation by applying negative pressure to the chest wall inside a tank (iron lung), outer shell (curaiss), or external garment ("pneumowrap"). Although these devices have the advantage of being noninvasive, they are bulky, uncomfortable, and often poorly tolerated. In addition, negative pressure ventilation is often complicated by development of intermittent upper airway obstruction and oxygen desaturation.

Intermittent positive pressure ventilation administered noninvasively by a nasal CPAP mask or face mask is becoming increasingly popular. Although some patients tolerate the mask poorly or find it difficult to synchronize spontaneous respiration with breaths imposed by the ventilator, noninvasive positive pressure ventilation is, in general, better tolerated than negative pressure ventilation. The usual goal is to provide ventilator assistance part-time, usually nocturnally, in anticipation that the physiological benefits will carry over during the day. Thus, the optimal candidate for this form of assisted ventilation is the patient who is reasonably stable and who can maintain adequate spontaneous ventilation for a major portion of the day.

Patients who do not tolerate or fail to improve with noninvasive ventilation, or are too ill to rely on even short periods of spontaneous breathing, require positive pressure ventilation through a tracheostomy. Placement of a tracheostomy permits continuous or intermittent ventilatory support with minimal discomfort. Potential complications of long-term tracheostomy include swallowing dysfunction, frequent lower respiratory tract infections, and tracheal stenosis. Other disadvantages include impaired speech and the need for frequent airway suctioning and maintenance. Some patients find tracheostomy cosmetically unacceptable.

Patients with adequate resources and psychosocial support and who are deemed suitable candidates may receive chronic ventilatory support at home. Long-term ventilatory systems in use today are highly portable and afford the patient a reasonably active life-style.

Phrenic nerve pacing is used occasionally for ventilatory assistance in patients with high cervical spinal cord lesions or central hypoventilation syndromes. This approach requires that radiofrequency-controlled electrodes be surgically implanted around the phrenic nerves in the neck; simultaneous bilateral stimulation of the phrenic nerves then causes contraction of the diaphragm. Minute ventilation can be controlled by varying the frequency and intensity of stimulation. However, like negative pressure ventilation, electrophrenic pacing may be complicated by intermittent upper airway obstruction.

BIBLIOGRAPHY

For a more detailed discussion, see Millman RP: Disorders of alveolar ventilation, in Fishman AP (ed), *Pulmonary Diseases and Disorders,* 2d ed. New York, McGraw-Hill, 1988, pp 1335–1345.

Douglas NJ: Nocturnal hypoxemia in patients with chronic obstructive pulmonary disease. Clin Chest Med 13:523–532, 1992.

Goldstein RS: Hypoventilation: Neuromuscular and chest wall disorders. Clin Chest Med 13:507–521, 1992.

Strumpf DA, Millman RP, Hill WS: The management of chronic hypoventilation. Chest 98:474–480, 1990.

Weese-Mayer DE, Silvestri JM, Menzies LJ, Morrow-Kenny AS, Hunt CE, Hauptman SA: Congenital central hypoventilation syndrome: Diagnosis, management, and long-term outcome in thirty-two children. J Pediatr 120:381–387, 1992.

Weinberger SE, Schwartzstein RM, Weiss JW: Hypercapnia. N Engl J Med 321:1223–1231, 1989.

Richard J. Schwab

Sleep is associated with a number of characteristic physiologic alterations in the control and mechanics of breathing. When abnormal or exaggerated, these sleep-induced changes can disrupt normal sleep architecture as well as contribute to the pathogenesis of cardiopulmonary disease, resulting in alveolar hypoventilation, hypoxemia, pulmonary hypertension, and cor pulmonale. This chapter reviews two primary disorders of sleep, central sleep apnea and obstructive sleep apnea, as well as a number of medical conditions whose manifestations and clinical course are worsened during sleep.

CENTRAL SLEEP APNEA

Central sleep apnea is defined as repeated episodes of apnea (cessation of airflow for 10 s or longer) during sleep in the *absence of any respiratory muscle effort.* Central sleep apnea is caused by transient interruption of central drive to the respiratory pump muscles. These apneic episodes can result in hypoxia, hypercapnia, and acidemia. Central sleep apnea may be idiopathic or associated with a number of neurologic conditions including Shy-Drager syndrome, myasthenia gravis, autonomic dysfunction, neuromuscular disease, bulbar poliomyelitis, brain-stem infarction, and encephalitis.

Clinical Presentation

Central sleep apnea can be separated into *hypercapnic* and *nonhypercapnic* categories.

Hypercapnic Central Sleep Apnea

In these patients, central sleep apnea is a manifestation of a persistent defect in the respiratory center or neuromuscular system. They are subject to recurrent episodes of respiratory failure and chronic alveolar hypoventilation. These patients manifest daytime hypoxemia and hypercapnia and, in the more severe cases, pulmonary hypertension, right heart failure, and polycythemia. Headache, most severe on arising in the morning, is characteristic; it is attributed to the cerebral vasodilation that results from the acute increase in the degree of hypercapnia that occurs during sleep. Symptoms of sleep fragmentation, including hypersomnolence and frequent nocturnal arousals, are common.

Nonhypercapnic Central Sleep Apnea

This is the more common category. It is due to the temporary loss of respiratory drive during sleep. Arterial blood-gas values are normal during wakefulness. These patients do not develop chronic pulmonary or cardiovascular sequelae. Manifestations of sleep fragmentation—daytime hypersomnolence, frequent nocturnal arousals, and fatigue—predominate.

Diagnosis

The definitive diagnosis of central sleep apnea requires polysomnography which demonstrates recurrent episodes of apnea in association with absence of respiratory efforts. Distinction between the hypercapnic and nonhypercapnic variants of central sleep apnea can be made on the basis of an arterial blood-gas sample drawn while the patient is awake.

Management

The treatment of patients with central sleep apnea depends on whether an underlying defect in respiratory drive or neuromuscular function is present, i.e., by the presence or absence of hypercapnia during wakefulness.

Hypercapnic Central Sleep Apnea

Treatment is directed toward relieving alveolar hypoventilation. In many of these patients, this can be accomplished by means of positive-pressure ventilation delivered via a nasal mask. Tracheostomy is reserved for those patients who fail or prove intolerant of the noninvasive methods of assisted ventilation. Respiratory stimulants, such as medroxyprogesterone and acetazolamide, are rarely of value in managing these patients.

Nonhypercapnic Central Sleep Apnea

Therapeutic interventions include acetazolamide, oxygen, and nasal continuous positive airway pressure (CPAP). CPAP is a reasonable first-line therapy. Although CPAP is often successful, the mechanism by which CPAP corrects central apneas remains unclear. Supplemental oxygen relieves the arterial hypoxemia associated with apnea but, in some patients, it increases the frequency and duration of apneic events. Therefore, supplemental oxygen should only be administered after it has been shown in the course of a sleep study to be helpful.

OBSTRUCTIVE SLEEP APNEA SYNDROME (OSAS)

Obstructive sleep apnea syndrome (OSAS) is defined as recurrent episodes of apnea during sleep due to upper airway occlusion. OSAS is a common clinical problem, occurring in at least 1 to 4 percent of the general population. In contrast to patients with central sleep apnea in whom central respiratory drive is impaired, patients with OSAS manifest no airflow (due to occlusion of the upper airway) despite persistent respiratory efforts (chest wall and abdominal wall movements). Disorders commonly associated with OSAS include obesity, nasal obstruction, facial bony abnormalities (retrognathia, micrognathia), macroglossia, acromegaly, hypothyroidism, hypertrophy of the uvula, and adenoidal/tonsillar enlargement.

Clinical Presentation

OSAS occurs in both sexes and in all age groups but is most common in middle-aged men. The cardinal symptoms are excessive daytime sleepiness and loud snoring. Patients may fall asleep at inappropriate times, such as at the dinner table or while driving an automobile. Indeed, the frequency of motor vehicle accidents in patients with OSAS is three to seven times as great as in normal subjects; the highest accident rates are seen in the patients with the most severe sleep apnea. Other common symptoms include personality changes (especially irritability), morning headaches, intellectual impairment, palpitations, and memory loss. In mild-to-moderate OSAS, the patients generally manifest obesity and mild hypertension. Severely affected patients manifest cardiac arrhythmias, polycythemia, pulmonary hypertension, right ventricular failure, and peripheral edema.

Diagnosis

The "gold standard" for the diagnosis of OSAS is the polysomnographic demonstration of repeated apneic episodes despite strenuous respiratory efforts, i.e., chest wall and abdominal wall movements. Arterial blood drawn during the episode reveals arterial hypoxemia and hypercapnia. The polysomnogram is also helpful in assessing the severity of disease, evaluating the degree of snoring, and determining whether the apneas are position dependent, i.e., occurring in the supine position but not in the lateral decubitus position. In addition, polysomnography provides information about other conditions that can cause excessive daytime sleepiness, e.g., nocturnal myoclonus. The use of oximetry throughout the night has been advocated as an inexpensive screening method for detecting recurrent bouts of oxyhemoglobin desaturation that are associated with the apneic periods. However, the accuracy and reliability of this test has not been fully evaluated. The severity of daytime sleepiness in these patients can be determined by using a Multiple Sleep Latency Test (MSLT) which entails a series of daytime naps: in the normal individual, the mean latency to stage 1 sleep during the naps of a MSLT exceeds 10 min; in the patient with sleep apnea, the mean latency is usually < 5 min.

Management

Both medical and surgical therapeutic options exist for patients with OSAS. All patients with OSAS should avoid alcohol and sedatives because these substances can exacerbate upper airway obstruction during sleep. Although weight loss can effectively decrease the severity of OSAS, sustained weight loss in this patient population is difficult to achieve. Sleeping in the lateral decubitus posture will often alleviate apneas in patients whose sleep apnea is position dependent. (Sewing pockets for one or two tennis balls in the back of the patient's nightshirt is a simple and effective means for preventing the patient from lying in the supine position.) Pharmacologic approaches, including acetazolamide, medroxyprogesterone, and protriptyline, have had only limited success and run the risk of significant side effects. Oxygen therapy has an unpredictable effect on obstructive apneas, abolishing these events in some patients and increasing their duration and frequency in others.

The treatment of choice for patients with OSAS is nasal CPAP therapy. This form of therapy substantially reduces the frequency of apneic episodes, prevents oxyhemoglobin desaturation, and alleviates daytime sleepiness. Nasal CPAP provides a pneumatic splint for the airway, thereby preventing collapse during sleep when the dilator muscle activity of the upper airway is low. The particular pressure necessary to abolish apneas varies from patient to patient and should be determined on the basis of a sleep study. As a rule, nasal CPAP therapy is well tolerated. Local problems such as rhinitis and nasal irritation may occur. They are related to high rates of airflow and to increased pressure. They can usually be treated by either humidification of the CPAP system or nasal decongestants.

Recently, a technique for delivering positive airway pressure has been developed that allows independent control of the inspiratory and expiratory positive airway pressures. This system, called BiPAP (bilevel positive airway pressure), is potentially more comfortable than CPAP since it can decrease the need for high levels of expiratory pressure while maintaining high levels of inspiratory pressure. Because it is more expensive than conventional CPAP therapy, BiPAP should be reserved for patients who do not tolerate CPAP, particularly for those who report difficulties with exhalation. Another new innovation available for CPAP is the option of "ramping up" to a prescribed CPAP pressure, i.e., of gradually increasing the CPAP pressure over a selected time interval. This permits the use of a lower, more comfortable level of pressure while the patient is falling asleep followed by a higher level after the patient is asleep.

In general, surgical therapy for patients with OSAS should be reserved for particular patients who fail CPAP therapy or for patients who have certain anatomic abnormalities. For example, nasal surgery can be helpful in relieving a local nasal obstruction or in correcting a troublesome deviation of the nasal septum. A procedure to promote mandibular advancement is indicated for patients with unequivocal cephalometric abnormalities, i.e., micrognathia, retrognathia. Similarly, patients with OSAS who have marked tonsillar or adenoidal hypertrophy may improve after surgical removal of these tissues.

Uvulopalatopharyngoplasty (UPPP) is the most common surgical procedure for OSAS. This procedure consists of removal of the tonsils and adenoids, uvula, distal margin of the soft palate, and any excessive pharyngeal tissue. The success rate of UPPP appears to be partially related to the site of obstruction; patients with oropharyngeal (retropalatal) obstruction have the best results, whereas results are less favorable in those with hypopharyngeal obstruction. In most patients with OSAS, the upper airway is narrowed in multiple sites, making it difficult to achieve success solely by UPPP. Many patients who undergo UPPP still require nasal CPAP therapy. UPPP has at least a 50 percent failure rate and is associated with several significant complications including oropharyngeal pain, infection, hemorrhage, nasopharyngeal reflux, and rhinolalia. UPPP should be reserved for specific patients with oropharyngeal obstruction who fail, or refuse, nasal CPAP therapy.

Tracheostomy is usually completely effective in relieving OSAS. However, it should only be considered for patients who, after failing medical or surgical therapy, are left with very severe disease that causes incapacitating hypersomnolence, malignant arrhythmias, or cardiac failure.

OTHER MEDICAL CONDITIONS ASSOCIATED WITH SLEEP-DISORDERED BREATHING

Asthma

Nocturnal exacerbation of asthma complicates the course of up to two thirds of asthmatics. In these asthmatic patients, peak flow and forced expiratory volume (FEV_1) can decrease by up to 50 percent during the night. The nocturnal asthmatic attacks are not related to any specific stage of sleep. At greatest risk for these episodes of nocturnal bronchoconstriction are patients recovering from recent asthmatic attacks and patients with poorly controlled daytime symptom. In this regard, it should be underscored that in asthmatic patients admitted to the hospital with an exacerbation, expiratory flow rates can be expected to decrease at night. As a corollary, attempts at weaning the asthmatic patient from a ventilator should be undertaken cautiously at night. Nighttime administration of long-acting bronchodilator preparations, e.g., oral theophylline or oral β-agonists, is sometimes effective in relieving nocturnal symptoms in these patients.

Chronic Pulmonary Disease

Sleep is associated with worsening hypoxemia and hypercapnia in some patients with chronic obstructive pulmonary disease (COPD). Deterioration in gas exchange is most pronounced during REM sleep. Contributing factors include sleep-associated decreases in minute ventilation and CO_2 responsiveness, cessation of the activity of the accessory respiratory muscles during REM sleep, and worsening of ventilation-perfusion mismatch. Bouts of hypoxemia in these patients can precipitate atrial and ventricular ectopy, myocardial ischemia, and increase pulmonary artery pressures. Noctural administration of oxygen can reverse these abnormalities and prolong survival.

Patients with other chronic lung diseases, e.g., interstitial lung disease, cystic fibrosis, and kyphoscoliosis, have been reported to develop hypoxemia during sleep. The impact of nocturnal hypoxemia on the natural history of these diseases and, conversely, the efficacy of nocturnal oxygen therapy in improving outcome remain to be determined. Overnight oximetry is useful in detecting the presence and degree of hypoxia during sleep.

Congestive Heart Failure

Patients with severe but stable congestive heart failure (New York Heart Association class 3 or 4) may demonstrate episodic hypoxemia during sleep even though arterial oxygenation is normal during wakefulness. These episodes of nocturnal hypoxemia relate to the occurrence of Cheyne-Stokes respiration during sleep, i.e., a pattern of periodic breathing characterized by intervals of apnea and hypopnea that alternate with hyperpnea. Hypoxemic events in these patients may not only further compromise myocardial function, but may disrupt the normal sleep pattern, with resultant frequent nocturnal arousals, insomnia, fatigue, and daytime hypersomnolence. Treatment of the heart failure is often successful in decreasing the frequency and severity of the episodes of nocturnal hypoxemia. Supplemental oxygen, and in some cases nasal CPAP, are also sometimes beneficial.

SLEEP IN THE INTENSIVE CARE UNIT

Sleep disruption is extremely common among critically ill patients in the intensive care unit (ICU) as a result of frequent diagnostic, therapeutic, and nursing interventions. Light and sound levels are often well above normal in this environment, resulting in sensory overload. In addition, crowding, pain, and frequent patient contact can disturb sleep patterns in patients in the ICU. Sensory overload and secondary sleep deprivation contribute to the development of the ICU syndrome or ICU psychosis. The clinical manifestations of this syndrome involve a spectrum of psychological reactions including depression, anxiety, hallucinations, delirium, fear, and disorientation. The ICU syndrome usually occurs on the third to seventh day after admission to the ICU, and can remit within 48 h of leaving the ICU or after the sleep deprivation is corrected. Polysomnographic studies of patients in the ICU demonstrate multiple abnormalities including decreased total sleep time, increased arousals with awakenings, loss of continuity of sleep stages, and decreased time in the deep stages of sleep including REM sleep.

Certain recommendations can be made to enhance the quality of sleep and minimize the risk of ICU syndrome.

1. Use individual patient rooms with observation doors and light dimmers to minimize noise and light.
2. Safe alarm systems must be developed which do not disturb sleep but will alert the staff to potential medical problems.
3. Procedures such as chest radiographs, phlebotomy, and frequent vital signs should be performed only if absolutely necessary during the night.

Unfortunately, many of these measures are difficult to achieve and patients often require sedation for sleep in the ICU. At present, benzodiazepines are the preferred agents for promoting and enhancing the quality of sleep in the ICU. These drugs exert multiple actions, including amnesia, anxiolysis, sedation, and muscle relaxation. Unfortunately, benzodiazepines blunt the central drive to breath and, in higher doses, can precipitate hypercapnia in patients with serious underlying lung disease. In addition, these agents affect the pattern of sleep: they reduce the time spent in the deeper stages of sleep and their effects often linger into the next day or night. The short-acting benzodiazepines (trizolam, midazolam, lorazepam) are the medications of choice to promote sleep in the ICU.

BIBLIOGRAPHY

For a more detailed discussion, see Millman RP, Fishman AP: Sleep apnea syndromes, in Fishman AP (ed), *Pulmonary Diseases and Disorders,* 2d ed. New York, McGraw-Hill, 1988, pp 1347–1361.

Bradley TD, Phillipson EA: Central sleep apnea. Clin Chest Med 13:493–505, 1992.

Hudgel DW: Mechanisms of obstructive sleep apnea. Chest 101:541–549, 1992.

Hudgel DW, Cherniack NS: Sleep and breathing, in Fishman AP (ed), *Update: Pulmonary Diseases and Disorders.* New York, McGraw-Hill, 1992, pp 249–261.

Kaplan J, Staats BA: Obstructive sleep apnea. Mayo Clin Proc 65:1087–1094, 1990.

Kryger MH: Management of obstructive sleep apnea. Clin Chest Med 13:481–492, 1992.

Aili Lazaar   Joseph Pilewski

Lung cancer is the leading cause of cancer mortality in the United States. Despite recent advances in the understanding of lung cancer tumorigenesis, long-term survival is uncommon.

EPIDEMIOLOGY

It is estimated that in 1991 there were 161,000 new cases of lung cancer and more than 140,000 deaths attributable to this disease. Although it has consistently been the leading cause of cancer deaths in men, mortality rates have begun to level off among middle-aged men. If current trends continue, the overall lung cancer death rate in men during this decade is expected to decrease. In contrast, deaths from lung cancer have increased sharply in women, largely the result of increased cigarette use over the past four decades. Indeed, lung cancer has recently surpassed breast cancer as the leading cause of cancer death in women.

Cigarette smoking is the major cause of lung cancer. The association between smoking and lung cancer has been appreciated since the 1950s, and a dose-response relationship between the number of cigarettes smoked and the development of lung cancer has been established. Moreover, the risk increases with earlier age of smoking initiation, the depth of inhalation, and the presence of chronic obstructive pulmonary disease. Although low tar cigarettes reduce the risk, tar level is less important than number of cigarettes smoked per day. After smoking cessation, relative risk decreases; at ten years, the risk of exsmokers approaches that of nonsmokers. Passive exposure to cigarette smoke has been reported to increase the risk of lung cancer, and it has been suggested that 25 percent of cases in nonsmokers are due to passive exposure.

Other established causes of lung cancer include asbestos and radon decay products. For both types of exposure, the relative risk is multiplicative for those also exposed to tobacco smoke. Recent attention has focused on household exposure to radon. About 10,000 lung cancer deaths per year have been attributed to radon, making it the second most important cause of lung cancer. The contributions of air pollution, genetic predisposition, and dietary deficiency, e.g., vitamin A, to the development of lung cancer remain speculative.

PATHOLOGY

Histologically, most cases of lung cancer can be classified into four major types: small cell (approximately 25 percent); squamous cell

(25 percent); adenocarcinoma (30 percent); and large cell (15 percent). Other, less common types include adenosquamous carcinoma, bronchial carcinoids, and mucoepidermoid tumors.

Small cell lung carcinoma (SCLC) is characterized histologically by small cells consisting almost entirely of nucleus with dispersed chromatin and few or no nucleoli. There is a tendency for one cell to indent the nucleus of another, known as "nuclear molding," and for cells to arrange around thin blood vessels into pseudorosettes. Mitoses are prominent and necrosis is common; released DNA imparts a dark stain to surrounding blood vessels.

Non-small cell lung cancer (NSCLC) includes squamous cell, adenocarcinoma, and large cell cancer. These cell types are considered together because staging and treatment are similar. However, the natural history and the clinical presentation of these various subtypes can differ considerably.

Squamous cell carcinoma develops after many years of change in the bronchial mucosa. Cytologic studies show progression from squamous metaplasia to carcinoma in situ before invasive cancer develops. Characteristic histologic features are keratinization and intercellular bridges; well-differentiated tumors produce keratin "pearls."

Adenocarcinomas are distinguished histologically by glandular formation and a tendency toward a papillary configuration. They may produce mucin. They often arise in areas of prior lung damage (scar carcinoma). They stain for carcinoembryonic antigen (CEA) and can be distinguished from mesothelioma on this basis. Bronchoalveolar carcinoma, a subtype of adenocarcinoma, characteristically lines the alveolar surface without invading or disrupting normal lung architecture.

Large cell carcinoma is a histologic subtype of exclusion. This category includes those non-small cell cancers with no evidence of squamous or glandular differentiation. Cells are anaplastic and undifferentiated and commonly accompanied by neutrophilic infiltration.

Histologic evidence suggests that all types of lung cancer originate from a common stem cell. A mixed cell type is often found in patients with SCLC, suggesting either different neoplasms or a common stem cell capable of differentiating histologically into squamous, glandular, and small cell cancers. The mixed histologic findings challenge the notion that small cell cancer arises from neuroendocrine cells.

CLINICAL MANIFESTATIONS

Five percent of patients are asymptomatic at the time of diagnosis. However, lung cancer usually evokes signs and symptoms attributable either to the primary tumor itself, to involvement of other intrathoracic structures, to distant metastases, or to paraneoplastic syndromes. Manifestations directly related to the tumor include cough, hemoptysis, and a dull, aching chest pain. Tumors that are centrally located and cause partial airway obstruction give rise to dyspnea, wheezing, or stridor; complete obstruction causes atelectasis or postobstructive pneumonitis. Peripheral tumors are less likely to be symptomatic; they often become clinically apparent when they involve pleura or chest wall, producing localized pleuritic chest pain or dyspnea due to a pleural effusion.

Intrathoracic spread of tumor to the mediastinum can produce an array of findings. Vocal cord paralysis, manifest clinically by the onset of hoarseness, signifies recurrent laryngeal nerve damage. An elevated hemidiaphragm suggests phrenic nerve paralysis. Dysphagia may be a symptom of either extrinsic esophageal compression or the formation of a bronchoesophageal fistula. Compression of the superior vena cava by tumor or enlarged lymph nodes can cause the superior vena cava syndrome, characterized by distended neck veins, facial and arm swelling, and prominent venous collaterals on the chest. Finally, pericardial extension of tumor may cause pericardial effusion that can, in turn, lead to cardiac tamponade.

Other intrathoracic symptoms relate to invasion of pleura, chest wall, and nerves. Pleural effusion, caused either by direct pleural involvement or by obstruction of lymphatics, is frequently accompanied by dyspnea. Tumors arising at the apex of the lung, commonly referred to as Pancoast tumors, have a particular predilection for involvement of the brachial plexus and sympathetic ganglia, resulting in a characteristic constellation of findings: shoulder pain radiating down the arm, corresponding to the distribution of the ulnar nerve, and Horner's syndrome (meiosis, ptosis, and ipsilateral anhydrosis).

Lung cancer can metastasize throughout the body to cause extrathoracic signs and symptoms. Neurologic deficits, such as hemiplegia, seizure, or behavioral abnormalities, may be a sign of intracranial metastases. Back pain, lower extremity weakness, and bladder or bowel dysfunction are highly suggestive of spinal cord compression and warrant rapid investigation and intervention. Metastatic spread to bone usually causes localized pain and may result in pathologic fractures. Although the liver, adrenal glands, and lymph nodes are common sites of metastases, involvement of these sites usually does not produce symptoms.

Paraneoplastic Syndromes

Lung cancers are associated with a diverse array of paraneoplastic syndromes, i.e., extrapulmonary and systemic abnormalities caused by biologically active factors produced either by, or in response to, the primary tumor. In some instances, the elaborated factor has been clearly identified. However, for a considerable number of systemic manifestations, no etiologic agent has yet been defined. The presence of one of these syndromes does not imply that the tumor is unresectable, because treatment of the primary tumor often results in complete resolution of the syndrome.

A comprehensive list of paraneoplastic manifestations of lung cancer appears in Table 28-1. The more common manifestations are discussed below.

Syndrome of inappropriate antidiuretic hormone secretion (SIADH) Arginine vasopression or antidiuretic hormone (ADH) controls the excretion of free water by the kidney. In a patient with a lung cancer,

TABLE 28-1 Paraneoplastic Manifestations of Lung Cancer

Endocrine	Hematologic
SIADH	Anemia
Cushing's syndrome	Hemolytic anemia
Hypercalcemia	Red cell aplasia
Neurologic	Thrombocytopenic purpura
Myopathy	Intravascular coagulopathy
Polymyositis	Hypofibrinogenemia
Myasthenia (Eaton-Lambert	Eosinophilia
syndrome)	Connective tissue
Carcinomatous neuromyopathy	Clubbing
Neuropathy	Hypertrophic pulmonary
Sensory, mixed	osteoarthropathy
Sensorimotor	Immunologic (?)
Encephalopathy	Dermatomyositis
Myelopathy	Systemic sclerosis
Thrombotic cerebral infarction	Membranous glomerulonephritis
Cerebellar degeneration	Rickets
Dementia	Retroperitoneal fibrosis
Psychosis	Chronic thyroiditis
Dermatologic	Proteinopathies
Pigmentation	Hypoalbuminemia
Pruritus	Hypergammaglobulinemia
Lanugo hirsutism	Amyloidosis
Acanthosis migrans	General systemic
Erythema gyratum nigricans	Pyrexia
Vascular	Anorexia
Thrombophlebitis migrans	Cachexia
Arterial thrombosis	Taste dysfunction
Nonbacterial thrombotic	
endocarditis	

SOURCE: Adapted from Ross EJ: Extrapulmonary syndromes associated with neoplasms of the lung, in Fishman AP (ed), *Pulmonary Diseases and Disorders*, 2d ed. New York, McGraw-Hill, 1988, p 1966.

excessive or inappropriate secretion of ADH is generally associated with small cell carcinoma. Elaboration of ADH by the tumor leads to the development of hyponatremia and hypotonicity of the extracellular fluid compartment. Clinically, this may be manifest as drowsiness, irritability, disorientation, seizure, or coma. Diagnosis requires demonstration of hyponatremia, low plasma osmolality, and inappropriately high urine osmolality and sodium excretion, despite euvolemia and normal renal, adrenal, and thyroid function. Immediate treatment consists of free water restriction and, if necessary, infusion of hypertonic (3%) saline. Long-term control can be achieved using demeclocycline, a tetracycline derivative, which antagonizes the action of ADH on the distal tubule.

Cushing's syndrome In the patient with a lung cancer, excessive ACTH secretion is most often associated with small cell carcinoma. Characteristic clinical manifestations include edema, hyperpigmentation, muscle weakness, mood disturbances, and hypertension. Centripetal obesity and striae are rare. Significant laboratory data include hypokalemic metabolic alkalosis, hyperglycemia, and persistently elevated plasma levels of corticotropin and cortisol. The excessive ACTH production is generally nonsuppressible, as evidenced by failure of exogenously administered dexamethasone to diminish urinary excretion of 17-hydroxycorticosteroids. When removal of the lung tumor is not possible, attempts to inhibit adrenal release of cortisol should be made using metyrapone in combination with mitotane or aminoglutethimide.

Hypercalcemia Abnormally high levels of calcium in serum are most often associated with squamous cell carcinoma. With mildly elevated levels, the patient may complain of increased thirst and polyuria; higher levels lead to nausea, vomiting, constipation, lethargy, and confusion. Hypercalcemia is due to the production by the tumor of a parathyroid hormone (PTH)-like factor which binds to the PTH receptor. Osteoclast-activating factor and prostaglandin E2, factors which cause hypercalcemia in other malignancies, do not contribute appreciably to hypercalcemia associated with lung cancer. Treatment includes vigorous hydration, diphosphonates, steroids, and mithramycin.

Other syndromes Nonmetastatic *neuromuscular* complications of lung cancer occur in up to 15 percent of patients and can precede the diagnosis of lung cancer by many months. The pathogenesis of these disorders remains obscure but is presumed to be related to elaboration of humoral substances by the tumor. The most common abnormalities include a peripheral polyneuropathy, usually with mixed sensorimotor involvement, and a nonspecific neuromyopathy involving the pelvic girdle and proximal limb muscles. A myasthenia-like disorder, the Eaton-Lambert syndrome, is seen in some patients with SCLC, apparently due to defective release of acetylcholine at the neuromuscular junction. Patients with this syndrome manifest weakness and aching of proximal muscles. The diagnosis is based on the electromyographic demonstration of a progressive increase in the amplitude of the muscle action potential with repetitive stimulation, a finding opposite to that seen in true myasthenia. Other neuromuscular syndromes include dementia, cerebellar degeneration, and polymyositis/dermatomyositis.

The most frequent *skeletal* abnormality, seen predominantly in patients with NSCLC, is clubbing of the digits. Clubbing is sometimes accompanied by hypertrophic osteoarthropathy, a syndrome of pain and tenderness involving the distal diaphyses of long bones, and characterized radiographically by periosteal elevation and new bone formation, i.e., periostitis. Bone scan results may be positive in the affected areas. Resection of the tumor can result in rapid regression of both clubbing and hypertrophic osteoarthropathy.

DIAGNOSIS

Chest radiograph There are no distinctive radiographic features by which the type of lung carcinoma can be made on the basis of a chest radiograph alone. Nonetheless, centrally located tumors are most apt to be squamous cell carcinoma or SCLC; cavitation of the mass is strongly suggestive of squamous cell carcinoma, whereas bulky mediastinal adenopathy is more consistent with SCLC. Peripherally located lesions are apt to represent adenocarcinoma or large cell cancer. A pattern of airspace consolidation, mimicking pneumonia, is suggestive of bronchoalveolar cell carcinoma.

Apical carcinomas (Pancoast tumors) present as an apical cap which may be easily overlooked or misinterpreted as residual changes of prior tuberculous infection. Lordotic views and computed tomography (CT) scans are helpful in documenting the presence of the tumor and defining its anatomic extent.

The chest radiograph is also invaluable in documenting the presence of tumor-related complications such as pleural effusion, rib destruction, atelectasis, and diaphragmatic paralysis.

Cytopathology Once a tumor is suspected by radiograph, it is imperative to obtain a pathologic diagnosis. Sputum cytology occasionally proves diagnostic in patients with proximal tumors and is a reasonable first step when sputum is easily obtained. Flexible fiberoptic bronchoscopy is an extremely useful tool for evaluating a patient with suspected lung cancer. Specimens are obtained by bronchial washings, brushings, forceps biopsy, and transbronchial needle aspiration. The diagnostic yield using a combination of these procedures is 70 to 95 percent, with the highest yield in proximal tumors. Transthoracic fine-needle aspiration under fluoroscopic guidance is also useful for diagnosis, particularly for peripheral lesions. Although the diagnostic yield may approach 90 percent, the false-negative rate is considerable. Diagnostic material may also be obtained from metastatic sites, including palpable lymph nodes, subcutaneous nodules, pleural effusions, or bone lesions.

STAGING AND TREATMENT

Once the diagnosis of lung cancer is established, the extent of local and metastatic spread of tumor should be defined, i.e., the tumor should be "staged," to determine appropriate therapy. Because of fundamental differences in the biologic behavior of NSCLC and SCLC, the staging systems and treatment modalities are distinct and will be discussed separately.

Staging and Treatment of NSCLC

A TNM staging system, based on characterization of the primary tumor (T), degree of regional node involvement (N), and presence or absence of distant metastases (M), is used in describing NSCLC (Tables 28-2 and 28-3).

Staging begins with a careful history and physical examination, paying special attention to systemic, cardiopulmonary, neurologic, and skeletal systems. Blood counts and chemistry studies are obtained to assess for bone marrow, liver, and cortical bone involvement. CT scanning of the chest and upper abdomen (to include the liver and adrenal glands) is performed to assess the extent of intrathoracic disease, as well as to look for metastases below the diaphragm. Although more accurate than plain radiograph, CT scanning of the mediastinum does not obviate the need to obtain tissue for histologic examination, because enlarged lymph nodes may not be cancerous, and normal-sized nodes may harbor tumor. Mediastinoscopy should be performed before committing to definitive surgery if suspicion is high that mediastinal nodes are involved. Bone scans should be obtained in all patients with musculoskeletal findings; CT of the brain should be done in all patients with neurologic manifestations. Because early metastases are sometimes asymptomatic, some clinicians recommend brain imaging and bone scan in patients with bulky tumors, with systemic symptoms such as weight loss, or when histology indicates adenocarcinoma or large cell.

Surgery Surgery is the mainstay of therapy for patients with stage I or II disease who have adequate pulmonary reserve. Lung resection is generally well-tolerated if the predicted postresection FEV_1, based

TABLE 28-2 New International Staging System for Lung Cancer: TNM Definitions

Primary Tumor (T)

TX   Tumor proven by the presence of malignant cells in bronchopulmonary secretions but not visualized radiographically or bronchoscopically, or any tumor that cannot be assessed as in a retreatment staging.

T0   No evidence of primary tumor.

TIS   Carcinoma in situ.

T1*   A tumor that is ≤ 3.0 cm in greatest dimension, surrounded by lung or visceral pleura, and without evidence of invasion proximal to a lobar bronchus at bronchoscopy.*

T2   A tumor > 3.0 cm in greatest dimension, or a tumor of any size that either invades the visceral pleura or has associated atelectasis or obstructive pneumonitis extending to the hilar region. At bronchoscopy, the proximal extent of demonstrable tumor must be within a lobar bronchus or at least 2.0 cm distal to the carina. Any associated atelectasis or obstructive pneumonitis must involve less than an entire lung.

T3   A tumor of any size with direct extension into the chest wall (including superior sulcus tumors), diaphragm, or the mediastinal pleura or pericardium without involving the heart, great vessels, trachea, esophagus, or vertebral body, or a tumor in the main bronchus within 2 cm of the carina without involving the carina.

T4†   A tumor of any size with invasion of the mediastinum or involving heart, great vessels, trachea, esophagus, vertebral body or carina or presence of malignant pleural effusion.*

Nodal Involvement (N)

N0   No demonstrable metastasis to regional lymph nodes.

N1   Metastasis to lymph nodes in the peribronchial or the ipsilateral hilar region, or both, including direct extension.

N2   Metastasis to ipsilateral mediastinal lymph nodes and subcarinal lymph nodes.

N3   Metastasis to contralateral mediastinal lymph nodes, contralateral hilar lymph nodes, ipsilateral or contralateral scalene or supraclavicular lymph nodes.

Distant Metastasis (M)

M0   No known distant metastasis.

M1   Distant metastasis present—specify site(s).

---

*The uncommon superficial tumor of any size with its invasive component limited to the bronchial wall which may extend proximal to the main bronchus is classified as T1.

†Most pleural effusions associated with lung cancer are due to tumor. There are, however, some few patients in whom cytopathologic examination of pleural fluid (on more than one specimen) is negative for tumor and in whom the fluid is nonbloody and is not an exudate. In such cases where these elements and clinical judgment dictate that the effusion is not related to the tumor, the patients should be staged T1, T2, or T3, excluding effusion as a staging element.

TABLE 28-3 New International Staging System for
Lung Cancer: Stage Groupings

Occult carcinoma	Stage IIIa
TX N0 M0	T3 N0 M0
Stage 0	T3 N1 M0
Carcinoma in situ	T1–3 N2 M0
Stage I	Stage IIIb
T1 N0 M0	Any T Any N3 M0
T2 N0 M0	T4 Any N M0
Stage II	Stage IV
T1 N1 M0	Any T Any N M1
T2 N1 M0	

on preoperative spirometry and quantitative ventilation-perfusion scans, exceeds 1 L (see Chap. 4). The extent of intrathoracic tumor spread noted at the time of surgery determines the operative procedure. Mediastinal lymph nodes are sampled at multiple levels, and lung resection, with or without resection of adjacent structures, proceeds if disease does not extend to contralateral or high paratracheal nodes. Lobectomy or pneumonectomy remain standard procedures with segmentectomy, wedge resection, bi-lobectomy, and sleeve resection as options in certain situations. The advantage of lobectomy over lesser operations that spare lung, such as wedge resection or segmentectomy, is under prospective investigation by the Lung Cancer Study Group. Five-year survival in patients who undergo surgical resection for stage I disease is approximately 60 percent. The outlook is somewhat less favorable for stage II disease, and is dictated, to some extent, by the histology of the tumor (Table 28-4).

Controversy exists concerning surgical resection in patients with ipsilateral mediastinal node involvement or chest wall invasion (stage IIIa). For direct extension into the chest wall, including Pancoast tumors that do not involve vertebral bodies or sympathetic

TABLE 28-4 Cumulative Proportion of Patients Surviving 5 Years
Following Apparent Complete Resection by Surgical-Pathologic Stage
and Cell Type

Stage	Squamous cell carcinoma, %	Adenocarcinoma and large cell carcinoma, %
I	56.0	61.2
II	37.1	26.0
IIIa	36.3	17.0

SOURCE: The University of Texas M. D. Anderson Hospital 1965–1982. Adapted from Mountain CF: Surgical treatment of non-small cell lung cancer. In: Fishman AP (ed), *Pulmonary Diseases and Disorders*, 2d ed. New York, McGraw-Hill, 1988, p 1997.

ganglia, en bloc resection with chest wall reconstruction is generally attempted; 5-year survival rates of up to 40 percent have been reported if surgical margins are free of tumor. Prognosis is worse for N2 nodal involvement, but stage IIIa patients appear to benefit if complete resection of mediastinal nodes can be accomplished. Patients with stages IIIb and IV disease are not candidates for surgical resection.

Radiotherapy Radiotherapy is used with curative intent in some patients with inoperable disease, as adjuvant therapy, and for palliation of tumor-related complications. Dysphagia secondary to esophagitis is a common side effect, but radiation pneumonitis is infrequent (< 10 percent).

High-dose radiotherapy administered with curative intent is sometimes used in inoperable patients, but its efficacy is unsupported by convincing clinical trials. For the individual with stage I disease who is inoperable because of advanced age, concomitant illness, or refusal to consent to surgery, radiotherapy with curative intent has been reported to be associated with long-term survival rates of up to 20 percent. In patients with more advanced disease, the success rates are marginal at best.

Adjuvant radiotherapy is commonly administered postoperatively in patients with N1-2 disease or with tumor involving the margins of resection. Although local recurrence rates are decreased by postoperative radiotherapy, survival appears to be unaffected. This is not surprising because about 80 percent of recurrences after surgical resection involve extrathoracic sites. Preoperative irradiation is used by some centers in the treatment of Pancoast tumors in an attempt to shrink the tumor and allow for complete resection.

Palliative radiotherapy is useful for the treatment of a number of intrathoracic complications including refractory cough, hemoptysis, atelectasis, postobstructive pneumonitis, and superior vena cava syndrome. Most patients with symptomatic brain metastases benefit from cranial irradiation as do patients with painful skeletal metastases who receive irradiation over the affected site.

Chemotherapy Chemotherapy for NSCLC does not improve survival, and associated toxicity is high.

Interventional bronchoscopy As a final therapeutic option for patients with inoperable NSCLC, bronchoscopic laser therapy or endobronchial radiation therapy (brachytherapy) may offer palliative relief of symptoms of tracheobronchial obstruction.

Staging and Treatment of SCLC

The TNM staging system, which provides detailed information about locoregional extent of tumor within the thorax, has not proven to be prognostically useful in SCLC. This is likely due to the systemic nature of SCLC, which precludes control of disease by local modalities alone, i.e., surgery and radiation. SCLC is, however, highly responsive to chemotherapy, and the ability to achieve sustained remission is best related to the presence or absence of extrathoracic disease. Thus, most investigators use a staging system which divides patients into two groups—limited and extensive disease. Limited disease (less than one third of patients) is confined to one hemithorax, with or without ipsilateral mediastinal, hilar, or supraclavicular lymph nodes. All other patients are considered to have extensive disease.

Staging of SCLC includes history and physical examination, blood count, and liver function studies. Because of the high incidence at presentation of metastatic disease involving bone (40 percent), liver (30 percent), bone marrow (15 to 25 percent), and brain (10 percent), initial evaluation routinely includes bone scan, CT scans of the liver and brain, and unilateral bone marrow aspirate and biopsy. The mediastinal lymph nodes are involved in most patients with SCLC. However, because this involvement falls within the limited-stage disease category, surgical staging by mediastinoscopy or mediastinotomy is not indicated.

The cornerstone of therapy for SCLC is combination chemotherapy. A variety of agents have proven activity against this tumor including cyclophosphamide, vincristine, cisplatin, etoposide, doxorubicin, methotrexate, and lomustine (CCNU). Conventional chemotherapy uses three or more agents for a minimum of 6 months. There is no convincing evidence that maintenance therapy alters survival.

Complete response, i.e., no clinical or radiographic evidence of tumor, can be achieved in > 50 percent of patients with limited disease and in > 20 percent with extensive disease. Median survival after treatment is 14 to 16 months and 6 to 8 months for limited and extensive disease, respectively. In contrast, the median survival in untreated patients is 3 months for limited disease and < 2 months for extensive disease. More importantly, long-term survival (> 5 years) has been reported in up to 12 percent of patients with limited disease treated aggressively with combination chemotherapy. Although this number is modest, it represents a significant achievement in a disease that previously was rapidly and uniformly fatal. Unfortunately, long-term survival has been achieved in only 1 to 2 percent of patients with extensive disease.

Because most patients with limited disease treated with chemotherapy alone will have relapse at the primary tumor site, many groups are reexamining the role of adjuvant modalities, e.g., radiotherapy or surgery, in enhancing locoregional control of disease. Several trials have demonstrated a survival benefit in patients with limited disease who receive both chemotherapy and local radiation to the chest, albeit at the expense of added toxicity. Preliminary evidence suggests a possible beneficial effect of surgical resection prior to chemotherapy in the < 10 percent of patients who present with the equivalent of TNM stage I or II disease. Importantly, there is no role for surgery in the treatment of patients with extensive stage disease, and radiation therapy in this group should be limited to palliation.

Another unsettled issue in the management of SCLC is the role of elective cranial irradiation. Central nervous system (CNS) metastases develop in up to 30 percent of patients during their course; this is attributed to the failure of most chemotherapeutic agents to cross the blood-brain barrier. It is generally agreed that cranial radiotherapy can reduce the incidence of brain metastases to 5 to 10 percent. Although this does not improve overall survival, the morbidity associated with brain metastases is lessened. Prophylactic cranial radiotherapy should be restricted to patients who achieve a complete response to chemotherapy because patients who are poorly responsive are likely to have disease progression outside the CNS before developing symptomatic brain metastases.

SCREENING

The natural history of lung cancer generally includes a long premalignant phase, which lasts from months to years and is potentially reversible. The preclinical period begins when cells undergo neoplastic transformation and continues until the cancer becomes detectable. The time required to develop from a single malignant cell to a clinically evident tumor depends on the rate of cell division, the doubling time. For lung cancers, the doubling time varies from about 30 days in SCLC to about 6 months for some adenocarcinomas. Detection of disease during the preclinical phase, before extrathoracic dissemination, is theoretically appealing because long-term survival for all types of lung cancer is better for those with limited-stage disease. However, several prospective controlled studies using sputum cytology and chest radiograph failed to demonstrate survival advantage in the group diagnosed by screening. The two screening techniques were complementary and detected earlier disease but did not reduce mortality rates. Mass screening of smokers does not, therefore, appear justified at this time.

BIBLIOGRAPHY

For a more detailed discussion, see Fishman AP: Epidemiology of cancer of the lung, in Fishman AP (ed), *Pulmonary Diseases and Disorders,* 2d ed. New York, McGraw-Hill, 1988, pp 1905–1912.

Dunn WF, Scanlon PD: Preoperative pulmonary function testing for patients with lung cancer. Mayo Clin Proc 68:371–377, 1993.

Garfinkel L, Silverberg E: Lung cancer and smoking trends in the United States over the past 25 years. Cancer 41:137–145, 1991.

Goodman GE, Livingston RB: Small cell lung cancer. Curr Prob Cancer 13:1–55, 1989.

Ihde NH, Minna JD: Non-small cell lung cancer. Curr Prob Cancer 15:63–104, 107–154, 1991.

Patel AM, Peters SG: Clinical manifestations of lung cancer. Mayo Clin Proc 68:273–277, 1993.

Alfred P. Fishman

Pulmonary nodules are circumscribed intrapulmonary nodules that are either spherical or oval in shape. By definition, they are sufficiently well delimited from surrounding lung parenchyma for their diameters to be measurable. The margins may be sharp or fuzzy. Distinction is made between a nodule and a mass: a nodule > 4 to 6 cm in diameter is called a *mass*. This distinction has diagnostic and prognostic implications because a mass is more apt to be neoplastic than is a nodule.

Pulmonary nodules may be solitary or multiple.

SOLITARY PULMONARY NODULE

The frequency with which solitary nodules prove to be malignant depends on the population under study. In parts of the country that are endemic for histoplasmosis and coccidioidomycosis, the incidence of malignant lesions in the general population is low, e.g., 10 to 15 percent. In surgical series that include a large number of heavy smokers, the incidence of malignant lesions will be much higher, e.g., 30 to 50 percent. With these reservations in mind, Table 29-1 provides some idea of the incidence of various disease processes as causes of solitary pulmonary nodules based on published reports.

Because the incidence of malignancy in solitary nodules is high (see Table 29-1), and because a malignant solitary nodule should be removed promptly if there is no evidence of local or distant spread, evaluation of a solitary nodule is pursued aggressively. Several criteria favor benignity: (1) the absence of risk factors, e.g., the patient is a nonsmoker; (2) the patient is < 35 years old; (3) the absence of current or prior primary extrapulmonary tumor; (4) a nodule that is small, circumscribed, and has not grown radiographically for 2 or more years; and (5) a distinctive pattern of calcification (see below). Although it is reasonable to use these criteria to determine the aggressiveness with which histologic proof of the nature of the lesion is sought, final proof of benignity often rests on histologic diagnosis.

Chest radiography Chest radiography is pivotal to the diagnosis and management of pulmonary nodules. Benign solitary nodules usually are small with distinct margins. Cavitation is uncommon. Calcification, if present, can be helpful in establishing the benign nature of the nodule. For example, central, laminated, diffuse, and popcorn patterns occur almost exclusively in benign lesions. Occasionally, calcification may be eccentric or have a multiple-fleck pattern.

TABLE 29-1 Causes of Solitary Pulmonary Nodules

	Incidence, %
Malignant Nodules	
Bronchogenic carcinoma	30
Bronchial adenoma	2
Metastasis	8
	Total 40%
Benign Nodules	
Infectious granulomas (tuberculoma, histoplasmoma, coccidioidoma, others)	50
Noninfectious granuloma (rheumatoid, Wegener's, paraffinoma)	3
Benign tumors (hamartoma, others)	3
Miscellaneous (pulmonary infarct, amyloidoma, hematoma, others)	4
	Total 60%

SOURCE: Modified after Table 124-1 of Lillington.

Unfortunately, the pattern of calcification is rarely absolute because similar patterns occur, albeit much less often, in malignancy.

The standard chest radiograph may fail to disclose calcification in a nodule. Computed tomography (CT) has largely replaced conventional chest tomography as a follow-up in the search for calcification. Not only is CT more effective in uncovering calcification, but it may also disclose other nodules that were indiscernible on the conventional chest radiograph. It also enables examination of the mediastinum and hilar areas for adenopathy and, if adenopathy is present, for staging.

Growth rate and doubling times The time that it takes for the nodule to double its volume (doubling time) is much slower for a benign than a malignant lesion, e.g., of the order of 20 to 400 days for a malignant lesion versus > 400 days for a benign lesion. (An acute infectious nodule may have a doubling time of 2 to 3 weeks or less.)

PRIMARY CARCINOMA OF THE LUNG AS SOLITARY NODULE

About 40 percent (see Table 29-1) of solitary nodules are malignant. Of these, about three quarters (30 percent) are bronchogenic carcinomas. Adenocarcinomas and squamous cell carcinomas are the more common and occur with about the same frequency; the incidence of large cell carcinomas is somewhat less. Small cell carcinomas and carcinoids rarely present as solitary nodules.

The guiding principle in dealing with a solitary nodule is that it must be promptly removed unless it can be proved to be benign. The criteria useful as a guide to benignity have been noted above.

However, if doubt remains, histologic proof is required. Bronchoscopy is often a preliminary if the nodule is located centrally, less
for histology than searching for airway lesions or extrinsic compression by cancerous nodes. Needle aspiration is much more rewarding,
i.e., it provides histologic diagnosis in 80 to 95 percent of malignant
nodules. Thoracoscopy and thoracotomy are the most reliable, but
also more invasive. Mediastinoscopy is generally reserved for those
patients; in-home CT suggests metastatic spread to the hilus or
mediastinum.

SOLITARY METASTATIC NODULE

About 5 to 10 percent of solitary pulmonary nodules are diagnosed
as metastatic (see Table 29-1). However, it is not always easy to
decide on histologic grounds about whether the neoplasm is primary
in the lungs or arises elsewhere. Adenocarcinomas are particularly
troublesome in this regard. In patients who are known to have
extrapulmonary primary neoplasm, the likelihood that a solitary
nodule is a metastasis to the lungs increases greatly, i.e., 25 to 50
percent of solitary nodules in these patients are metastatic. Surgical
resection is commonly done for a solitary metastatic nodule, but
the influence of this intervention on the course of the disease is
unclear.

BENIGN SOLITARY NODULE

About 50 percent of all solitary nodules are infectious granulomas
(see Table 29-1). The major interest in these lesions is to prove that
they are not neoplastic. Often this can be done by taking into
account the history of exposure, e.g., coccidioidomycosis; by skin
testing, e.g., tuberculosis; and by serial chest radiographs, e.g., at
monthly intervals to determine rate and pattern of growth or
resolution. However, as noted above, histologic evidence (obtained
by bronchoscopy, by needle or thoracoscopic biopsy, or by thoracotomy), is often required to prove that the lesion is benign. Of
these procedures, bronchoscopy is least likely to establish that a
lesion is benign and needle biopsy is apt to provide proof of
benignity in only about 50 percent of patients. Thoracoscopy and
thoracotomy are much more rewarding.

MULTIPLE PULMONARY NODULES

A wide variety of etiologies can cause multiple pulmonary nodules
(Table 29-2). However, widespread metastatic carcinoma is the most
common cause. Cavitation is common. Usually, metastatic nodules
are peripheral or subpleural in location. Both lungs are usually
involved and the lesions are more often at the bases. As a rule, the
primary extrapulmonary site is known or materializes in the course

TABLE 29-2 Causes of Multiple Pulmonary Nodules

Malignant Nodules
  Metastatic malignancy
  Alveolar cell carcinoma of lung, multicentric
  Lymphomas
  Multiple primary neoplasms (bronchogenic carcinomas, adenomas)
  Plasmacytomas
  Lymphomatoid granulomas
Benign Nodules
  Neoplasms
    Hamartomas
    Juvenile papillomatosis
    Chondromas
    Benign metastasizing leiomyomas
  Other benign lesions
    Infectious granulomas (tuberculosis, atypical mycobacterial infection, histoplasmosis coccidioidomycosis)
    Pyogenic abscesses
    Noninfectious granulomas (sarcoid, Wegener's, rheumatoid nodules, paraffinomas, lymphomatoid granulomatosis)
    Vasculitis
    Parasitic (paragonimiasis, hydatid cysts, dirofilariasis)
    Pneumoconioses
    Bronchial lesions (cystic bronchiectasis, mucoid impaction syndrome, allergic bronchopulmonary aspergillosis)
    Rheumatoid nodules
    Multiple mycetomas
    Multiple amyloidomas
    Arteriovenous malformations
    Sjögrens disease (pseudolymphomas)
Combinations (neoplastic and inflammatory)

SOURCE: Modified after Table 124-2 of Lillington.

of work-up or serial observations. However, in some instances, despite intensive search, an extrapulmonary site cannot be identified.

In metastatic lesions, the nodules usually grow rapidly and new nodules generally appear in the course of serial radiographs. CT scanning can reveal multiple nodules that are not evident on the chest radiograph. However, CT can be a mixed blessing. Indeed, it has the potential for creating ambiguity by uncovering not only malignant lesions, but also artifacts and residua of old inflammatory processes that may be indistinguishable from neoplastic nodules. Histologic evidence obtained by biopsy is prerequisite for treatment of malignant lesions.

BIBLIOGRAPHY

For a more detailed discussion, see Lillington GA: Systematic diagnostic approach to pulmonary nodules, in Fishman AP (ed), *Pulmonary Diseases and Disorders,* 2d ed. New York, McGraw-Hill, 1988, pp 1945–1954.

Caskey CI, Templeton PA, Zerhouni EA: Current evaluation of the solitary pulmonary nodule. Radiol Clin North Am 28:511–521, 1990.

Miller DL, Allen MS, Deschamps C, Trastek VF, Pairolero PC: Video-assisted thoracic surgical procedure: Management of a solitary pulmonary nodule. Mayo Clin Proc 67:462–464, 1992.

Viggiano RW, Swenson SJ, Rosenow EC III: Evaluation and management of solitary and multiple pulmonary nodules. Clin Chest Med 13:83–95, 1992.

Robert Walker

A multitude of primary neoplasms and cysts may arise in the mediastinum. Also, a wide assortment of malignant lesions may involve the mediastinum either by metastases or by direct extension; these often include tumors of the lung, esophagus, trachea, and heart as well as lymphoreticular malignancies.

EPIDEMIOLOGY

The incidence of primary mediastinal tumors is about 1/100,000 persons per year, affecting all age groups, with an equal male to female incidence. Approximately half of mediastinal tumors occur in the anterior mediastinum; the remainder are equally divided between the middle and posterior compartments (Table 30-1). In adults, about 25 percent of mediastinal lesions are malignant; in children this figure is higher, i.e., of the order of 50 percent. Taken together, thymomas, neurogenic tumors, developmental cysts, and lymphomas account for nearly 70 percent of all primary mediastinal lesions.

CLINICAL MANIFESTATIONS

As a general rule, asymptomatic lesions, e.g., those that are detected incidentally on the chest radiograph, are benign: up to 50 percent of all patients with primary mediastinal tumors are asymptomatic when first seen; 80 to 90 percent of these tumors are benign. In contrast, more than 50 percent of the lesions that cause symptoms ultimately prove to be malignant.

Symptoms and signs evoked by mediastinal tumors can be categorized as intrathoracic or systemic.

Intrathoracic manifestations Many of the intrathoracic signs and symptoms are the result of compression or invasion of adjacent structures. Among the more common manifestations are cough, dyspnea, chest pain, dysphagia, hoarseness (caused by vocal cord paralysis), and recurrent pneumonias (caused by airway obstruction). Occasionally, the superior vena cava syndrome, Horner's syndrome, phrenic nerve dysfunction, and spinal cord compression, occur. On rare occasion, anterior mediastinal lesions cause pericarditis and pericardial tamponade, whereas middle mediastinal lesions obstruct right ventricular outflow to cause cor pulmonale.

Systemic manifestations An impressive array of systemic manifestations can be elicited by mediastinal tumors (Table 30-2). The relationship between thymomas and myasthenia gravis is well

TABLE 30-1 Relative Frequencies of Mediastinal Masses

Compartment	Lesion	Incidence, %
Anterior	Thymoma	20
	Lymphoma	13
	Germ cell neoplasm	11
	Endocrine	6
	Primary carcinoma	4
	Mesenchymal	6
Middle	Pericardial cyst	6
	Bronchogenic cyst	6
	Enteric cyst	2
Posterior	Neurogenic	20

SOURCE: Adapted from Davis et al: Ann Thorac Surg 1987.

TABLE 30-2 Systemic Syndromes Associated with Primary Mediastinal Lesions

Syndrome	Neoplasm
Myasthenia gravis	Thymoma (usually benign)
Collagen vascular disease	Thymoma
Hypoglycemia	Mesothelioma, teratoma, neurosarcoma, neurilemmoma
Hypercalcemia	Parathyroid adenoma, lymphoma
Hypertension	Pheochromocytoma, ganglioneuroma, chemodectoma
Cushing's disease	Carcinoid, thymoma
Diarrhea	Ganglioneuroma
Hypertrophic osteoarthropathy	Neurofibroma, neurilemmoma, mesothelioma, thymoma
Hypogammaglobulinemia	Thymoma
Red blood cell aplasia	Thymoma
von Recklinghausen's disease	Neurofibroma
Vertebral anomalies	Enteric cysts
Whipple's disease	Thymoma
Megaesophagus	Thymoma
Gynecomastia	Germ cell tumor
Peptic ulcer	Neurilemmoma, enteric cysts

established. Much more subtle can be the relationship between systemic effects that result from the elaboration by certain mediastinal tumors of circulating hormones or other biologically active materials.

DIAGNOSTIC TESTS

Although the patient usually comes to medical attention because of an abnormality on the chest radiograph, it is uncommon for the chest radiograph, per se, to be diagnostic. Other imaging techniques can be helpful both with respect to etiology and intervention. These include computed tomography (CT), magnetic resonance imaging (MRI), radiographic swallowing studies, radionuclide scanning, angiography, and myelography. In some instances, assays for hormones, e.g., catecholamines or specific tumor markers, can be helpful.

Special diagnostic evaluation Most benign lesions are removed surgically because of the long-term risks of compression, rupture, hemorrhage, infection, and, rarely, of malignant degeneration. Therefore, diagnostic biopsy of a mediastinal mass is reserved for suspected metastatic or unresectable localized disease, for suspected systemic diseases such as lymphoma and sarcoid, and for suspected malignant germ cell tumors where nonsurgical treatment will be used. Mediastinal sampling can usually be performed by percutaneous or transbronchoscopic fine-needle aspiration, mediastinoscopy, or mediastinotomy. Because of anatomic considerations due to the arching aorta and pulmonary trunk, left-sided mediastinal lesions are approached by mediastinotomy rather than mediastinoscopy. If lymphoma is the most likely diagnosis on clinical grounds, a biopsy procedure that will disclose architecture is far superior to aspiration that will yield individual cells.

DIFFERENTIAL DIAGNOSIS

As a rule, primary mediastinal tumors and cysts can be categorized according to the compartment of the mediastinum in which they arise, i.e., anterior, middle, or posterior (Fig. 30-1). However, exceptions do occur, e.g., lesions that usually occur in the anterior or middle mediastinum occasionally appear as a posterior mediastinal mass, or vice versa.

Anterior Mediastinum

Thymoma

Typically, a thymic tumor appears as a round, lobulated mass on the chest radiograph, near the junction of the heart and great vessels, often filling in the retrosternal air space. Calcifications may be present. Thymic tumors include benign and malignant thymomas, thymic cysts, and thymic hyperplasia; they account for about 20 percent of mediastinal lesions in adults.

On the CT scan, thymoma often appears as irregular soft tissue masses in the anterior compartment, sometimes compressing the heart and great vessels and partially compressing the trachea. Gross invasion of mediastinal structures may also be evident.

Whether a thymoma is benign or malignant is generally decided at the time of surgery by whether it has extended, grossly or microscopically, beyond its capsule rather than by its cell type:

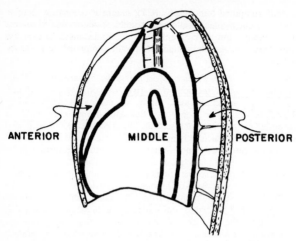

ANTERIOR	MIDDLE	POSTERIOR
Thymoma	Cysts	Neurogenic tumors
Lymphoma	Pericardial	(schwannoma,
Germ cell tumors	Bronchogenic	neurofibroma)
Teratomas	Noncystic lesions	
Seminomas	Lymphoma	Lymphoma
Dysgerminomas	Miscellaneous	
Mixed		
Endocrine tumors		
(thyroid;		
parathyroid;		
carcinoids)		
Miscellaneous		

FIG. 30-1 Neoplasms and cysts of the mediastinum according to the compartments in which they commonly occur. (Modified after Tables 134-1 and 134-2 of Lyerly HK, Sabiston DC Jr.)

lymphocytic, epithelial, or mixed. This determination is usually made at the time of surgery. Histologically, a thymoma may be difficult to distinguish from other tumors such as lymphoma, seminoma, or carcinoid. Electron microscopy may then be helpful in identifying a thymoma by revealing well-formed desmosomes and bundles of tonofilaments. The peak incidence of thymomas is in the fourth to sixth decades, whereas thymic cysts and thymic hyperplasia occur predominantly in childhood. Approximately two thirds of patients with thymoma have either intrathoracic or systemic complaints, e.g., cough, chest pain, superior vena cava syndrome, or a "parathymic" syndrome.

Myasthenia gravis occurs as a "parathymic" syndrome in up to 50 percent of patients with thymoma. In contrast, in only 8 to 15 percent of patients with myasthenia gravis is there an associated thymoma; coexistent myasthenia gravis and a thymoma portend a poorer prognosis. For reasons that are unclear, thymectomy is of greater benefit in patients with myasthenia gravis who do not have a thymoma.

Other "parathymic" syndromes include hematologic alterations (red blood cell aplasia, pancytopenia, polycythemia, leukemia), autoimmune disorders (lupus erythematosus, rheumatoid arthritis, hypogammaglobulinemia, dermatomyositis, Whipple's disease), and miscellaneous other conditions (megaesophagus, Cushing's disease, and granulomatous myocarditis).

When possible, treatment of thymoma involves complete surgical resection via a median sternotomy. Lesions that appear invasive are often associated with distant metastases and a 15-year survival rate of only 10 to 15 percent; in contrast, 50 percent of patients without invasive tumors survive for 15 years. Invasive lesions are currently treated by resecting as much of the tumor as possible followed by postoperative radiation therapy. Some investigators favor this adjunctive radiation therapy even for noninvasive tumors. The use of chemotherapy for invasive thymoma remains investigational.

Lymphoma

Lymphomas are the second most common tumors of the anterior mediastinum. They account for approximately 13 percent of primary mediastinal lesions in adults, two thirds of which are of the non-Hodgkin's type. As a rule, in the patient with lymphoma, the mediastinum is involved as part of a systemic disease. In only 5 to 10 percent is the mediastinum the only site of involvement ("primary mediastinal lymphoma").

Primary mediastinal lymphoma usually affects patients in the third and fourth decades. Common signs and symptoms include chest pain, cough, dyspnea, fever, fatigue, and weight loss. The superior vena cava syndrome and tracheal obstruction sometimes occur. Chest radiography reveals lymphadenopathy that is irregularly shaped in the anterior mediastinum. Open biopsy is often required to obtain sufficient tissue to reveal the distinctive cellular architecture. Treatment of primary mediastinal lymphoma is dictated by the same considerations as for lymphoma that arises at other sites.

Germ Cell Tumors

The mediastinum is the most frequent site of origin of extragonadal germ cell tumors. These neoplasms of the mediastinum account for about 11 percent of mediastinal masses. They are presumed to derive from primitive germ cells that migrated to the mediastinum during embryogenesis. However, because of the possibility that a mediastinal germ cell tumor does, in fact, represent metastasis, full staging should be performed with particular attention to the testes and retroperitoneum.

Mediastinal germ cell tumors can be classified into five major groups: (1) teratomas; (2) seminomas; (3) dysgerminomas or embryonal cell carcinomas; (4) choriocarcinomas; and (5) mixed germ cell tumors. A combination of embryonal cell carcinoma and a teratoma is called a teratocarcinoma.

Teratomas Teratomas occur most often in adolescents and young adults; the gender distribution is equal. They contain a disorganized mixture of ectodermal, mesodermal, and endodermal derivatives. A benign cystic teratoma ("dermoid cyst") may include skin, teeth, hair, cartilage, bone, intestinal and respiratory epithelium, and neurovascular tissue. About 80 percent of teratomas are benign. Malignant teratomas occur almost exclusively in men.

Nearly two thirds of patients with teratomas present with intrathoracic symptoms. Occasionally, a lesion ruptures into a bronchus causing the patient to expectorate hair, sebaceous material, or blood. Rupture into the pericardial and pleural spaces can lead to cardiac tamponade or pneumothorax, respectively. Teratomas have also been associated with recurrent attacks of hypoglycemia that remit after the tumor is resected.

Benign cystic teratomas ("dermoid cyst") appear on the chest radiograph as smooth, well-rounded masses, often protruding into one hemithorax. The radiographic presence of teeth is essentially diagnostic of a "dermoid cyst," whereas solid teratomas are often lobulated and asymmetric. Malignant teratomas are usually accompanied by increased serum levels of certain polypeptide hormones which act as tumor markers, i.e., α-fetoprotein, carcinoembryonic antigen, or human chorionic gonadotropin.

Teratomas should be completely resected, not only for the sake of removing or preventing malignancies, but also to avoid unpleasant side effects of benign masses. Complete resection of malignant teratomas is usually curative. However, at times, complete resection is not possible because of local invasion or distant metastases. Except for an occasional report indicating that chemotherapy may prolong survival, neither chemotherapy nor radiation therapy is generally considered to be beneficial.

Seminomas These are aggressive tumors that both extend locally and metastasize. They usually occur in young men in their late 20s to early 30s. Often they are asymptomatic when diagnosed. When present, symptoms may include chest pain, hoarseness, superior vena cava syndrome, fever, and weight loss. The prognosis is poorer for those > 35 years old, those with fever, those with adenopathy in the hilar, cervical, or supraclavicular beds, and those with the superior vena cava syndrome.

Despite their aggressive nature, seminomas are very radiosensitive; they may also be very chemosensitive, even when metastatic. The 5-year survival rate for treated mediastinal seminoma is 75 percent.

Dysgerminomas (embryonal cell carcinomas) and choriocarcinoma

These are referred to collectively as nonseminomatous germ cell tumors. They are also highly malignant, aggressive tumors. Embryonal cell tumors often elaborate α-fetoprotein, carcinoembryonic antigen, or both, whereas choriocarcinomas usually produce human chorionic gonadotropin. Therefore, these markers may be helpful diagnostically and in following the efficiency of treatment. Recently, intensive cisplatin-based induction chemotherapy has been used to normalize tumor markers before surgical resection of residual tumor. This approach has improved survival rates, i.e., 5-year survival rates approaching 60 percent have been reported in selected cases. The prognosis for nonseminomatous germ cell tumors is less favorable than for seminomas.

Mixed germ cell tumors All of these tumors derive from totipotential germ cells. Therefore, it is not surprising that different histologic patterns often coexist and that metastatic lesions may differ in histologic appearance from the primary neoplasm. Mixed germ cell tumors may have a variety of combinations, e.g., teratoma, embryonal carcinomas, yolk cell tumor, and human chorionic gonadotropin syncytiotrophoblast may exist all in one. As noted above, a combination of embryonal cell carcinoma and a teratoma is called a *teratocarcinoma*.

Endocrine Tumors

The thyroid and parathyroid glands can give rise to mediastinal neoplasms.

Thyroid A cervical goiter is a common lesion of the mediastinum. The great majority arise in the neck and descend into the superior part of the anterior mediastinum, carrying along its blood supply from vessels in the neck. In contrast, a primary mediastinal thyroid neoplasm is exceedingly rare and its blood supply is from thoracic vessels. Although most thoracic goiters are in the anterior mediastinum, a few occur in the posterior mediastinum.

Mediastinal thyroid tumors usually occur in middle-aged or older women. As a rule, they are asymptomatic. However, occasionally they compress airways and vascular structures eliciting one or more of a variety of clinical signs: cough, hoarseness, upper airway obstruction, facial and upper extremity swelling, esophageal compression (dysphagia), and nerve compression (neurologic signs). Most patients are euthyroid. Palpation sometimes reveals a cervical goiter or a mass in the suprasternal notch. Diagnosis of a mediastinal thyroid can be made readily by radionuclide scanning with ^{131}Iodine. If a mediastinal thyroid is found, a cervical thyroid scan is done (along with thyroid function tests) to determine if the mediastinal thyroid is the only functional thyroid tissue in the body. Usually no specific treatment is required unless signs and symptoms caused by compression of adjacent structures calls for resection.

Parathyroid Approximately 5 to 10 percent of all parathyroid adenomas that cause hyperparathyroidism occur in the anterior mediastinum, usually imbedded in the thymus gland to which the inferior parathyroid glands are related embryologically. Because mediastinal parathyroid adenomas are usually active, they are manifest clinically by evidence of excessive secretion of parathormone. Diagnosis can be made by CT scans of the mediastinum, radionuclide scanning, arteriography, and selective sampling of cervical and thyroid veins for parathyroid hormonal levels. Surgical resection is required for a hormonally active mediastinal adenoma. This operation is usually curative, but 10 percent of patients may develop permanent postoperative hypoparathyroidism.

Carcinoids Carcinoid tumors of the mediastinum are usually large, solid, lobulated tumors. Unlike thymomas, they do not undergo cystic degeneration. They are believed to arise from Kulchinsky cells in the thymus. These tumors most commonly occur in men in their 40s who may present with cough, chest pain, or dyspnea. About 50 percent of patients develop endocrine abnormalities including Cushing's syndrome, syndrome of inappropriate antidiuretic hormone secretion (SIADH), or hyperparathyroidism. Mediastinal carcinoids may also be one component of multiple endocrine adenomatosis. Treatment for noninvasive tumors is surgical resection. Invasive carcinoids are usually treated with chemotherapy, radiotherapy, or a combination of the two.

Miscellaneous anterior mediastinal lesions Up to 10 percent of neoplasms that originate in the mediastinum are carcinomas for which no extramediastinal source can be found. These so-called primary carcinomas of the mediastinum typically occur in men in their fourth through sixth decades. They are associated with manifestations of an expanding intrathoracic neoplasm and systemic effects: weight loss, cough, hoarseness, and chest pain. These neoplasms are extremely aggressive and usually unresectable because of either local extension or distant metastases. Histologically, they are poorly differentiated and respond poorly to chemotherapy and radiotherapy.

Mesenchymal elements in the mediastinum may also give rise to tumors in the anterior mediastinum. They include lipomas, fibromas, lymphangiomas, their sarcomatous counterparts, mesotheliomas, and other rare tumors.

Middle Mediastinum

Developmental Cysts

Developmental cysts arise from anomalies of the developing foregut, tracheobronchial tree, and pericardium. They account for approximately 15 percent of primary mediastinal lesions in both the adult and pediatric populations. They are benign, usually asymptomatic, and most often discovered incidentally on the chest radiograph. Pericardial and bronchogenic cysts are the more common mediastinal cysts.

Pericardial cysts Pericardial cysts are believed to arise from remnants of the developing embryonic pericardium. Adults in their fourth and fifth decades are the most frequently affected. For unknown reasons, the right cardiophrenic angle is the most common site for pericardial cysts. Rarely, pericardial cysts are acquired later in life as a sequel of pericarditis or other inflammatory process. Pericardial cysts are usually spherical and unilobular, contain a transudative fluid, and may measure up to 30 cm in diameter. Their radiographic appearance is that of a smooth, well-demarcated, ovoid density. Approximately 10 percent actually communicate with the pericardial space. Definitive diagnosis can sometimes be made on the basis of chest CT. Although the cysts are almost invariably benign, they are usually excised.

Bronchogenic cysts Bronchogenic cysts result from abnormal branching of the tracheobronchial tree during embryogenesis. They are spherical, a few cm in diameter, uni- or multiloculated, and lined by respiratory epithelium. They are usually found on the chest radiograph in adults in their third and fourth decades. Radiographically, bronchogenic cysts appear as round or ovoid masses with sharp borders closely associated with a large airway, often just posterior to the carina. Fluoroscopy may reveal changes in the shape of the cyst related to respiration.

Because of their relationship to airway structures, bronchogenic cysts occasionally produce symptoms such as wheezing and cough; sometimes they cause bronchial stenosis. Communication with an airway produces an air-fluid level in the cyst; secretions may then accumulate in the cul de sac, serving as a good medium for bacterial growth and possibly infection. For this reason, it is advisable to resect these lesions even though they are benign.

Enteric cysts are similar in location and radiographic appearance to bronchogenic cysts, but are lined instead with digestive epithelium. They are much more common in children than adults; they are often associated with vertebral abnormalities.

Noncystic middle mediastinal lesions Adenopathy in the paratracheal, subcarinal, or hilar lymph beds may account for abnormal mediastinal widening on the chest radiograph. The etiology of this adenopathy is usually lymphoma, metastatic cancer, or granulomatous inflammation. Vascular enlargements involving the aorta, pulmonary arteries, superior vena cava, and azygous vein can also present as mediastinal masses, e.g., aneurysms, coarctation of the aorta, and nonspecific dilatations. Although CT and MRI scans may be useful diagnostically, angiography remains the definitive test.

Diaphragmatic hernias of the stomach or intestine through the foramen of Morgagni usually present as a right-sided mass in the cardiophrenic angle. In contrast, diaphragmatic hernias through the foramen of Bochdalek are frequently left sided and in the posterior mediastinum. An air-fluid level on the upright chest radiograph is characteristic of these lesions.

Posterior Mediastinum

Tumors of the posterior mediastinum are almost always either neurogenic or esophageal in origin. Esophageal tumors include leiomyoma, fibroma, lipoma, sarcoma, and carcinoma. Bronchogenic and enteric cysts may also occur in the posterior mediastinum.

Neurogenic tumors may account for more than 20 percent of mediastinal tumors, making them, along with thymomas, one of the more common mediastinal neoplasms. Radiographically, they usually appear in the paravertebral sulcus as well-circumscribed tumors. Approximately one quarter are malignant in adults, one half in children. Many are asymptomatic and are discovered on a routine chest radiograph. However, some patients, especially children, present with the consequences of local growth and compression: cough, chest pain, stridor, or recurrent pneumonias on the one hand, or a variety of neurologic syndromes on the other. For example, the release of catecholamines may occur, not only with pheochromocytomas of the mediastinum, but also with ganglioneuromas and nonchromaffin paragangliomas. Hypoglycemia sometimes accompanies insulin-producing neurilemmomas and neurosarcomas.

Neurogenic tumors can be classified according to their tissue of origin (Table 30-3): peripheral nerve; sympathetic ganglia; or paraganglionic tissue.

TABLE 30-3 Classification of Neurogenic Tumors by Tissue of Origin

Peripheral nerves	Sympathetic ganglia	Paraganglionic tissue
Neurofibroma	Ganglioneuroma	Pheochromocytoma
Neurilemmoma	Ganglioneuroblastoma	Paraganglioma
Neurosarcoma	Neuroblastoma	
	Sympathicoblastoma	

Peripheral nerves Primary neurogenic neoplasms of the mediastinum commonly arise form peripheral nerves. They include neurofibromas, neurilemmomas (or schwannomas), and neurosarcomas.

Neurofibromas often become quite large. They contain both nerve and nerve sheath cells. Their appearance in the mediastinum may be a manifestation of widespread neurofibromatosis (von Recklinghausen's disease); in 10 to 15 percent of such individuals, the tumor may develop into a neurosarcoma.

Neurilemmomas arise exclusively from nerve sheath cells, are well encapsulated, and do not invade other structures. However, they do have a propensity for extending into the intervertebral foramina and assuming a "dumbbell" configuration while compressing the spinal cord. High levels of blood insulin are also associated with this tumor. Neurilemmomas or neurofibromas, especially in generalized neurofibromatosis, undergo malignant degeneration. These neurosarcomas have a poor prognosis.

Sympathetic ganglia Ganglioneuromas are neurogenic tumors that arise from sympathetic ganglia. They include benign ganglioneuromas, which occur primarily in children, and malignant neuroblastomas, ganglioneuroblastomas, and sympatheticoblastomas. These tumors typically elaborate catecholamines resulting in diarrhea, flushing, abdominal distention, palpitations, diaphoresis, hypertension, fever, anorexia, and weight loss.

Paraganglionic tissue This type of tissue, e.g., as found in chemoreceptors, can give rise to pheochromocytomas and paragangliomas (or chemodectomas). Although these tumors are benign in > 95 percent of patients, they may elaborate vasoactive catecholamines resulting in the endocrine syndrome described under sympathetic ganglia. Complete surgical resection is usually curative.

BIBLIOGRAPHY

For a more detailed discussion, see Rosenberg JC, Bowles AL Sr: Nonneoplastic disorders of the mediastinum, in Fishman AP (ed), *Pulmonary*

Diseases and Disorders, 2d ed. New York, McGraw-Hill, 1988, pp 2069–2086.

Lyerly HK, Sabiston DC Jr: Primary neoplasms and cysts of the mediastinum, in Fishman AP (ed), *Pulmonary Diseases and Disorders,* 2d ed. New York, McGraw-Hill, 1988, pp 2087–2116.

Pearson FG (ed): Mediastinal tumors. Sem Thorac Cardiovasc Surg 4:1–70, 1992.

Rice TW: Benign neoplasms and cysts of the mediastinum. Semin Thorac Cardiovasc Surg 4:25–33, 1992.

Alfred P. Fishman

Among the more common nonneoplastic disorders of the mediastinum are acute and chronic infections, mediastinal emphysema, and mediastinal hemorrhage. Each of these entities is considered in turn below.

INFECTIONS OF THE MEDIASTINUM

Acute Mediastinitis

Acute mediastinitis is a fulminant process that can rapidly become life threatening. Causes of acute mediastinitis are listed in Table 31-1. The most common cause is esophageal perforation. Next in incidence is rupture of the trachea or a bronchus. Once an infection gains access to the mediastinum, the mediastinal pleura only affords a temporary barrier to spread into one or both pleural spaces. The pressure gradient from atmosphere to mediastinum also forces air between fascial planes that run between deep cervical compartments and the mediastinum.

Clinical picture Crepitus of the subcutaneous tissues of the upper thorax and neck is usually an early sign, often appearing before chest radiography reveals air in the mediastinum. Sepsis usually becomes manifest within 24 h after perforation. Heart sounds may be distant. A Hamman's sign (a "washing machine" murmur synchronous with the heart beat) may be heard in the upright position.

In some instances, acute mediastinitis gives rise to a localized abscess. Immunosuppressed patients are particularly vulnerable to this complication. Often the localized abscess is visible on the chest radiograph as a circumscribed mass that compresses adjacent structures. Surgical drainage is mandatory.

Chest radiography After esophageal perforation, the mediastinum is widened and air can be seen in the mediastinum. A perforation of the lower esophagus is often associated with a left pleural effusion. The site of perforation can usually be demonstrated by an esophagram using water-soluble contrast material.

Treatment The therapeutic challenge is formidable: combat sepsis and restore hemodynamic stability; vent, debride, and drain the closed space in which an aggressive purulent infection is threatening vital structures; close the communication between esophagus or trachea and the mediastinum; and control the infection. With rare

TABLE 31-1 Causes of Acute Mediastinitis

Causes	Comment
Perforation of esophagus	Most often during endoscopy; also during dilation of esophageal stricture, endotracheal intubation, foreign body, trauma, ruptured suture line
Rupture of esophagus	During violent vomiting (Boerhaave's syndrome)
Infection after median sternotomy	Usual organisms: pseudomonas; staphylococci
Tear of tracheobronchial tree	Usually after chest trauma; occasionally after bronchoscopy
Ulcerating carcinoma of esophagus	May also follow esophageal resection and leaky anastomosis
Oropharyngeal suppuration	Secondary to dental infection and Ludwig's angina; uncommon since antibiotics
Direct extension from lungs or pleura, chest cage, vertebrae	Rare

SOURCE: Modified after Table 133-2 of Rosenberg JC, Bowles AL Sr.

exception (see below), prompt surgical intervention is essential to close the communication between the perforated viscus and the mediastinum and to decompress and drain the mediastinum. The mortality rate for those operated on within 24 h is about 6 percent; after 24 h, the mortality is of the order of 9-fold greater. Before surgical intervention, supportive measures, i.e., fluids, are given intravenously to counter hemodynamic instability and shock. Because the organisms are often a mix of gram-positive and gram-negative aerobic and anaerobic organisms, antibiotic coverage is broad, e.g., penicillin and an aminoglycoside in full dosage. In patients who survive, recovery is usually complete.

Not all patients with acute mediastinitis require surgical intervention. For example, a small esophageal perforation may close spontaneously in response to antibiotics and supportive measures. In contrast, a large esophageal tear, brought on by vomiting, almost invariably requires surgical intervention to close the communication.

One infrequent but troublesome complication of median sternotomy is infection with atypical mycobacteria, i.e., *Mycobacterium chelonei* and *Mycobacterium fortuitum*. The infection is manifested by failure of the wound to heal and continued drainage from the incision site. As a rule, these infections are much more indolent than those caused by a perforated viscus. Treatment consists of antituberculous therapy (isoniazid, rifampin, and ethambutol) in conjunction with debridement.

A rare cause of acute mediastinitis is anthrax. If not promptly recognized and treated, the mediastinal infection spreads hematogenously to become widespread and life threatening. Cardinal clues are a relevant history of exposure and widening of the mediastinum on the chest radiograph. Early antibiotic treatment, e.g., penicillin or tetracycline, can be lifesaving.

Chronic Mediastinal Infections

An uncommon cause of chronic mediastinitis is delayed, or inadequately treated, acute mediastinitis. A common cause of chronic mediastinitis is *granulomatous inflammation* of the mediastinal lymph nodes, particularly tuberculosis or histoplasmosis. A third, and much more unusual, form of chronic mediastinitis is *idiopathic fibrosing mediastinitis.* Chronic mediastinal infections are usually clinically silent until they cause obstruction of a mediastinal structure, e.g., esophagus, airway, or superior vena cava.

Granulomatous Inflammation of the Mediastinal Lymph Nodes

Chronic granulomatous inflammation of mediastinal lymph nodes, especially that due to histoplasmosis or tuberculosis can be sorted into three related, and often sequential, categories: *mediastinal granulomatous adenitis, mediastinal granuloma,* and *mediastinal fibrosis.*

Mediastinal granulomatous adenitis This category is exemplified by the Ghon complex of primary tuberculosis in which mediastinal granulomatous adenitis accompanies granulomatous infection of the lungs. The lymphadenitis is confined to the affected lymph nodes and does not involve adjacent mediastinal structures. Histoplasmosis and coccidioidomycosis can give rise to a similar primary infection. In addition to fungal infections (including *Actinomyces, Nocardia,* and *Aspergillus* as well as *Histoplasma*), mediastinal granulomatous adenitis may be part of sarcoidosos. It may also be a consequence of neoplastic invasion or of a drug reaction, e.g., methysergide.

As a rule, the enlarged nodes cause no symptoms except for a "brassy" cough. Uncommonly, enlarged nodes obstruct a bronchus leading to distal infection and bronchiectasis. The bronchus to the right middle lobe is particularly vulnerable because of a collar of lymph nodes. Obstruction due to infection and swelling of these nodes can cause recurrent pneumonias of the right middle lobe, partial collapse of the lobe, and bronchiectasis. Occasionally, a calcified node breaks into the bronchus and may be expectorated as a broncholith.

Mediastinal granuloma This category is distinguished from *mediastinal granulomatous adenitis* by the presence of an encapsulated fibrous mass around caseating lymph nodes. The fibrous mass represents extension of the granulomatous inflammatory process into surrounding tissue (a periadenitis) while the core of the lesion undergoes caseation necrosis. As a result of the invasive periadenitis, adjacent structures are involved, directly or indirectly, in the inflammatory process, resulting in distortions, scarring, and the formation of masses. For example, involvement of the esophagus can give rise to a traction diverticulum. Also, a fibrotic reaction in the right paratracheal area can obstruct the superior vena cava. The airways are less susceptible to distortion and obstruction because of their cartilaginous backbones.

Medical treatment, except in the case of tuberculosis, has little to offer. Surgical exploration discloses the etiology in about two thirds of patients with mediastinal granuloma. Antifungal agents, such as amphotericin B, have no proven value in infection with *Histoplasma capsulatum.* Steroids run the risk of disseminating the infection.

Mediastinal fibrosis Histoplasmosis is the most common cause of this entity. By a process of continuing periadenitis, mediastinal structures undergo progressive scarring and contraction ("sclerosing mediastinitis").

Clinical syndromes resulting from granulomatous inflammation of the mediastinal lymph nodes Distinctive clinical syndromes can result from compression, invasion, distortion, or entrapment of mediastinal structures. Among the more common syndromes are superior vena caval obstruction (much more rarely due to granulomatous inflammation than to carcinoma of the lung), bronchial obstruction (a cause of the right middle lobe syndrome), pulmonary venous obstruction (the clinical picture resembles mitral stenosis), and pulmonary arterial obstruction (more common in mediastinal histoplasmoma than in other causes of mediastinal fibrosis).

Idiopathic Fibrosing Mediastinitis

Idiopathic fibrosing mediastinitis resembles retroperitoneal fibrosis. Lymphatic obstruction by the fibrosis seems to set up a viscious cycle in which the obstruction causes transudation of protein-rich lymph fluid which, in turn, stimulates further proliferation of fibrous tissue. In contrast to the granulomatous inflammatory processes, the fibrosis does not invade, compress, or distort adjacent tissues. Instead, the fibrosis is usually localized to the periaortic areas. Occasionally, it may extend upward, along the aorta, to trap the superior vena cava or a tributary.

MEDIASTINAL EMPHYSEMA (PNEUMOMEDIASTINUM)

Air gains access to the mediastinum through (1) an esophageal perforation or tear; (2) a tracheobronchial perforation or tear; or (3) an alveolar rupture that allows alveolar air to make its way

TABLE 31-2 Common Causes of Pseudomediastinum

Alveolar tear due to chest compression, coughing, straining
Complication of pulmonary disease
Barotrauma by mechanical ventilation
Perforation of the esophagus
Rupture of tracheobronchial tree
Dental extractions
Improper ascent from deep dive

SOURCE: Modified after Table 133-5 of Rosenberg JC, Bowles AL Sr.

toward a surface of the lung via a peribronchovascular sheath. Frequently, mediastinal emphysema is accompanied by a pneumothorax, unilateral or bilateral, or subcutaneous emphysema (see Chapter 55).

Mediastinal emphysema can be triggered in a variety of ways (Table 31-2). Symptoms are generally absent or mild unless considerable air is pumped into the mediastinum. The increased pressure may elicit severe pericardial pain indistinguishable from that of myocardial infarction or compress blood vessels in the deep cervical fascia. Crepitation may be palpable in the suprasternal notch often in association with subcutaneous emphysema. Hamman's sign may be heard. The chest radiograph, particularly the left lateral view, shows air in the mediastinum.

Treatment is unnecessary unless pain and dyspnea are severe and evidence appears of hemodynamic compromise. Needle aspiration may relieve the manifestations. Occasionally, mediastinotomy, involving an incision above the suprasternal notch (as for tracheotomy), may be required.

MEDIASTINAL HEMORRHAGE

Bleeding into the mediastinum is the result of rupture of a major blood vessel. A common cause is blunt or penetrating trauma to the chest. Frequently, the cause is iatrogenic, e.g., catheterization of a subclavian vein. Other causes include coagulopathies, uremia, neoplasia, and dissecting aneurysm. Bleeding into the mediastinum is manifested by radiographic evidence of acute mediastinal widening.

As a rule, venous bleeding is without symptoms and stops spontaneously. However, a large hemorrhage can cause dyspnea and substernal pain. The patient prefers to sit upright. If cardiorespiratory compromise is threatening, blood can be aspirated at the level of the suprasternal notch. A thoracotomy is only done if the situation becomes life threatening.

BIBLIOGRAPHY

For a more detailed discussion, see Rosenberg JC, Bowles AL Sr: Nonneoplastic disorders of the mediastinum, in Fishman AP (ed), *Pulmonary*

Diseases and Disorders, 2d ed. New York, McGraw-Hill, 1988, pp 2069–2086.

Byl B, Jacobs F, Antoine M, Depierreux M, Serruys E, Primo G, Thys JP: Mediastinitis caused by *Aspergillus fumigatus* with ruptured aortic pseudoaneurysm in a heart transplant recipient: Case study. Heart Lung 22:145–147, 1993.

Dunn EJ, Ulicny KS Jr, Wright CB, Gottesman L: Surgical implications of sclerosing mediastinitis. A report of six cases and review of the literature. Chest 97:338–346, 1990.

Gregory SA, Grippi MA: The clinical diagnosis of drug-induced pulmonary disorders. J Thorac Imaging 6:8–18, 1991.

Lyerly HK, Sabiston DC Jr: Primary neoplasms and cysts of the mediastinum, in Fishman AP (ed), *Pulmonary Diseases and Disorders,* 2d ed. New York, McGraw-Hill, 1988, pp 2087–2114.

Smith BA, Ferguson DB: Disposition of spontaneous pneumomediastinum. Am J Emerg Med 9:256–259, 1991.

Sridhar KS, Hussein AM, Patten JE: Spontaneous pneumomediastinum in esophageal carcinoma. Am J Clin Oncol 13:527–531, 1990.

Wheatley MJ, Stirling MC, Kirsh MM, Gago O, Orringer MB: Descending necrotizing mediastinitis: Transcervical drainage is not enough. Ann Thorac Surg 49:780–784, 1990.

Robert Walker

Normally, the pleural spaces are moist with no detectable free fluid on either physical examination or chest radiography. A pleural effusion represents excess and evident fluid in the pleural space. Regardless of etiology, pleural effusions manifest certain diagnostic features, especially when large. For example, in moderate to large effusions, dyspnea is a common complaint and physical findings are distinctive.

For proper management, two diagnostic elements are essential: (1) identification of etiology; and (2) distinction between transudate and exudate. Fortunately, the distinction can usually be made by applying a few criteria (Table 32-1).

TRANSUDATES

Definition

A *transudate* is an ultrafiltrate of plasma. It is highly fluid, low in protein, and virtually devoid of inflammatory cells or formed cell elements. It can be distinguished from an exudate on the basis of protein and lactose dehydrogenase (LDH) concentrations listed in Table 32-1.

Etiologies

The common causes of transudates are listed in Table 32-2.

Pathophysiology

Transudates have one physiologic feature in common: an upset in the balance of forces in Starling's law of transcapillary exchange. These include hydrostatic and oncotic pressures within the pleural capillaries on the one hand, and within the pleural space(s) on the other; and pleural capillary permeability. Among the forces commonly affected that lead to transudates are abnormally high pleural capillary pressures, as in congestive heart failure; abnormally low intrapleural pressures, as in stiff lungs; and abnormally low capillary oncotic pressure due to hypoalbuminemia as in nephrosis or hepatic cirrhosis.

Pulmonary mechanics and gas exchange are little affected by a pleural effusion until it is large enough to compress appreciable amounts of underlying pulmonary parenchyma. At this juncture, lung volumes begin to decrease, dyspnea appears on exertion, a restrictive pattern is found on pulmonary function testing, and hypoxemia results from ventilation-perfusion inhomogeneities.

TABLE 32-1 Transudates versus Exudates

Measurement	Transudate	Exudate
Pleural fluid: Serum protein ratio	< 0.5	> 0.5
Pleural fluid: Serum LDH ratio	< 0.6	> 0.6
LDH concentration	< ⅔ upper limit of normal for serum	> ⅔ upper limit of normal for serum

LDH = lactic dehydrogenase

TABLE 32-2 Common Causes of Transudative Effusions

Cause	Comment
Congestive heart failure	Causes > 70% of transudates
Nephrotic syndrome	Hypoalbuminemia is important factor
Hepatic cirrhosis	Hypoalbuminemia is important factor
Ascites	Fluid crosses diaphragm via defects or lymphatics
Peritoneal dialysis	Fluid crosses diaphragm via defects or lymphatics
Urinary tract obstruction	Urothorax via peritoneum either across diaphragm or via retroperitoneal dissections
Meigs' syndrome	Benign ovarian tumor, ascites, and pleural effusion (usually right sided)

Dyspnea in patients with pleural effusion is rarely due to hypoxemia. Instead, it stems from abnormal mechanics of breathing; enlargement of the thoracic cage by the effusion causes breathing to occur at a less favorable position than normal on the thoracic length-tension curve, thereby compromising the efficiency of breathing and increasing the work (and oxygen cost) of breathing.

Clinical Manifestations

Patients with small transudative pleural effusions are more apt to have symptoms arising from the underlying disease than from the effusion. For example, in heart failure, dyspnea on exertion and orthopnea usually stem from congested lungs. Also, in patients with cirrhosis and ascites, pleural manifestations are generally minor compared to the symptoms of hepatic disease. Pleural effusions in congestive heart failure tend to be right sided or bilateral. In patients with the nephrotic syndrome, effusions tend to be bilateral and equal in size. A large pleural effusion sometimes follows peritoneal dialysis: it usually occurs on the right side, within 48 h after the start of dialysis and is accompanied by marked dyspnea. The effusion is due to passage of dialysate across the diaphragm, from the peritoneal cavity into the pleural space.

Pleural effusions < 300 ml are difficult to detect on physical examination.

Usual Diagnostic Tests

Chest radiography Not only the conventional posteroanterior (PA) and lateral views, but also the decubitus projection may be helpful in delineating and quantifying a suspected pleural effusion. Early in the accumulation of pleural fluid (up to about 100 ml), blunting of the costophrenic angle on the lateral chest radiograph may reveal the presence of excess fluid. Larger amounts (on the order of 200 ml) become visible as blunting of the costophrenic angle on the PA view. Still larger amounts obscure the boundary between diaphragm and overlying lung while a broad-sweeping meniscus outlines the top of the effusion. Lateral decubitus views are helpful in demonstrating the redistribution of the transudate under the influence of gravity and provide a picture of the underlying lung.

Because of the free-flowing nature of a transudate, more sophisticated radiographic examinations are rarely needed. Ultrasound is occasionally helpful in localizing loculated fluids, e.g., in a fissure, and in guiding the thoracentesis needle. Computed tomography (CT) is of more value in dealing with exudates than transudates.

Thoracentesis

Noninvasive tests will not distinguish a transudate from an exudate. Nearly all patients with a significant amount of free pleural fluid should undergo a diagnostic thoracentesis. One exception to this rule is the patient in overt congestive heart failure.

On gross inspection, transudates are clear or have a slightly yellow tint, whereas exudates are generally more turbid and deeper in color. In cirrhosis, the pleural fluid may be blood tinged or even frankly bloody, possibly due to an associated coagulopathy.

If the LDH and protein concentrations indicate that the effusion is a transudate (see Table 32-1), no further evaluation of the fluid need be done, and attention should be turned to treatment of the underlying condition.

Natural History and Prognosis

Most transudative effusions resolve if the underlying medical condition is managed successfully. In an occasional patient, the transudate is refractory to therapy and may require specific therapy directed at the effusion (see below). A small number of transudative effusions may become secondarily infected, either by extension from another site, or by contamination during the thoracentesis. A previously evaluated transudate that increases in size despite medical therapy of the underlying disorder or that becomes associated with localized pain or fever, warrants a second diagnostic thoracentesis to rule out a superimposed process.

EXUDATES

Definition

An exudate is caused by increased permeability of the microcirculatory vessels, i.e., capillaries, arterioles, and venules. The vessels usually become "leaky." An exudate differs from a transudate in that it is rich in protein, cells, and cellular debris. Its distinctive features are listed in Table 32-1.

Etiology

The common causes of nonneoplastic exudative effusions are listed in Table 32-3. Most exudates are associated with pulmonary infections. But a variety of other intrathoracic, abdominal, and systemic disorders may also lead to the formation of exudates.

PARAPNEUMONIC EFFUSIONS AND EMPYEMA

Definition

A *parapneumonic effusion* is a sterile exudate associated with an inflammatory focus in the lung, usually bacterial pneumonia, abscess, or bronchiectasis.

    Empyema refers either to pus in the pleural space or to an exudate that contains organisms on Gram stain. Most empyemas are parapneumonic in origin. However, 25 percent follow surgery or trauma; 10 percent occur without evident cause; some are subdiaphragmatic in origin.

    Three stages have been described in the evolution of an empyema: (1) the *exudative* stage, characterized by a sterile, free-flowing effusion; (2) the *fibropurulent* stage, characterized by an increasing

TABLE 32-3 Common Causes of Nonneoplastic Exudative Effusions

Parapneumonic effusions
Empyema
Tuberculous pleurisy
Gastrointestinal process, e.g., esophageal perforation, pancreatitis, abdominal abscesses, surgery
Collagen vascular disease
Postcardiac injury syndrome
Pulmonary embolism
Benign asbestos effusion
Chylothorax
Hemothorax

volume of fluid that contains bacteria, polymorphonuclear leukocytes and cellular debris; pleural fluid pH and the concentration of
glucose levels are low, and the concentration of LDH is abnormally
high. Loculation begins; and (3) the *organizing phase,* is marked by
the formation of a pleural peel that entraps the lung preventing it
from full expansion.

Etiology

Parapneumonic effusions occur in 40 to 60 percent of all cases of
pneumococcal and staphylococcal pneumonia. However, in patients
with pneumococcal pneumonia, the effusions are almost always
sterile (> 95 percent) whereas in staphylococcal pneumonia, cultures
are positive. *Haemophilus* flu, *Escherichia coli,* and *Pseudomona*
organisms are responsible for > 70 percent of all culture-positive
gram-negative effusions. Pleural effusion occurs in 50 percent of
patients with *Legionella* pneumonia.

Empyemas are often polymicrobial anaerobic (35 percent) or
mixed aerobic/anaerobic (40 percent). In patients younger than 18
years of age, coagulase-positive staphylococcus is the predominant
causative organism. Ten to 20 percent of empyemas are culture
negative despite repeated attempts to isolate organisms.

Clinical Manifestations of Parapneumonic Effusions and Empyema

The clinical manifestations of a parapneumonic effusion depend
heavily on the source of the infection and the infecting organism.
For example, a parapneumonic effusion in association with an
underlying aerobic infection presents clinically as an aerobic bacterial pneumonia. In contrast, an anaerobic bacterial infection of the
pleural space usually is more insidious in onset, e.g., loss of weight,
and is likely to occur in an individual with poor dentition, a history
of chronic alcoholism, and often an episode that predisposes to
aspiration, e.g., a period of unconsciousness.

An empyema is a parapneumonic effusion with positive bacterial
cultures as well as a considerable increase in white blood cells, e.g.,
> 15,000 wbc/mm³. Empyema is not infrequent after pneumonec-
tomy. If the empyema *does not* communicate with the airways, the
signs are those of pus in a closed cavity, i.e., fever, systemic toxicity.
If the empyema *does* communicate via a bronchopleural fistula,
systemic toxicity is apt to be minimal but pleural fluid is expectorated and an air-fluid level can be seen on the chest radiograph.

Usual Diagnostic Tests

The initial evaluation of a pleural effusion should include PA and
lateral chest radiographs. If blunting of a costophrenic angle is seen

on either view, a decubitus film is in order; if the distance between the chest wall and the lung is < about 1 cm, the effusion is probably of no grave concern, i.e., it can be expected to resolve in response to antibiotic therapy. However, if this distance is > about 1 cm, diagnostic thoracentesis should be done and the fluid evaluated for color, turbidity, and odor; the concentrations of protein, LDH, glucose, and amylase; cell count and differential; Gram stain; and cultures, including aerobic, anaerobic, fungal, and mycobacterial.

Ultrasound is sometimes helpful in detecting loculations of fluid or pus or pleural thickening; it is sometimes helpful in directing thoracentesis. In some instances, fiberoptic bronchoscopy and CT help to uncover related endobronchial or peribronchial disease that is causing postobstructive pneumonia complicated by pleural effusion.

Considerable effort is warranted to identify the bacteria responsible for the underlying pneumonia and the pleural effusion. Gram stain of the sputum and culture are an important first step. If the chest radiograph identifies an infiltrate and the patient cannot expectorate spontaneously, sputum induction, using aerosolized hypertonic saline, can be tried. If these procedures are unsuccessful, transthoracic needle aspiration or bronchoscopy may be rewarding.

Treatment

Antibiotics and adequate drainage of infected fluid are the mainstays of therapy. The initial choice of antibiotics is guided by Gram stains of the sputum and of the empyema fluid.

If thoracentesis reveals pus or if the pleural fluid gram stain is positive, a chest tube is placed immediately. In the absence of gross pus or positive Gram stain, the decision about placing a chest tube is based on the pleural fluid pH and the concentrations of glucose, and LDH. For example, drainage is not required if the pH is > 7.20, glucose is > 40 mg/dl, and LDH is < 1000 IU/L; 90 percent of these effusions will resolve in response to antibiotics alone. Conversely, if the pH is < 7.0 or the glucose is < 40 mg/dl, then the effusion is a "complicated effusion" and warrants immediate chest tube drainage. If the results fall between these limits, thoracentesis is repeated every 12 to 24 h until a pattern evolves on which to base management.

For chest tube drainage, a large-caliber tube is placed in the dependent part of the effusion and connected to underwater seal or suction. If clinical or radiographic improvement fails to occur after 48 h of drainage, the tube position and antibiotic regimen have to be reviewed. A chest ultrasound examination is helpful in finding loculations that do not communicate with the tube; if one or more loculations are found, additional chest tubes or surgical intervention may be required. The chest tube is removed when the following criteria are met: control of infection and absence of fever, < 100 ml of chest tube drainage per day, re-expansion of the lung, and closure of a preexisting bronchopleural fistula.

Approximately 20 to 30 percent of patients fail to respond to antibiotics and closed chest drainage as manifested by persistent fever and continued purulent drainage. In these individuals, the therapeutic options include the intrapleural installation of fibrinolytic agents, e.g., streptokinase, leaving the chest tube in place; chronic open drainage which entails rib resection and the creation of a skin-lined tract (Eloesser flap); and decortication of the lung, a major surgical procedure with high mortality (10 to 50 percent).

BIBLIOGRAPHY

For a more detailed discussion, see Winterbauer RH: Nonneoplastic pleural effusions, in Fishman AP (ed), *Pulmonary Diseases and Disorders,* 2d ed. New York, McGraw-Hill, 1988, pp 2139–2157.

Henschke Cl, Davis SD, Romano PM, Yankelevitz DF: The pathogenesis, radiologic evaluation, and therapy of pleural effusions. Radiol Clin North Am 27:1241–1255, 1989.

Hughes CE, Van Scoy RE: Antibiotic therapy of pleural empyema. Semin Respir Infect 6:94–102, 1991.

Kendall SW, Bryan AJ, Large SR, Wells FC: Pleural effusions: Is thoracoscopy a reliable investigation? A retrospective review. Respir Med 86:437–440, 1992.

Light RW: Pleural diseases. Dis Mon 38:261–331, 1992.

McLoud TC, Flower CD: Imaging the pleura: Sonography, CT, and MR imaging. AJR Am J Roentgenol 156:1145–1153, 1991.

Strange C, Sahn SA: The clinician's perspective on parapneumonic effusions and empyema. Chest 103:259–261, 1993.

Paul Richman

As a cause of exudative pleural effusions, those due to neoplasms (malignant pleural effusions) are seen less frequently than parapneumonic effusions. A small number of histologic types account for the bulk of neoplastic pleural effusions: adenocarcinomas from different sites, especially the lung and breast, account for about 50 percent of neoplastic pleural effusions; lymphomas are next in frequency. In up to 10 percent, the primary site of the neoplasm escapes detection.

PATHOPHYSIOLOGY

Ninety percent of malignant effusions are exudative. A bloody pleural exudate in a patient with a known adenocarcinoma, e.g., breast, lung, or ovary, almost always signifies metastatic tumor implants on the pleura, implying advanced (stage IV) disease. However, in a patient who is known to have a carcinoma, a pleural exudate need not be a sign of metastasis. For example, in primary carcinoma of the lung that obstructs a bronchus, the distal lung is often atelectatic, leading to abnormally low pleural pressures and accumulation of pleural fluid. Other nonmetastatic causes of pleural effusion in patients with cancer include pulmonary embolism and parapneumonic effusions.

In 5 to 10 percent of patients with malignant lymphoma, a pleural effusion is present at the time of diagnosis. However, in only 25 percent of patients with Hodgkin's disease can malignant cells be demonstrated in the pleural fluid. In these patients, the effusions are presumably due to enlargement of mediastinal lymph nodes that obstruct pleural lymphatic drainage. In contrast, the yield in non-Hodgkin's lymphoma is much greater: malignant cells are obtained 75 percent of the time on thoracentesis because the neoplasm infiltrates the pleura directly. Frequently, a pleural effusion due to a lymphoma is chylous secondary to obstruction of the thoracic duct by the neoplasm.

CLINICAL MANIFESTATIONS

Dyspnea is the most common presenting complaint. It occurs in 50 percent of patients with a malignant pleural effusion. Gnawing chest pain occurs less often (25 percent); some patients describe a sense of something "moving around" in the chest.

Physical examination reveals evidence of pleural fluid, generally on one side. Usually, a pleural friction rub is not heard. Occasionally localized chest pain can be elicited, indicating chest wall involvement, e.g., invasion of a rib by the neoplasm. A chest radiograph reveals the effusion, which may be small or large enough to opacify an entire hemithorax. When the chest radiograph shows ipsilateral loss of lung volume, and the mediastinum is pulled toward the effusion, the primary tumor is almost certainly a lung carcinoma that is obstructing a bronchus.

ROUTINE DIAGNOSTIC STUDIES

To prove that a pleural effusion is neoplastic, malignant cells must be demonstrated either by cytologic examination of the pleural fluid, or by histologic examination of the pleura.

Thoracentesis is diagnostic 40 to 80 percent of the time, revealing malignant cells in the pleural fluid. The diagnostic yield is greater when either a large volume of fluid or multiple specimens are obtained. Closed needle biopsy of the pleura combined with pleural fluid cytology increases the diagnostic yield to 67 to 90 percent.

The composition of the pleural fluid is that of an exudate, but the findings are nonspecific: the concentration of lactate dehydrogenase (LDH) in the pleural fluid is abnormally high, usually > 12 μkat/L. The pH and glucose concentration act in parallel. A pH < 7.30 and a glucose concentration < 60 mg/dl are signs of extensive pleural involvement and such values generally accompany positive cytology. These low values suggest that the disease is in a preterminal stage with little likelihood of successful tetracycline pleurodesis. Chromosomal analysis of pleural fluid cells to look for polyploidy and aberrant chromosomal structure is recommended by some, especially in those patients in whom the fluid cytology is benign but in whom lymphoma or mesothelioma is suspected on clinical grounds.

FURTHER DIAGNOSTIC EVALUATION

Occasionally, despite a high level of clinical suspicion that the patient has a treatable malignancy, e.g., Hodgkin's disease, two serial thoracenteses with pleural biopsy fail to confirm the diagnosis. A surgical pleural biopsy, either by thoracoscopy or thoracotomy is then in order. If the diagnosis of malignancy is not established but the patient has a positive purified protein derivative skin test, it is advisable to treat for active tuberculosis while the acid-fast bacilli cultures of pleural biopsy specimens are pending. When a less treatable form of malignancy is suspected, less invasive screening examinations may suffice. Notable among this group are adenocarcinomas that metastasize to pleura.

TREATMENT

In patients in whom the primary malignancy can be treated with systemic chemotherapy, the chemotherapy frequency controls the effusion. However, chemotherapy is often not feasible. In some patients, severe dyspnea is relieved by drainage thoracentesis only to recur when the fluid reaccumulates; in others, removal of even modest quantities of pleural fluid affords temporary relief. If fluid reaccumulates, chemical pleurodesis may be advisable (see Chapter 35). Unfortunately, one requirement for successful chemical pleurodesis is that the pleural space be completely drained to enable apposition of the visceral and parietal pleura. This is particularly difficult to achieve in patients with multiloculated effusions and in patients in whom an obstructing bronchial carcinoma causes pulmonary atelectasis. In patients carefully selected to satisfy the criteria for successful pleurodesis, the success rate is 75 to 85 percent.

Radiation therapy is ineffective in treating malignant pleural implants, but it occasionally can shrink mediastinal lymph nodes that have interrupted the thoracic duct. In one series of such patients with chylothorax due to mediastinal carcinoma, radiation was effective in 50 percent. Because the patient with untreatable cancer metastatic to the pleura will have a short survival, aggressive procedures are only justified for relief of distressing symptoms.

BIBLIOGRAPHY

For a more detailed discussion, see Sahn SA: Malignant pleural effusions, in Fishman AP (ed), *Pulmonary Diseases and Disorders,* 2d ed. New York, McGraw-Hill, 1988, pp 2159–2170.

Keller SM: Current and future therapy for malignant pleural effusion. Chest 103 (1 Suppl):63S–67S, 1993.

Light RW: Pleural diseases. Dis Mon 38:261–331, 1992.

Sahn SA, Good JT: Pleural pH in malignant effusions. Ann Intern Med 108:345–349, 1988.

Alfred P. Fishman

Normally, the pleural space is gas free. Pneumothorax simply signifies gas in the pleural space. Air can gain entrance into the pleural space in one of three ways: (1) by way of the airways and alveoli via a tear in the visceral pleura; (2) by way of the chest wall, diaphragm, mediastinum, or esophagus, e.g., after perforating chest trauma; or (3) from gas-producing microorganisms in the pleural space.

High transpulmonary pressures are usually involved in the pathogenesis of a pneumothorax. Under normal circumstances, pleural pressures are negative, ranging from -3 to -5 cmH$_2$O. Peak negativity is reached at end-inspiration. Entry of air into the pleural space raises intrapleural pressures toward atmospheric; the lung collapses because of its natural elastic recoil. A *tension pneumothorax* results when the accumulation of air in the pleural space causes pleural pressures to exceed atmospheric, as by a flap-valve that opens during coughing or positive pressure breathing. High intrapleural pressures, i.e., > 15 to 20 cmH$_2$O, displace the mediastinum into the contralateral chest and impede systemic venous return to the thorax.

SPONTANEOUS PNEUMOTHORAX

Distinction is made between a *primary* (simple) spontaneous pneumothorax, which is usually a benign condition that occurs in individuals who are otherwise healthy, and *secondary* (complicated) spontaneous pneumothorax, which occurs in patients with underlying pulmonary disease and is generally much more serious and occasionally life threatening.

Primary (Simple) Spontaneous Pneumothorax

This disease occurs predominantly in young men between 20 and 35 years of age. As a rule, the affected individuals are tall, slender, and otherwise healthy.

Etiology and pathogenesis The usual cause of this type of pneumothorax is the rupture of a bleb or cyst in an upper lobe near the apex. This preferential location is generally attributed to the formation of blebs as a result of more negative pleural pressures at the apexes of the lungs than at the bases. About 25 to 30 percent of these individuals will experience one or more recurrences, the great majority on the same side, but not infrequently on the opposite side. Intervals between recurrence are also variable, on the average between 1.5 and 2.5 years. Each occurrence favors subsequent recurrence. Cigarette smoking is strongly related to the occurrence of primary spontaneous pneumothorax.

Physiologic consequences The effects of a pneumothorax depend on its volume and the degree to which it raises intrapleural pressures. In a normal individual, a small pneumothorax, e.g., which raises pleural pressure from -5 cmH$_2$O to -2.5 cmH$_2$O is well tolerated even though pulmonary function tests become abnormal: the vital capacity and the arterial P$_{O_2}$ decrease and the alveolar-arterial difference in P$_{O_2}$ (AaΔP$_{O_2}$) widens. In contrast, in the patient with secondary spontaneous pneumothorax, even a modest pneumothorax often precipitates respiratory failure.

Clinical manifestations The onset is usually at rest with pain, dyspnea, and cough. The pain lessens as air accumulates and separates the pleural surfaces. In some patients, the only complaint is malaise, so that visit to a physician is delayed.

Physical examination reveals an enlarged hemithorax and diminished excursion on the affected side along with diminished breath sounds and tactile fremitus. A large pneumothorax is generally associated with increased resonance on the affected side.

The chest radiograph is diagnostic; it reveals a partially collapsed lung outlined by the visceral pleural line. Frequently, a small pneumothorax may be visualized only on a chest radiograph made during a forced expiration or in the lateral decubitus position. In some instances, a small amount of fluid, often but not invariably blood, may be seen. A tension pneumothorax is suggested by a mediastinal shift toward the unaffected side. The chest radiograph is often used to estimate the volume of the pneumothorax by relating the volume of the collapsed lung to the volume of the hemithorax. However, even in the hands of experts, this approach is far from infallible.

The electrocardiogram, often taken because of chest pain, shows changes (rightward shift of the QRS axis, decreases in voltage and inversion of T waves across the pericardium) that can be misinterpreted as a subendocardial myocardial infarction.

Management How the pneumothorax is handled depends on its size and course. A small pneumothorax (< 10 to 20 percent of the hemithorax on the chest radiograph) in an asymptomatic patient generally needs no intervention because the air can be expected to resorb in 1 to 2 weeks. Breathing of O$_2$-enriched air hastens the rate at which the pneumothorax is absorbed.

Larger pneumothoraxes require aspiration. The choice is between needle aspiration or a chest tube (tube thoracostomy). Needle aspiration is tried first; a 16-gauge needle is used to introduce a polyethylene catheter into the pleural space. If large volumes, e.g., 4 to 5 L are withdrawn from the pleural space without encountering resistance, aspiration is discontinued, and a chest tube is placed. The chest tube is connected to an underwater seal or a flutter valve. A chest tube is also called for in patients with tension pneumothorax or in those who are very symptomatic. The tube is left in place for a few days, generally for 24 h after the lung has fully re-expanded, and there is no evidence of air leak.

About 40 percent of patients with primary spontaneous pneumothorax experience a recurrence after treatment either without intervention or by tube thoracostomy. Therefore, a *sclerosing agent* to prevent recurrence, is being used increasingly as part of management. Of the various agents that have been tried, tetracycline seems to be the most effective. Unfortunately, introduction of tetracycline into the pleural space is extremely painful. Xylocaine, 250 mg injected intrapleurally, and parenteral analgesics are administered to blunt the pain. The patient is positioned to promote contact between the tetracycline (20 mg/kg) and the apical pleura.

Open thoracotomy is considered as a last resort, i.e., if the air leak persists or if the lung fails to re-expand after 5 days of chest tube drainage. It is also indicated in the patient with recurrent pneumothorax after pleural instillation of tetracycline. This procedure permits oversewing of the air leak (usually apical pleural blebs) and scarification of the pleura. Although this procedure is almost uniformly successful in eliminating the air leak and in preventing recurrence, it does entail major surgery for a disorder that rarely causes death and from which 50 percent have no recurrence after the initial episode.

Thoracoscopic examination and treatment have, at some clinics, virtually replaced open thoracotomy for persistent air leaks. It enables elimination of pleural blebs and bullae, pleurectomy, or the introduction of a sclerosing agent to effect pleurodesis. This intervention is much less traumatic than open thoracotomy and is becoming increasingly popular at centers where thoracoscopy is practiced.

Secondary (Complicated) Spontaneous Pneumothorax

This type of pneumothorax occurs in patients with underlying pulmonary disease. It is more threatening than primary spontaneous pneumothorax because it compromises further pulmonary function that is subnormal to begin with.

Etiology and pathogenesis The most common underlying pulmonary disease is chronic obstructive pulmonary disease (COPD). In addition to COPD, secondary spontaneous pneumothorax can be a complication of interstitial fibrosis, sarcoidosis, cystic fibrosis, and a bevy of less common lung diseases, many of which are characterized by widespread interstitial fibrosis. In addition, secondary pneumothorax occurs in patients with a variety of neoplasms, infections, and the adult respiratory distress syndrome. On rare occasion, it can complicate endometriosis (catamenial pneumothorax).

In the patient with acquired immunodeficiency syndrome, *Pneumocystis carinii* pneumonia is the most likely cause. It does so by rupturing pneumatoceles or foci of pulmonary necrosis. Sometimes, the cause is iatrogenic, i.e., in the course of transbronchial biopsy or bronchoalveolar lavage. Occasionally, it is precipitated by strong coughing in the course of treatment with aerosolized pentamidine.

Physiologic consequences Because of the underlying lung disease, physiologic derangements in secondary spontaneous pneumothorax are generally severe and often life threatening. Arterial hypoxemia and hypercapnia are generally marked.

Clinical features Although these vary somewhat with the underlying disease, respiratory distress is the rule and clinical deterioration is rapid.

Dyspnea generally increases markedly, usually accompanied by chest pain on the affected side. Sudden death may occur before chest tubes can be placed. Respiratory failure can occur within hours after the tubes are inserted. Massive gastrointestinal bleeding is another complication. The mortality rate associated with secondary spontaneous pneumothorax is high, i.e., about 15 percent. The recurrence rate for secondary spontaneous pneumothorax is about the same as for primary, about 40 to 50 percent.

Chest radiography usually clinches the diagnosis. However, in contrast to primary spontaneous pneumothorax, the visceral pleural line in secondary spontaneous pneumothorax may be more difficult to see because of underlying hyperlucent lung which may obscure distinction between pneumothorax and emphysematous lung, particularly a large bulla. This distinction is critical if placing a chest tube is under consideration, i.e., placement of a chest tube in a bulla can be catastrophic. The shape of the pleural line can provide an important clue in distinguishing between a pneumothorax and a bulla: the pleural line demarcating a bulla is concave toward the lateral chest wall, whereas it is convex when a pneumothorax is present. If chest radiography is equivocal, computed tomography easily makes the distinction.

Management The therapeutic options for the patient with secondary spontaneous pneumothorax are the same as those for primary spontaneous pneumothorax, but the circumstances are much more urgent. Even a small pneumothorax may be life threatening for the patient with underlying lung disease. Consequently, virtually all patients with secondary spontaneous pneumothorax are treated with chest tubes (tube thoracostomy). If the patient is undergoing positive pressure ventilation, tube thoracostomy is mandatory to avoid expansion of the pneumothorax. If the lung fails to expand and the air leak persists due to a bronchopleural fistula, ventilation has to be adjusted to compensate for the loss of part of each tidal volume into the pleural space. A variety of strategies are available to deal with severe leaks, e.g., high frequency, low pressure ventilation.

Tube thoracostomy is less effective in secondary than in primary spontaneous pneumothorax. Often, multiple chest tubes are required and longer delays are encountered in expanding the lung. To avoid recurrences, tetracycline is commonly used after the lung has expanded.

Chest tubes should not be placed in patients with carcinoma of the lung in whom the pneumothorax is a complication of bronchial obstruction and total collapse of the lung. The absence of an air bronchogram is an important clue to the presence of an endobronchial obstructing lesion which has led to lung collapse.

Complications relating to tube thoracostomy are not uncommon. These include bleeding, infection of the pleural space, re-expansion pulmonary edema, and injury of the underlying lung by the chest tube.

TRAUMATIC PNEUMOTHORAX

Trauma to the chest, either penetrating or nonpenetrating, may introduce air into the pleural space. Air may enter directly through an opening in the chest wall, by alveolar rupture secondary to chest compression and alveolar overdistention, or by direct laceration of the lung by either a foreign body or a fractured rib. Chest compression, by raising alveolar pressure abruptly, can cause alveoli to rupture and force air into the pulmonary interstitium. This air dissects its way toward either the visceral pleura or mediastinum. Any break in the visceral or mediastinal pleura can then cause a pneumothorax.

Traumatic pneumothorax calls for tube thoracostomy. A second chest tube is required if blood, as well as air, accumulates in the pleural space. As a rule, the air leak closes and the lung expands within 72 h.

If the air leak is large, either the trachea or a large bronchus may have been lacerated. The likelihood of this complication is increased if one or more of the upper three ribs is fractured or the patient coughs up blood. The occurrence of a hydropneumothorax after a closed chest injury raises the suspicion of a ruptured esophagus. This diagnosis is substantiated by a high concentration of amylase in the pleural fluid.

IATROGENIC PNEUMOTHORAX

This type of pneumothorax has grown increasingly common as the number of diagnostic and therapeutic interventions has increased, particularly in the intensive-care setting. Accidental laceration or puncture of the visceral pleura is a common cause. This complication has to be kept in mind while placing a central venous line or performing a thoracentesis, closed pleural biopsy, or percutaneous lung aspiration. It also can occur in the course of bronchoscopic biopsy and in the course of procedures that cause alveolar overdistention, such as cardiopulmonary resuscitation, mechanical ventilation, or anesthesia. Frequently, it is detected in an asymptomatic patient in the routine chest radiograph following a procedure. However, if the pneumothorax is large and progressive, it may cause respiratory distress or hemodynamic deterioration.

CATAMENIAL PNEUMOTHORAX

Spontaneous pneumothorax, usually on the right side, sometimes occurs in women in association with menstruation. As a rule, it affects women 25 to 30 years of age. Its mechanism is unclear, but it is commonly attributed to minute endometrial implants on the surface of the lung. The spontaneous pneumothorax generally occurs within 48 h of the start of the menstrual period. Treatment consists of the use of ovulation-suppressing drugs because of the tendency of the condition to recur. If these agents are not successful, surgical exploration is required. Chemical pleurodesis is often the treatment of choice, particularly in women who wish to bear children.

BRONCHOPLEURAL FISTULA AND PULMONARY BAROTRAUMA

A persistent pneumothorax may be the result of a bronchopleural fistula. Persistent air leaks have become increasingly common in patients with the adult respiratory distress syndrome who are intubated and ventilated using high peak pressures. In some of these patients, not only barotrauma, but also a necrotizing bacterial pneumonia, can cause air leaks. Once an air leak is established, positive pressure mechanical ventilation drives air continuously into the pleural space. In some patients, a tension pneumothorax may develop. The first evidence of a bronchopleural fistula secondary to barotrauma may be provided by the chest radiograph. Sometimes pneumomediastinum and subcutaneous emphysema accompanies the pneumothorax.

A bronchopleural fistula in a patient with the adult respiratory distress syndrome is a serious complication. Management while the patient is on mechanical ventilation is difficult. A high-frequency jet ventilator has been introduced in an attempt to diminish the air leak by resorting to lower airway pressures. In some instances, pleurodesis has been undertaken but not always with success.

BIBLIOGRAPHY

For a more detailed discussion, see Anthonisen NR, Filuk RB: Pneumothorax, in Fishman AP (ed), *Pulmonary Diseases and Disorders,* 2d ed. New York, McGraw-Hill, 1988, pp 2171–2182.

Engdahl O, Toft T, Boe J: Chest radiograph—a poor method for determining the size of a pneumothorax. Chest 103:26–29, 1993.

Inderbitzi RG, Furrer M, Striffeler H, Althaus U: Thoracoscopic pleurectomy for treatment of complicated spontaneous pneumothorax. J Thorac Cardiovasc Surg 105:84–88, 1993.

Light RW: *Pleural Diseases,* 2d ed. Philadelphia, 1990, pp 237–262.

Wait MA, Estrera A: Changing clinical spectrum of spontaneous pneumothorax. Am J Surg 164:528–531, 1992.

Mitchell Margolis

DEFINITION

Malignant pleural mesothelioma (MPM) is a cancerous proliferation of mesothelial cells that usually involves a large extent of the pleural cavity.

PATHOLOGY

In its earliest stages, the lesions appear as multiple small nodules on visceral or parietal pleura. The tumor nodules then spread along the pleural surfaces, eventually forming a thick irregular peel that compresses the underlying lung. In its late stages, MPM invades the subjacent lung parenchyma, ribs, and intercostal and subcutaneous tissues and may metastasize to regional lymph nodes, contralateral lung, liver, brain, bone, and elsewhere. However, metastatic disease is seldom clinically apparent during life or the cause of death. The macroscopic features can be as important in diagnosis as the microscopic appearance, which is variable and difficult to distinguish from metastatic adenocarcinoma in some cases and from several types of reactive mesothelial proliferation and pleural fibrosis in others. This histologic diversity results from the ability of mesothelial cells to differentiate into mesenchymal and papillary epithelial elements. Most pathologists recognize three predominant types: epithelial, fibrosarcomatous, and mixed (biphasic) forms, with a relative frequency of 2:1:1. Some include an undifferentiated polygonal variant. A better prognosis has been ascribed to the epithelial subtype. Ultimately, the diagnosis of this malignancy rests on a combination of macroscopic and microscopic findings in a compatible clinical setting, rather than on any one morphologic feature.

ETIOLOGY

A landmark study of South African asbestos miners published in 1960 strongly suggested a relationship between occupational asbestos exposure and the subsequent development of MPM. Since then, the causal association between asbestos exposure and MPM has been established experimentally and epidemiologically. However, in patients with MPM, pulmonary asbestosis tends to be mild or even absent. The latency period between the first occupational exposure and diagnosis usually ranges from 30 to 45 years.

Different types of asbestos fibers vary in their ability to induce MPM, presumably because of divergencies in their aerodynamic qualities. Long, thin fibers (with a high length-to-diameter ratio) are probably inhaled more deeply and penetrate to the pleura more efficiently. Thus, crocidolite is especially hazardous, whereas workers exposed the comparatively short, blunt fibers of chrysotile and anthophyllite are much less likely to develop MPM. Curiously, the long, thin fibers of erionite, chemically distinct from those of asbestos, can also cause MPM.

Although a dose-response relationship is generally believed to exist between asbestos exposure and the incidence of MPM, frequently MPM has occurred in individuals with brief, nonoccupational exposures, including wives of asbestos workers. Indeed, in some reports, no exposure to asbestos could be identified in one third or more of patients with MPM. In these instances, it is likely that other, as yet unknown, cocarcinogens or genetic factors are at work. For example, typical mesotheliomas have been induced in chickens using strain MC20 avian leukosis virus. Cigarette smoking does not appear to be a cofactor.

EPIDEMIOLOGY

The incidence of MPM is currently on the rise in the United States. This may reflect the latency period following exposure of many workers to high levels of asbestos in the 1940s and 1950s. Still, MPM is an uncommon tumor, with a yearly incidence of 11.4/1,000,000 population in men and 2.8/1,000,000 in women. The highest rates often occur in coastal cities with large shipbuilding industries. Other workers at high risk are asbestos miners and millers, pipefitters, insulation workers, roofers, and those who repair brake linings. However, even those who launder asbestos-contaminated clothing or live near asbestos mines or factories may also be at increased risk. Clusters of cases have been noted among Pueblo Indians who use asbestos in the manufacture of silver jewelry and whitening of moccasins and in the village of Karain, Turkey, where erionite is mined extensively. The median age at diagnosis is between 50 and 60 years, but the range extends from childhood to old age. Men outnumber women by 2 to 6:1, probably reflecting greater occupational asbestos exposure.

CLINICAL MANIFESTATIONS

History The cardinal symptoms are chest pain and progressive dyspnea, which usually develop insidiously over months. The pain is usually localized over the involved hemithorax but may radiate to the arm, neck, or shoulder. It tends to be constant and sometimes acquires a neuritic quality due to infiltration of intercostal nerves. Some patients complain of only mild discomfort, whereas in others the pain is incapacitating, among the most distressing encountered in chest medicine. Cough, weight loss, fever, malaise, sweats, weakness, and hemoptysis (slight and probably due to lung invasion) occur in a few patients. On rare occasion, MPM is discovered in an asymptomatic patient; an occasional patient presents with the acute onset of pain and dyspnea caused by either hemothorax or spontaneous pneumothorax.

Physical examination The only consistent physical findings are dullness and diminished breath sounds and fremitus over the involved hemithorax due to pleural fluid or the tumor mass. Cachexia occurs in some patients. Clubbing, lymphadenopathy, and friction rubs are unusual. A large pleural mass can depress the liver or spleen, giving the false impression of hepatomegaly or splenomegaly. In patients with advanced disease, a variety of other manifestations can be encountered: decreased mobility of the affected hemithorax, chest wall masses, vocal cord paralysis, Horner's syndrome, anesthesia of the overlying skin, superior vena cava syndrome, or tumor growth along the track of thoracentesis or the site of thoracotomy.

USUAL DIAGNOSTIC TESTS

Chest radiography The chest radiograph most often shows a unilateral pleural effusion, which is often massive. Effusion is absent in about 20 percent of patients. Bilateral effusions are present in < 5 percent of patients when they are first seen. The mediastinum may be shifted to the contralateral side or "frozen" in the midline. In advanced cases, massive pulmonary encasement by the neoplasm may draw the mediastinum toward the ipsilateral hemithorax. Chest radiographs may also demonstrate nodular pleural thickening, but this characteristic finding is often somewhat obscured by the overlying effusion. Radiographic evidence of contralateral asbestosis or pleural plaques are seen in about one third of patients and may be helpful in suggesting the diagnosis of MPM. Late in the course of MPM, the chest radiographic findings include rib destruction, mediastinal widening, and an enlarged cardiac silhouette due to pericardial effusion.

Chest computed tomography Scanning is extremely useful for demonstrating extensive nodular pleural thickening, pleural effusion, and pleuropulmonary changes in the opposite hemithorax. This test frequently demonstrates more extensive disease than does the chest radiograph and clarifies the pathologic anatomy in the involved hemithorax.

Pulmonary function tests Pulmonary function tests usually show progressive restrictive disease. Arterial blood gases remain normal until late in the disease when hypoxemia and respiratory failure supervene.

Routine blood tests Routine blood tests are usually unrevealing. Thrombocytosis was a prominent feature in one study and abnormally high levels of hyaluronic acid in the serum in another.

SPECIAL DIAGNOSTIC EVALUATION

Thoracentesis In general, pleural fluid findings can only suggest a diagnosis of MPM. Diagnostic thoracentesis discloses straw-colored fluid in early disease but serosanguineous or frankly bloody fluid later on. As the tumor bulk increases, pleural fluid formation may actually lessen. Marked resistance may be encountered during thoracentesis as the needle traverses the overlying mass to enter the pleural space. The pleural fluid is an exudate with a leukocyte count usually < 5000/ml. The pH and the glucose concentration may be low, and the concentration of hyaluronic acid may be high (normal level ≤ 0.2 ng/ml). A very high level of hyaluronic acid in the pleural fluid may impart a viscid quality to the fluid but does not constitute a specific or sensitive test for MPM. Pleural fluid cytology is said to be diagnostic in only about 10 percent of cases; it is difficult to distinguish benign from malignant mesothelial cells by this technique.

Pleural biopsy Specimens for histologic diagnosis are best obtained by open pleural biopsy. Thorascopic biopsy may also be useful early in the disease before pleural symphysis has occurred. Both sampling techniques provide ample specimens and allow visual recognition of typical gross features, consisting of multiple pleural masses or a thick irregular pleural peel. Specimens obtained by percutaneous closed pleural biopsy tend to be small, physically difficult to obtain, and insufficient for diagnosis.

DIFFERENTIAL DIAGNOSIS

Adenocarcinoma involving the pleura is most apt to be mistaken for MPM, particularly the epithelial type. The adenocarcinoma may arise from a peripheral lung cancer or from metastases from a remote visceral malignancy. In fact, it may be impossible to differentiate between MPM and adenocarcinoma by history, physical examination, chest radiograph, or pleural fluid chemistry and cytology. Even an open biopsy routinely stained for histology can fail to make the distinction. In such cases, special stains or electron microscopy can sometimes be helpful. For example, the demonstration of neutral mucins by the periodic acid-Schiff stain after diastase digestion strengthens the diagnosis of adenocarcinoma. However, many adenocarcinomas lack this feature. Also helpful in diagnosing adenocarcinoma may be immunocytochemical staining using monoclonal antibodies directed against carcinoembryonic antigen, Leu-M1, or B72.3. Immunochemical stains are usually negative in MPM, with the exception of anti-MS. Acid mucins may be demonstrated in MPM by alcian blue staining. In MPM, electron microscopy often identifies the numerous long microvilli and desmosomes of mesothelial cells. Although immunohistochemical and electron-microscopic data may support one diagnosis over the other, these studies are rarely definitive. Because treatment options for both entities are extremely limited at present, the importance of making an unequivocal distinction can be questioned.

The second most difficult differential diagnosis is benign asbestos pleurisy. This entity can mimic MPM in that it occurs in asbestos workers, causes chest pain, and sometimes produces a bloody exudative effusion. Further confusion arises from the fact that a few patients develop MPM years after an episode of benign asbestos pleurisy. In attempting to distinguish between the two entities, it is helpful to keep in mind that benign asbestos pleurisy is more likely to develop in the first 20 years after asbestos exposure, is more often asymptomatic, and tends to cause only small, nonprogressive effusions. An episodic, recurrent course is common, and the pleural fluid cytology may be eosinophilic. Many believe that the diagnosis of benign asbestos pleurisy can only be made with certainty after a very lengthy follow-up to ensure that MPM has not developed.

Benign fibrous mesothelioma is more likely to cause nosologic rather than clinical confusion. This is an often asymptomatic, encapsulated tumor which is amenable to surgical resection. It may be associated with hypertrophic osteoarthropathy and hypoglycemia but is not related to asbestos exposure. The typical chest radiograph shows a well-marginated solitary pleural mass, but pleural effusion is distinctly uncommon. In some patients cough, chest pain, dyspnea, and fever occur.

Many other pleural lesions can be initially mistaken radiographically for MPM. These include rounded atelectasis, large irregular hyaline plaques, and various types of pleural fibrosis and reactive proliferative mesothelial lesions. Usually the relentless clinical advancement of MPM distinguishes it from these nonprogressive, often asymptomatic lesions.

PROGNOSIS AND TREATMENT

With rare exception, MPM is currently incurable. Indeed, a strong case can be made for withholding treatment except for research protocols or to provide symptomatic relief. Widely divergent views of the current roles of surgery, radiotherapy, and chemotherapy are held at different centers.

Surgery, radiotherapy, and chemotherapy individually and in combination have been tried. Despite treatment, the clinical course is usually one of progressive dyspnea, chest pain, and inanition, with death occurring from respiratory failure, infection, pulmonary embolism, or arrhythmias secondary to pericardial invasion. Median survival times generally vary from 7 to 20 months.

Perhaps the most informative and sizable study is that of Law and coworkers, who prospectively assigned comparable patients to receive either nonradical parietal pleurectomy with decortication, combination chemotherapy, high-dose megavoltage radiotherapy, or no treatment. No significant difference was noted in survival between treatment groups or between treated and untreated patients. Median survival in all groups ranged from 18 to 20 months. Variability in the natural history of MPM was underscored by the finding in the untreated group of 31 percent 2-year survival and 11 percent 4-year survival. These survival rates approach or exceed those of several series in which radical surgery was performed.

It is important to emphasize that palliative measures can be helpful in dealing with progressive symptomatic MPM. Narcotic analgesics can be given both around-the-clock and as needed. Limited surgery and radiotherapy can lessen pleural fluid formation, pain, and dyspnea. Nutritional supplementation, palliative thoracentesis, psychological counseling, and oxygen are among the many other supportive measures that may benefit individual patients. In one report, prednisolone was helpful in alleviating fever and sweats.

BIBLIOGRAPHY

For a more detailed discussion, see Kleinerman JI: Neoplasms of the pleura, chest wall, and diaphragm, in Fishman AP (ed), *Pulmonary Diseases and Disorders,* 2d ed. New York, McGraw-Hill, 1988, pp 2033–2044.

Collins CL, Ordonez NG, Schaefer R, Cook CD, Xie SS, Granger J, et al: Thrombomodulin expression in malignant pleural mesothelioma and pulmonary adenocarcinoma. Am J Pathol 141:827–833, 1992.

Keller SM: Current and future therapy for malignant pleural effusion. Chest 103:63S–67S, 1993.

Law MR, Gregor A, Hodson ME, Bloom HJ, Turner-Warwick M: Malignant mesothelioma of the pleura: A study of 52 treated and 64 untreated patients. Thorax 39:255–259, 1984.

Light RW: Malignant and benign mesotheliomas, in Light RW (ed), *Pleural Diseases,* 2d ed. Philadelphia, Lea and Febiger, 1990, pp 117–128.

Ramael M, Lemmens G, Eerdekens C, Buysse C, Deblier I, Jacobs W, et al: Immunoreactivity for p53 protein in malignant mesothelioma and non-neoplastic mesothelium. J Pathol 168:371–375, 1992.

Ruffie PA: Pleural mesothelioma. Curr Opin Oncol 3:328–334, 1991.

X | PULMONARY INFECTIONS

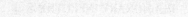

Wallace T. Miller, Jr.

The chest radiograph continues to be a powerful and cost-effective tool in the evaluation of pneumonia. This chapter focuses on the radiographic patterns associated with particular infectious agents.

When evaluating for a potential pneumonia, every attempt should be made to obtain a posteroanterior (PA) and lateral chest radiograph rather than rely on a portable chest radiograph. PA and lateral films are produced under a standard set of conditions, using optimal technique. This is not true of portable chest radiographs which, therefore, are often of inferior quality.

Radiographic abnormalities of the lungs can be divided into two broad categories: alveolar disease and interstitial disease.

Alveolar disease results in filling of the alveoli. This filling may be by fluid, i.e., pulmonary edema, blood (alveolar hemorrhage), pus (pneumonia), or tumor (alveolar cell carcinoma). The characteristic radiographic appearance is one of confluent opacities in the lung, often with air bronchograms. In contrast, in *interstitial disease,* the radiographic hallmarks are numerous fine lines or nodules of millimeter dimensions. Care must be taken to avoid overreading interstitial disease; normal interstitial markings can become more prominent in underexposed and expiratory radiographs.

Interstitial or alveolar disease should be further characterized as *focal* or *diffuse.* In most instances, this distinction is easy. However, a *focal* disease may occasionally be widespread and resemble a diffuse disease, e.g., widespread aspiration pneumonia. *Diffuse* diseases are usually distributed quite symmetrically, either throughout both lungs or in a zone of the lungs, i.e., basilar, mid-lung, or apical. In contrast, widespread focal diseases are usually not symmetrical; instead, areas of greater and lesser disease are disposed haphazardly.

BACTERIAL PNEUMONIA

The characteristic appearance of acute bacterial pneumonia is that of alveolar disease, usually confined to a single lobe or part of a lobe. With few exceptions, specific bacterial organisms do not elicit distinctive radiographic appearances. However, the clinical history may suggest the type of organism, e.g., community-versus hospital-acquired pneumonias.

The radiographic appearance of a pneumonia may lag behind the clinical presentation. Therefore, a normal chest radiograph does not exclude the clinical diagnosis of pneumonia. However, a follow-up chest radiograph should confirm the diagnosis of pneumonia. If radiographs taken in a few days fail to reveal an alveolar infiltrate, then a diagnosis other than bacterial pneumonia should be considered.

Although the radiographic findings of pneumonia may persist for 6 to 8 weeks despite clinical resolution of symptoms, radiographic infiltrates should not increase beyond the first few days once treatment is begun. If the infiltrates become more extensive, then either the pneumonia is being inadequately treated by the antibiotics, or a process other than pneumonia should be considered as a possible cause of the infiltrates. Also, if the radiographic abnormalities persist beyond 1 or 2 months, then alternate diagnoses should be considered.

All pneumonias, particularly those in patients > 40 years old, should be followed by serial chest radiographs until resolution is complete to exclude structural causes of pneumonia, especially carcinoma of the lung, but also other endobronchial lesions. Because recurrent pneumonias in the same lobe or segment often can be a clue to an endobronchial lesion, bronchoscopy is indicated to evaluate persistent or recurrent pneumonias. In individuals in whom bronchoscopy is not feasible, thin section computed tomography (CT) through the bronchus in question (at 5-mm contiguous intervals) has nearly the same sensitivity as does bronchoscopy for the detection of endobronchial disease. Unfortunately, unlike bronchoscopy, it affords less specificity because bronchoscopy can obtain material for histologic and cytologic evaluation.

A pleural effusion on the same side as the pneumonia is a common finding. Because such effusions are usually exudative, they are often partially or completely loculated. Persistence of loculated fluid, despite clearance of the alveolar infiltrate, may indicate an empyema. When the effusion is small, ultrasound examination may help in identifying an appropriate site for thoracentesis. The combination of a pleural effusion and alveolar infiltrate often raises two diagnostic possibilities: a pneumonia with a parapneumonic effusion versus an effusion accompanied by passive atelectasis. In this situation, the dominant radiographic feature generally indicates the primary process. If the consolidation is more conspicuous than the effusion, then the primary process is apt to be pneumonia accompanied by a parapneumonic effusion. Oppositely, if the effusion is the more prominent process, the consolidation is more likely to be passive atelectasis, secondary to the effusion.

Multilobar pneumonias constitute a distinct class of acute pneumonias. The most common cause of multilobar pneumonia is aspiration (Table 36-1). Another characteristic feature of aspiration pneumonia is the rapid radiographic onset of disease, i.e., within the first few hours of the aspiration. In contrast to the usual bacterial pneumonia in which alveolar infiltrates are largely a result of the inflammatory response of the host, the infiltrates in aspiration pneumonia result from the aspirated fluid itself, in addition to pulmonary edema caused by the gastric acid and inflammatory response.

Legionella pneumonia is also multilobar in 50 to 65 percent of patients (see Table 36-1). However, unlike aspiration pneumonia, which is often multilobar from the onset, legionella pneumonia is usually unilobar at presentation, but progresses to a multilobar pattern when the disease is at its peak.

Viral pneumonias, which may also be multilobar, are considered below.

SEPTIC EMBOLI

Radiographically, septic emboli are a type of bacterial pneumonia in which distinct or indistinct nodules, approximately 1 to 3 cm in size, are randomly scattered throughout the lungs. These frequently cavitate within a few days of presentation. This pattern is distinctive and often suggests the diagnosis.

ATYPICAL PNEUMONIA

Primary atypical pneumonia is usually suspected on clinical grounds: low-grade fever, nonproductive cough often with myalgias, and other constitutional symptoms. The etiologies for atypical pneumonias includes *Mycoplasma,* viruses, and *Chlamydia.*

Mycoplasma

Mycoplasma pneumonia produces several radiographic patterns. Typically, it elicits a solitary lobar infiltrate identical to that of bacterial pneumonias. Most often, the alveolar consolidation involves one lobe, occasionally several; the consolidation may be patchy or uniform. In patients with the pattern of alveolar consolidation, the onset of symptoms is relatively acute, similar to that of a bacterial pneumonia. The pulmonary infiltrates usually resolve in the course of a few weeks in response to appropriate antibiotic therapy.

The second (less common) pattern of disease is that of diffuse reticulonodular interstitial infiltrates distributed widely throughout

TABLE 36-1 Multilobar Alveolar Infiltrates

Aspiration pneumonia	Predilection for dependent regions of lung
Legionella pneumonia	May start unifocal and progress to multifocal
Viral pneumonia	Variable appearance depending on organism but most commonly resembles other community-acquired pneumonias

the lungs; these persist without progression to alveolar disease. This pattern is usually associated with a more insidious onset of cough and dyspnea, often without fever. The radiographic changes are slow to clear and may take several months.

Viral Pneumonia

Influenza pneumonia (an uncommon manifestation of influenza) presents radiographically with alveolar consolidation. Typically, this consolidation is nonconfluent at presentation, but becomes confluent during the next few days. In approximately one half the patients, the consolidation is unilateral, and in the others, bilateral. About one half the bilateral consolidations are diffuse and resemble severe pulmonary edema. Although pneumonia is a relatively uncommon manifestation of influenza viral infection, it can be rapidly progressive and fatal; bacterial superinfection is common. Unfortunately, because the virus itself produces alveolar infiltrates, it is difficult to detect superinfection radiographically.

Varicella and measles pneumonias have a characteristic radiographic appearance which, in the appropriate clinical setting, often suggest the diagnosis. Numerous small (5 to 10 mm), irregular alveolar nodules are scattered uniformly throughout the lungs, i.e., a "rash" in the lungs that parallels the skin manifestations. Radiographic clearance of these small infiltrates may take days to many months. On rare occasions, these pneumonias progress to the adult respiratory distress syndrome.

Chlamydial Pneumonia

The chlamydial pneumonias—psittacosis, Q fever, and others—do not have distinctive radiographic features. In general, they appear as nonspecific alveolar infiltrates.

CHRONIC PULMONARY INFECTIONS

Unlike the acute pneumonias, chronic pulmonary infections often elicit characteristic radiographic appearances which suggest the diagnosis.

Tuberculosis

Tuberculosis is the most common of the chronic pneumonias encountered in North America.

Primary infection follows inhalation of *Mycobacterium tuberculosis* after exposure to an individual with active tuberculosis. Because the symptoms of the primary infection are mild and assumed to be a "cold" or viral upper respiratory infection, the primary infection is rarely recognized clinically, and therefore is rarely imaged. On the chest radiograph, a primary infection is manifested as a focal alveolar infiltrate which is indistinguishable from the more common bacterial pneumonias. However, the infiltrate is frequently associated with hilar or mediastinal adenopathy, a rare finding in pneumonias except for those caused by granulomatous infections, i.e., mycobacteria and fungi (Table 36-2). In the normal host, the alveolar infiltrate and adenopathy resolve during the next few months. As the alveolar consolidation resolves, it contracts slowly and centrifugally, sometimes forming a solitary pulmonary nodule which can be confused with primary or metastatic carcinoma. Over several months to a year, this nodule either contracts to form a small calcified granuloma that is approximately 5 to 10 mm in size, or disappears completely. While the primary focus is resolving, the adenopathy also shrinks and often calcifies. This combination of a peripheral granuloma and central calcified lymph nodes, known as a Ranke's complex, is a sign of prior granulomatous infection, most often tuberculosis. The parenchymal nodule is known as a Ghon's focus.

In certain individuals with diminished immune function, e.g., the very young and very old or in the patient with chronic illness, the primary infection is not contained by the immune system. Radiographically, the areas of consolidation increase and often spread to the contralateral lung, by a bronchogenic route, producing a widespread, asymmetric, patchy alveolar consolidation. This is called *progressive primary tuberculosis.*

Postprimary or reactivation tuberculosis characteristically involves the upper portions of the lung: the apical and posterior segments of the upper lobes and the superior segments of the lower lobes (Table 36-3). The appearance is that of irregular dense strands mixed with small (5 to 10 mm) nodules which is often described as "fibronodular, apical infiltrates." The more alveolar the appearance of these infiltrates,

TABLE 36-2 Mediastinal and Hilar Adenopathy

Common	
Primary tuberculosis	Primary infection only; not seen in reactivation
Acute histoplasmosis	Often seen with alveolar infiltrate or
Primary coccidioidomycosis	nodule indicating the parenchymal focus of infection
Atypical mycobacteria	Seen predominantly in immunocompromised hosts, particularly AIDS
Cryptococcosis	
Rare	
Epstein-Barr virus (infectious mononucleosis)	Adenopathy usually isolated

AIDS = acquired immunodeficiency syndrome

TABLE 36-3 Apical Lung Disease

Infectious causes	Radiographic features
Common	
Tuberculosis	Fibronodular stranding, alveolar infiltrates, cavitation
Semi-invasive aspergillosis	Thick pleural rind, mycetoma
Bacterial pneumonia	Alveolar infiltrates, rapid changes on serial chest radiograph, acute symptoms
Uncommon	
Atypical mycobacterium	Resembles tuberculosis
Rare	
Histoplasmosis	Resembles tuberculosis
Coccidioidomycosis	Resembles tuberculosis
Noninfectious causes	
Bronchogenic carcinoma	More nodular appearance

the more likely is the infection to be active. Cavitation of the infiltrate almost always indicates active infection. Although the only definitive way of determining the activity of a tuberculous infiltrate is sputum culture, changing infiltrates on serial radiographs often indicate activity. In most instances, if the infiltrate remains unchanged for 6 months or more, the tuberculosis is inactive.

In advanced reactivation tuberculosis, spread may occur to the opposite lung by a bronchogenic route. This mode of spread is uncommon in infections other than tuberculosis.

Miliary tuberculosis occurs as a result of hematogenous infection, particularly in severely immunocompromised hosts. Radiographically, the appearance is that of tiny interstitial nodules. These nodules at times are so fine that they are easily overlooked. Miliary tuberculosis may be a manifestation of either primary or reactivation tuberculosis, usually of primary disease.

Atypical Mycobacterial Pneumonias

Mycobacterium avium-intracellulare and *Mycobacterium kansasii* are the most common causes of atypical mycobacterial pneumonias. The radiographic appearance of this infection differs according to the clinical characteristics of the individual in whom it occurs. The classic appearance is that of cavitary fibronodular infiltrates which resemble reactivation tuberculosis. This pattern is seen predominantly in elderly men with chronic lung disease, especially chronic obstructive pulmonary disease (COPD). It is also seen in individuals with certain extrapulmonary diseases, e.g., cancer and collagen vascular diseases.

Another pattern of disease is seen in elderly individuals without significant systemic disease. In these individuals, usually women, the radiographic manifestation is that of an indistinct infiltrate in one or several subsegmental areas. The infiltrate may be interstitial or alveolar in character; occasionally the appearance may resemble that of bronchiectasis. Characteristically, the infiltrates evolve slowly over several years.

In patients with AIDS, atypical mycobacterial infection assumes an entirely different radiographic pattern. Invariably, the mycobacterial infection is widely disseminated throughout the body. In the chest, the most common appearance is that of isolated mediastinal and hilar adenopathy. Small subsegmental areas of consolidation are also common and may occur with, or without, adenopathy.

Adenopathy within the abdomen and retroperitoneum is also common in AIDS patients infected with atypical mycobacteria. This adenopathy can be detected by CT and, in some instances, the nodules have characteristic hypodense centers which may suggest the diagnosis of atypical mycobacterium infection. However, this pattern has also been seen in AIDS patients with tuberculosis, histoplasmosis, and lymphoma.

Fungal Pneumonias

The nonopportunistic fungal pneumonias incident to histoplasmosis, coccidioidomycosis, and blastomycosis have both acute and chronic manifestations. In some instances, the fungi responsible for these diseases can act as opportunistic invaders and span all varieties of pneumonias.

Histoplasmosis Infection of the lung by *Histoplasma capsulatum* is usually asymptomatic or elicits such minor symptoms that the patient does not seek medical attention. Therefore, the most common radiographic manifestation of histoplasmosis is one or more calcified granulomas associated with calcified mediastinal or hilar lymph nodes, the residuum of a remote previous infection. This finding is particularly common in the midwestern United States where histoplasmosis is endemic. If a chest radiograph is obtained during the acute infection, one or several ill-defined subsegmental regions of consolidation may be detected, often with enlarged hilar or mediastinal lymph nodes.

On rare occasion, acute histoplasmosis presents with symptoms of fever, headache, chills, and cough, presumably due to a larger inoculum. Radiographically, large nonsegmental regions of consolidation are present, often accompanied by hilar and mediastinal adenopathy. In the absence of adenopathy, the differential diagnosis includes acute bacterial and viral pneumonia.

In some patients who have received a large inoculum, disseminated nodular opacities are scattered throughout the lungs (Table 36-4). These opacities range in size from several millimeters to several centimeters. Although this pattern may resemble miliary tuberculosis, the nodules are larger than those of tuberculosis.

A *histoplasmoma,* which appears radiographically as a pulmonary nodule, probably represents the chronic residuum of the acute infiltrate. Histoplasmomas may be single or multiple and may shrink, remain stable or, on rare occasion, grow over time. The presence of central or ringlike calcifications within the nodule are virtually pathognomonic of the disease. In the absence of calcification, the differential diagnosis includes all other causes of solitary or multiple pulmonary nodules (Table 36-5). Calcified hilar lymph nodes are associated with most histoplasmomas; in their absence, the diagnosis of histoplasmoma is unlikely.

A chronic form of histoplasmosis occurs predominantly in patients with COPD. The radiographic characteristics are similar to those of reactivation tuberculosis with segmental or subsegmental regions of consolidation in the apices of the lungs. Progressive scarring and loss of volume may be seen on successive chest radiographs. Cavitation may also occur.

Sclerosing mediastinitis refers to the exuberant mediastinal fibrosis

TABLE 36-4 Diffuse Nodules—Infectious Causes

Tuberculosis	Usually very tiny nodules (1–2 mm)
Histoplasmosis	Indistinct nodules (2–5 mm or sometimes larger)
Coccidioidomycosis	Similar to tuberculosis
Cryptococcosis	Similar to tuberculosis
Varicella pneumonia	Larger indistinct nodules (5–10 mm); associated rash
Measles pneumonia	Similar to varicella

TABLE 36-5 Pulmonary Nodules—Single or Multiple—Infectious Causes

Tuberculoma	Usually solitary, asymptomatic, or mildly symptomatic
Histoplasmoma	Often multiple, can be solitary, midwestern United States, asymptomatic
Coccidioidoma	Most likely to cavitate [especially likely if thin (1–2 mm) wall], southwestern United States
Cryptococcoma	Single or multiple; multiple more common in immunocompromised hosts (except AIDS where nodules are rare)
Septic emboli	Acute symptoms, ill-defined edges, usually cavitate within 2–5 days of radiographic presentation, usually multiple
Abscess	Cavitary, air-fluid levels
(Round pneumonia)	Will change radiographic appearance over days to a few weeks

that is secondary to mediastinal involvement in histoplasmosis. It is a rare disorder that can cause pericardial tamponade, the superior vena caval syndrome, pulmonary hypertension, bronchial obstruction, and esophageal stenosis or diverticula by strangulating the various mediastinal structures by the extensive fibrosis. The presence of calcification in the mediastinal lymph nodes coupled with the appropriate clinical manifestations generally suggests this diagnosis. Further support of the diagnosis is provided by CT or magnetic resonance imaging, which may demonstrate narrowing of vascular or bronchial structures or pericardial thickening. Barium swallow examination demonstrates the esophageal changes.

Coccidioidomycosis This fungal infection, endemic to the southwestern United States, radiographically mimics tuberculosis in many ways. Primary infection is characterized by a patchy area of alveolar consolidation usually about a segment in size. In approximately 20 percent of patients, hilar adenopathy is also present. In another 20 percent, a small pleural effusion is present. In a few patients, as in those with tuberculosis, the primary infection persists and spreads to large areas of the remaining lung, producing a widespread focal pattern of disease. These individuals are usually symptomatic and occasionally develop respiratory failure and die.

As in the other granulomatous infections, coccidioidomycosis can persist as a chronic nodular focus, a *coccidioidoma*. These may be single or multiple, usually present in the upper lobes, and are one half to several centimeters in size. Coccidioidomas are more likely to cavitate than are the other granulomatous infections. Thin walls (< 1 cm thick) are a hallmark of cavitary coccidioidomas and suggest the diagnosis; however, occasionally, the walls of the cavity are thick.

Coccidioidomycosis may resemble tuberculosis by producing a chronic fibronodular cavitary infiltrate of the upper lobe. Like tuberculosis, this is thought to represent reactivation of dormant organisms at a time when resistance of the host is low. Unlike tuberculosis, this infiltrate may involve the anterior segment of the upper lobe. Also, unlike tuberculosis, it is a rare phenomenon, occurring in < 1 percent of patients.

Hematogenous dissemination, with a miliary pattern on the chest radiograph, can occur in the course of primary or reactivation disease.

North American blastomycosis This is an unusual fungal infection that occurs in the midwestern region of the United States. It is usually associated with time spent in wooded areas. The radiographic appearance is relatively nonspecific, showing a large confluent area of consolidation that resembles bacterial pneumonia. Rounded regions of consolidation are also common and may mimic pulmonary malignancies. Cavitation, adenopathy, and pleural effusions are rare. Thickening of the pleura adjacent to the pneumonia is common and may suggest the diagnosis. Blastomycosis may invade the chest wall and destroy adjacent ribs. This finding is strongly suggestive of blastomycosis; the major differential diagnosis is actinomycosis and lung cancer.

Actinomycosis and Nocardiosis

Radiographically, actinomycosis most often appears as a focal area of alveolar consolidation resembling a usual bacterial pneumonia. In the absence of particular features that point to another type of pneumonia, chronicity of the infiltrate should raise the suspicion of actinomycosis. Cavitation is common and occurs in up to one third of patients. The alveolar infiltrates of actinomycosis may also appear masslike and simulate lung carcinoma (Table 36-6). If left untreated or inadequately treated, actinomycosis often invades the pleura and chest wall, resulting in pleural effusion, pleural thickening or bone destruction, and occasionally, a palpable chest wall mass (Table 36-7). This progression usually takes months or years. Chest wall involvement is a feature of actinomycosis that is strongly suggestive of the disease. Cross-sectional imaging often provides additional detail concerning chest wall involvement.

TABLE 36-6 Pneumonia That Simulates a Pulmonary Mass

Common	
Unspecified bacterial pneumonia	An infrequent manifestation of bacterial pneumonia but statistically among the most common causes of this finding because of the relative frequency of bacterial pneumonia
Uncommon	
Actinomycosis	Common features of uncommon pneumonias.
Nocardiosis	These are more commonly confused with
Blastomycosis	pulmonary neoplasms because the infiltration tends to be more chronic than bacterial pneumonias

TABLE 36-7 Chest Wall Invasion from Lung Focus (Often with Rib Destruction)

Infectious Causes	
Actinomycosis	Chronic infiltrate, sporadic
Blastomycosis	Midwestern United States, time spent in wooded environment
Tuberculosis	Rare manifestation of tuberculosis
Noninfectious Causes	
Bronchogenic carcinoma	Most common cause of this pattern
Lymphoma	Most commonly seen in region adjacent to mediastinum

The radiographic patterns of nocardial pneumonia are similar to those of actinomycosis. Chronic infiltrates are the most common manifestation. It may also appear masslike and often cavitates. However, chest wall involvement is rare. Although this pathogen may be found in any patient, it has a predilection for individuals with diseases of the reticuloendothelial system and for those with pulmonary alveolar proteinosis.

OPPORTUNISTIC INFECTIONS

Pneumocystis Pneumonia

With the advent of the AIDS epidemic and the widespread use of immunosuppressive agents, pneumocystis pneumonia is now among the most common opportunistic infections. Characteristically, it appears as a fine diffuse interstitial process, relatively uniformly spread throughout the lungs. When severe, this pneumonia can become a diffuse alveolar process which resembles pulmonary edema. Most often the differential diagnosis includes cytomegalovirus (CMV) pneumonia on the one hand, and interstitial or alveolar pulmonary edema secondary to congestive heart failure on the other (Table 36-8). Interstitial edema can usually be excluded by repeating the chest radiograph following diuresis. In patients with long-standing AIDS, a mild baseline interstitial lung disease is present which can be confused with an acute widespread pneumonia, i.e., "nonspecific interstitial pneumonitis." Therefore, previous chest radiographs are often helpful in determining whether a diffuse interstitial pattern is new and presumably a pneumonia, or old and represents chronic interstitial scarring.

Pneumocystis pneumonia sometimes assumes more unusual appearances, e.g., solitary or multiple regions of focal alveolar consolidation. This is particularly true in the AIDS population. In some patients with pneumocystis pneumonia, the initial chest radiograph may be normal. Therefore, in the appropriate clinical setting, a normal chest radiograph does not exclude the diagnosis of pneumocystis pneumonia.

In patients receiving prophylactic aerosolized pentamidine, the

TABLE 36-8 Fine Diffuse Interstitial Infiltrates (Linear Pattern)

Infiltrates	Population
Pneumocystis pneumonia	AIDS
	Lymphoproliferative disorders
	Transplants
CMV pneumonia	AIDS
	Lymphoproliferative disorders
	Transplants
Interstitial edema from congestive heart failure	

interstitial infiltrates of pneumocystis pneumonia may be confined to the upper zones of the chest radiograph. This is thought to be due to the preferential deposition of pentamidine in the dependent portions of the lungs. Some affected individuals develop numerous small cystic spaces in the upper lung zones. These are attributed to a low-grade chronic infection by *Pneumocystis carinii;* they are characteristically distributed peripherally and are best demonstrated by CT.

Cytomegalovirus Pneumonia

CMV pneumonia infects the same population of patients and has the same radiographic appearance as does pneumocystis pneumonia, i.e., diffuse linear interstitial infiltrates which, in more severe cases, may progress to a diffuse alveolar infiltrate resembling pulmonary edema. Unlike pneumocystis pneumonia, CMV pneumonia is virtually always a diffuse process.

Cryptococcosis

In non-AIDS immunocompromised patients, the most common radiographic appearance is that of a solitary nodule or of multiple pulmonary nodules. However, patchy nonsegmental alveolar infiltrates are also seen in about one third of such patients. Pleural effusions are rare and usually a sign of disseminated disease. Compared to other mycoses, adenopathy is relatively uncommon, i.e., it occurs in approximately 10 to 30 percent.

In patients with AIDS, pulmonary nodules are distinctly uncommon as a manifestation of cryptococcosis. Mediastinal and hilar adenopathy and focal or diffuse interstitial infiltrates together, or in isolation, account for most of the radiographic manifestations.

Aspergillosis

Aspergillus infection can be manifested clinically in a variety of ways. These are generally sorted into three categories: *noninvasive, semi-invasive,* and *invasive aspergillosis.* The form that is expressed depends on the immune status of the host.

Noninvasive aspergillosis is a saprophytic infestation of preexisting pulmonary cavities that usually are the residua of prior infection by other organisms, e.g., tuberculosis. Radiographically, a mycetoma or fungus ball is seen within the cavity. The mycetoma appears as a mobile round or oval density within the lucency of the cavity. Mobility of the mycetoma can be demonstrated by chest radiographs taken in both the erect and decubitus positions; the mycetoma moves to the most dependent position within the cavity. In some instances, the mycetoma is difficult to recognize on the chest radiograph. In this circumstance, CT imaging in the erect and supine positions can be useful in showing the mobility of the mycetoma. Noninvasive aspergillosis is often found unexpectedly in a healthy individual.

Semi-invasive aspergillosis is most often encountered in patients with diseases that cause mild degrees of immunosuppression. It is a particularly common complication of severe sarcoidosis and also occurs in alcoholics and, occasionally, in patients with COPD or disseminated cancer. Semi-invasive aspergillosis often resembles noninvasive aspergillosis in that it is manifested as a mycetoma within a thick-walled cavity. However, unlike noninvasive aspergillosis, semi-invasive aspergillosis is a gradual process which progressively destroys the pulmonary parenchyma. The cavities involved in semi-invasive aspergillosis are invariably located in the apices of the lungs. Extensive pleural thickening is a common feature of this disease, a characteristic which helps distinguish it from reactivation tuberculosis where pleural thickening is less common. The apical disease is often bilateral but usually asymmetrically.

On a single chest radiograph it may be impossible to distinguish noninvasive from semi-invasive aspergillosis, although semi-invasive aspergillosis is typically associated with a more exuberant degree of surrounding pulmonary consolidation. The two entities are best distinguished by following the radiographic picture over time; radiographic progression favors semi-invasive disease. In contrast, noninvasive aspergillosis is a saprophytic infestation and does not change with time, except for changes in the size of the mycetoma.

Invasive aspergillosis occurs in severely immunocompromised patients, in patients with lymphoproliferative disorders, and in patients with neutropenia. Characteristically, a few scattered, small subsegmental regions of alveolar consolidation develop soon after the white blood cell count reaches its nadir. As the white blood cell count rebounds, these infiltrates cavitate spontaneously to produce an "air-crescent sign." This is a small sickle-shaped lucency usually at the superior aspect of the infiltrate. At times, this appearance resembles a mycetoma within a cavity. However, the central density does not move with gravity. *Aspergillus* species are angioinvasive and may produce pulmonary infarction. The presence of infarction may be suggested by the rapid development of an area of consolidation in a vascular territory.

Candida Pneumonia

Candida pneumonia is often part of a systemic infection involving many organs. The radiographic appearance is usually that of patchy alveolar disease. Usually the disease is widespread and bilateral, but it is unilateral in approximately 20 percent of patients. In approximately one half the patients, there is an associated interstitial component. This infection is not radiographically distinctive. Therefore, the diagnosis depends on clinical suspicion reinforced by culture of sputum or biopsy.

BIBLIOGRAPHY

For a more detailed discussion, see Swartz MN: Approach to the patient with pulmonary infections, in Fishman AP (ed), *Pulmonary Diseases and Disorders,* 2d ed. New York, McGraw-Hill, 1988, pp 1375–1410.

Brown ST, Almenoff PL: Pulmonary mycobacterial infections associated with neoplasia. Semin Respir Infect 7:104–113, 1992.

Fraser RG, Peter Paré JA, Paré PD, Fraser RS, Genereux GP: *Diagnosis of Diseases of the Chest,* 3d ed. Philadelphia, WB Saunders, 1989, 2:774–1176.

Levine SJ: An approach to the diagnosis of pulmonary infections in immunosuppressed patients. Semin Respir Infect 7:81–95, 1992.

Lynch DA, Armstrong JD II: A pattern-oriented approach to chest radiographs in atypical pneumonia syndromes. Clin Chest Med 12:203–222, 1991.

Rubin SA, Gefter WB, Goodman PC, Reed JC (eds): Pneumonia in patients with normal immunity. J Thorac Imaging 6:1–88, 1991.

37

Guide to Antimicrobial Therapy for Respiratory Tract Infections and Selected Adverse Effects of Frequently Used Antimicrobials

John E. Connors

Guide to Antimicrobial Therapy for Respiratory Tract Infections*

Organism	Bacterial infections Therapy of choice
Gram-positive Aerobes	
Actinomyces israelii	Penicillin G
Bacillus anthracis	Penicillin G
Nocardia asteroides	Co-trimoxazole
Staphylococcus aureus	
Nonpenicillinase producing	Penicillin G or V
Penicillinase producing	β-Lactamase stable penicillin‡
Methicillin resistant	Vancomycin
Streptococcus pneumoniae	
Penicillin sensitive (MIC < 0.1 μg/ml)	Penicillin G or V
Intermediate penicillin resistance (MIC = 0.1–1.0 μg/ml)	Cefotaxime or ceftriaxone
High level penicillin resistance (MIC ≥ 2.0 μg/ml)	Vancomycin
Streptococcus pyogenes	Penicillin G or V
Gram-negative Aerobes	
Acinetobacter species	Imipenem
Aeromonas hydrophilia	Ciprofloxacin or ofloxacin
Bordetella pertussis	Erythromycin
Brucella species	Doxycycline plus rifampin
Citrobacter freundii	Imipenem
Eikenella corrodens	Ampicillin
Enterobacter species	Imipenem +/– aminoglycoside§
Escherichia coli	Third-generation cephalosporin‖
Flavobacterium meningosepticum	Vancomycin
Francisella tularensis	Streptomycin or gentamicin
Haemophilus influenzae	Third-generation cephalosporin‖
Klebsiella pneumoniae	Third-generation cephalosporin‖
Legionella species	Erythromycin +/– rifampin
Moraxella catarrhalis	Co-trimoxazole
Neisseria meningitidis	Penicillin G
Pasteurella multocida	Penicillin G
Proteus mirabilis	Ampicillin
Proteus species (indole +)	Third-generation cephalosporin‖
Pseudomonas aeruginosa	Antipseudomonal penicillin** + aminoglycoside§

Alternatives

Doxycycline
Erythromycin, a tetracycline[†]
Sulfisoxazole, minocycline

β-Lactamase stable penicillin[‡], first-generation cephalosporin,
vancomycin, clindamycin, imipenem, amoxicillin/clavulanate,
ticarcillin/clavulanate, ampicillin/sulbactam
First-generation cephalosporin, vancomycin, clindamycin, imipenem,
amoxicillin/clavulanate, ticarcillin/clavulanate, ampicillin/sulbactam
Teicoplanin[††], ciprofloxacin

Ampicillin, amoxicillin, cefazolin, erythromycin, clarithromycin,
clindamycin, cefaclor, loracarbef, cefpodoxime
Vancomycin

Ceftriaxone, cefotaxime, ceftizoxime

Other β-lactams, erythromycin, clindamycin, vancomycin

Ticarcillin or mezlocillin or piperacillin plus amikacin, co-trimoxazole,
ticarcillin/clavulanate
Co-trimoxazole, aminoglycoside[§], imipenem
Co-trimoxazole
Co-trimoxazole plus rifampin
Ciprofloxacin, ofloxacin, aminoglycoside[§]
Erythromycin, doxycycline, amoxicillin/clavulanate
Antipseudomonal penicillin[**] + aminoglycoside[§], co-trimoxazole,
ticarcillin/clavulanate, ciprofloxacin, ofloxacin
Antipseudomonal penicillin[**], aminoglycoside[§], amoxicillin/clavulanate,
ticarcillin/clavulanate, ampicillin/sulbactam, co-trimoxazole, imipenem,
other cephalosporins, aztreonam, ciprofloxacin, ofloxacin
Co-trimoxazole, rifampin
Doxycycline, chloramphenicol
Cefuroxime, co-trimoxazole, amoxicillin/clavulanate, ciprofloxacin,
ofloxacin, cefaclor, cefixime, clarithromycin
Ciprofloxacin, ofloxacin, aminoglycoside[§], ticarcillin/clavulanate,
ampicillin/sulbactam, antipseudomonal penicillin[**], co-trimoxazole,
imipenem, aztreonam, amoxicillin/clavulanate
Clarithromycin, azithromycin, co-trimoxazole, ciprofloxacin, ofloxacin
Doxycycline, amoxicillin/clavulanate, third-generation cephalosporin[//],
clarithromycin, cefprozil, loracarbef
Third-generation cephalosporin[//], cefuroxime, chloramphenicol, a
sulfonamide
Doxycycline, ceftriaxone, amoxicillin/clavulanate
A cephalosporin, co-trimoxazole, aminoglycoside[§], aztreonam,
antipseudomonal penicillin[**], imipenem, ciprofloxacin, ofloxacin
Imipenem, aminoglycoside[§], aztreonam, ciprofloxacin, ofloxacin
Ceftazidime or imipenem or ticarcillin/clavulanate plus an
aminoglycoside[§], ciprofloxacin

Bacterial infections

Organism	Therapy of choice
Pseudomonas cepacia	Co-trimoxazole
Pseudomonas pseudomallei	Ceftazidime
Serratia marcescens	Third-generation cephalosporin//
Xanthomonas maltophilia	Co-trimoxazole
Yersinia enterocolitica	Co-trimoxazole
Yersinia pestis	Streptomycin
Anaerobic Lung Infection	Clindamycin
Bacteroides melaninogenicus	
Fusobacterium nucleatum	
Peptostreptococci	
Acid-fast Bacteria	
Mycobacterium avium complex	Clarithromycin + rifampin + ethambutol
Mycobacterium kansasii	Rifampin + isoniazid + ethambutol
Mycobacterium tuberculosis	Isoniazid + rifampin for 6 months with pyrazinamide +/− ethambutol‡‡ for first 2 months
Other Bacteria	
Chlamydia psittaci	Tetracycline
Chlamydia trachomatis	Erythromycin
Chlamydia pneumoniae (TWAR)	Doxycycline or tetracycline
Coxiella burnetii	Doxycycline
Mycoplasma pneumoniae	Erythromycin or a tetracycline†
Rickettsia species	Doxycycline

Viral infections

Organism	Therapy of choice
Influenza viruses	Amantadine (type A)
Respiratory syncytial virus	Ribavirin
Herpes simplex	Acyclovir
Cytomegalovirus	Ganciclovir or foscarnet
Varicella	Acyclovir

Protozoan infections

Organism	Therapy of choice
Entamoeba histolytica (amebiasis)	Metronidazole followed by iodoquinol
Pneumocystis carinii	Co-trimoxazole or pentamidine (IV)
Toxoplasma gondii	Pyrimethamine + sulfadiazine + folinic acid

Fungal infections

Organism	Therapy of choice
Aspergillus species	Amphotericin B
Blastomyces dermatitidis	Ketoconazole, amphotericin B
Candida species	Amphotericin B
Coccidioides immitis	Ketoconazole, amphotericin B

Alternatives

Ceftazidime, follow in vitro susceptibility data
Ceftazidime plus co-trimoxazole, chloramphenicol plus doxycycline plus co-trimoxazole, amoxicillin/clavulanate
Gentamicin, imipenem, ciprofloxacin, ofloxacin, aztreonam
Ticarcillin/clavulanate, ciprofloxacin, minocycline
Ciprofloxacin, aminoglycoside[§], third-generation cephalosporin[//], tetracycline
A tetracycline[†], chloramphenicol
Ticarcillin/clavulanate, imipenem, cefoxitin, ampicillin/sulbactam

Isoniazid plus ethambutol plus rifampin plus streptomycin; substitute or add ciprofloxacin, rifabutin, amikacin, cycloserine
Streptomycin, ethionamide, cycloserine, clarithromycin

Ethambutol, streptomycin, cycloserine, ethionamide, ciprofloxacin, ofloxacin

Chloramphenicol
Doxycycline, sulfonamide
Erythromycin, azithromycin, clarithromycin
Erythromycin
Clarithromycin
Chloramphenicol

Viral infections

Prophylaxis

Amantadine (type A), rimantadine[††], vaccine

Ganciclovir, acyclovir (transplant patients)
Varicella-zoster immune globulin

Protozoan infections

Alternatives

Dehydroemetine followed by chloroquine plus iodoquinol

Dapsone plus trimethoprim, clindamycin plus primaquine, atovaquone

Clindamycin plus pyrimethamine plus folinic acid

Fungal infections

Alternatives

Itraconazole
Itraconazole
Fluconazole
Itraconazole

Organism	Fungal infections Therapy of choice
Cryptococcus neoformans	Amphotericin B +/ – flucytosine
Histoplasma capsulatum	Amphotericin B, ketoconazole
Mucormycosis	Amphotericin B
Sporothrix schenckii	Amphotericin B

*When an organism is susceptible to multiple agents, consideration should be given to selecting an antimicrobial regimen that has a narrower spectrum of activity and is less expensive.

†A tetracycline includes demeclocycline, doxycycline, minocycline, and tetracycline.

‡β-Lactamase stable penicillins include cloxacillin, dicloxacillin, methicillin, nafcillin, and oxacillin.

§ Systemic aminoglycosides include amikacin, gentamicin, netilmicin, and tobramycin.

// Parenteral third-generation cephalosporins include cefotaxime, ceftazidime, ceftizoxime, and ceftriaxone.

** Antipseudomonal penicillins include carbenicillin, ticarcillin, mezlocillin, azlocillin, and piperacillin.

†† Investigational in the United States.

‡‡ Ethambutol is added for suspected isoniazid resistance.

+/– With or without.

+ Combine all.

Alternatives
Fluconazole
Itraconazole
Itraconazole

Selected Adverse Effects of Frequently Used Antimicrobials

Aminoglycosides	
Amikacin	Ototoxicity (eighth cranial nerve damage)
Gentamicin	*Vestibular symptoms: dizziness, vertigo, nystagmus, and ataxia*
Kanamycin	
Netilmicin	*Auditory symptoms: roaring in ears, tinnitus, loss of hearing (may be permanent)*
Streptomycin	
Tobramycin	*Nephrotoxicity: nonoliguric azotemia, ↑ BUN and serum creatinine, ↓ urine specific gravity*
	Neuromuscular blockade (most likely in patients receiving general anesthetics or who have neuromuscular disease such as myasthenia gravis), peripheral neuropathy or encephalopathy
Amphotericin B	Nephrotoxicity
	Fever, chills, nausea, vomiting
	Phlebitis at the IV site
	Hypokalemia, hypomagnesemia, anemia
Aztreonam	Transient eosinophilia and transiently ↑ ALT, AST, and alkaline phosphatase
Cephalosporins	
General adverse effects	Positive direct and indirect Coombs' test
	Transient ↑ BUN and serum creatinine
	Transient ↑ AST, ALT, alkaline phosphatase, LDH, and bilirubin
	Nausea, vomiting, diarrhea
Cefaclor	Serum sickness
Cefamandole	Hypoprothrombinemia
Cefixime	Abdominal pain, anorexia, flatulence, dry mouth, and ↑ serum amylase
	Headache, dizziness, nervousness, insomnia, somnolence, malaise, and fatigue
Cefmetazole	Hypoprothrombinemia
Cefonicid	↑ Platelet count, eosinophilia
Cefoperazone	Hypoprothrombinemia with or without bleeding, diarrhea, and slight ↓ in Hgb and Hct
Ceftazidime	Eosinophilia, thrombocytosis, metallic taste, ↑ GGT
Ceftizoxime	Eosinophilia and thrombocytosis
Ceftriaxone	Eosinophilia, thrombocytosis, leukopenia, diarrhea, and biliary sludging or cholelithiasis
Cefuroxime	Bitter taste when oral tablets are crushed, gastrointestinal effects more common with oral dosage form
	↓ Hgb and Hct, transient eosinophilia
Moxalactam	Transient neutropenia, leukopenia, granulocytopenia, anemia, eosinophilia, thrombocytopenia, or thrombocytosis
	Hypoprothrombinemia and/or inhibition of platelet function may result in clinical bleeding

Selected Adverse Effects of Frequently Used Antimicrobials *(Continued)*

Chloramphenicol	Aplastic anemia, leukopenia, thrombocytopenia, and anemia
	Gray syndrome and optic neuritis
Clarithromycin	Diarrhea, nausea, abnormal taste, dyspepsia, abdominal pain, headache
	↑ BUN
Clindamycin	Nausea, vomiting, diarrhea, and abdominal pain
	Pseudomembranous colitis
	Generalized morbilliform rash
Co-trimoxazole	Nausea, vomiting, anorexia
	Skin reactions including rash, Stevens-Johnson syndrome and erythema multiforme
	Frequency of some adverse effects is higher in patients with AIDS
	Anemia, neutropenia, and thrombocytopenia
Erythromycin salts	Abdominal cramping and pain, nausea, vomiting, and diarrhea
	Hepatic dysfunction, cholestatic hepatitis (estolate and ethylsuccinate salts), and reversible ototoxicity
Fluoroquinolones	
Ciprofloxacin	
Ofloxacin	Seizures, toxic psychosis, and hallucinations have been reported
	Administration to immature animals has resulted in arthropathy. Therefore, it is recommended that these agents not be administered to pregnant women and children < 18 years old
	Phototoxicity
	Nausea, diarrhea, vomiting, abdominal pain, headache, restlessness, and increased AST and ALT (ciprofloxacin)
	Nausea, headache, insomnia, dizziness, and diarrhea (ofloxacin)
Imipenem/cilastatin	Nausea, diarrhea, vomiting, eosinophilia, positive Coombs' test, seizures, transient ↑ BUN, serum creatinine, AST, ALT, and alkaline phosphatase
	Transient leukopenia, neutropenia, agranulocytosis, thrombocytopenia, and thrombocytosis
Penicillin derivatives	
Penicillin G and V	Serum sickness-like reaction, positive direct Coombs' test, and seizures
	Nausea, vomiting, diarrhea, and epigastric pain
	Jarisch-Herxheimer reaction (when treating syphilis)

Selected Adverse Effects of Frequently Used Antimicrobials *(Continued)*

Penicillinase-resistant penicillins	
Cloxacillin	Nausea, vomiting, diarrhea, epigastric pain and
Dicloxacillin	flatulence
Methicillin	Acute interstitial nephritis with methicillin
Nafcillin	Hepatic dysfunction with IV oxacillin
Oxacillin	
Aminopenicillins	
Amoxicillin	Generalized maculopapular rash occurring
Amoxicillin/clavulanate	3–14 days after starting therapy
Ampicillin	(ampicillin/amoxicillin rash)
	High incidence of rash when administered to
	patients with a viral infection
	Nausea, vomiting, diarrhea, anorexia,
	epigastric distress
	Frequency of nausea, vomiting, diarrhea:
	Ampicillin > amoxicillin/clavulanate > amoxicillin
Extended-spectrum penicillins	
Carbenicillin	Prolonged bleeding time and abnormal
Ticarcillin	platelet function: carbenicillin, ticarcillin >
Azlocillin	azlocillin, mezlocillin, piperacillin
Mezlocillin	Loose stools/diarrhea
Piperacillin	Hypokalemia
Ticarcillin/clavulanate	
Tetracycline derivatives	
Doxycycline	Nausea, vomiting, diarrhea, anorexia,
Tetracycline	epigastric pain
	Oral and vaginal candidiasis
	Photosensitivity reactions
	A reversible Fanconi-like syndrome has
	occurred following administration of outdated
	or deteriorated tetracycline derivatives
Vancomycin	Ototoxicity and nephrotoxicity
	IM administration may result in necrosis
	Red man's syndrome from rapid IV infusion
	(flushing and/or rash, +/– hypotension)

AIDS = acquired immunodeficiency syndrome; ALT = alanine aminotransferase; AST = aspartate aminotransferase; BUN = blood urea nitrogen; GGT = γ-glutamyltransferase; Hct = hematocrit; Hgb = hemoglobin; LDH = lactic dehydrogenase

DEFINITION

Pneumonia is designated as *community-acquired* if it develops outside of the hospital. Because relatively few microorganisms account for the vast majority of cases of community-acquired pneumonia, this designation is useful clinically both in predicting the most likely pathogens and in selecting appropriate antibiotic coverage. The major organisms responsible for community-acquired pneumonia, as well as their characteristic clinical, radiographic, and diagnostic features are summarized in Table 38-1.

PATHOGENESIS

Pneumonia may develop because of an overwhelming of host defenses by either a large inoculum of pathogenic organism(s) or a particularly virulent organism, or because of impaired defense mechanisms. Host defenses may be impaired by a variety of factors such as a loss of consciousness, cigarette smoke, hypoxemia, alcohol, corticosteroids and other immunosuppressive agents, and malnutrition. Organisms may gain access to the lungs by aspiration of oropharyngeal secretions, inhalation of airborne bacteria, or by the blood stream.

EPIDEMIOLOGY AND ETIOLOGY

In up to 70 percent of patients, the organism(s) responsible for an acute community-acquired pneumonia can be identified. The most common bacterial pathogen is the "pneumococcus" *(Streptococcus pneumoniae)*, which is responsible for > 50 percent of community-acquired pneumonias. The frequency with which other pathogens are the cause depends on the specific host and the environmental conditions. For example, in young adults, *Mycoplasma pneumoniae* is a common cause, whereas in the elderly, it accounts for only a small percentage of community-acquired pneumonias. *Haemophilus influenzae* and *Staphylococcus aureus* cause 5 to 10 percent of cases of community-acquired pneumonia, *S. aureus* with greater frequency in the elderly and in patients recovering from influenza. Nonetheless, despite the association of *S. aureus* with postinfluenzal pneumonia, *S. pneumoniae* is still the most common etiologic agent for postinfluenza pneumonia. Recently, *Moraxella catarrhalis* has been reported as a cause of community-acquired pneumonia, particularly in patients with chronic obstructive pulmonary disease

TABLE 38-1 Differential Diagnosis of Community-Acquired Pneumonia

Etiologic agent	Clinical features	Chest radiograph	Diagnosis
S. pneumoniae ("pneumococcus") *H. influenzae* Gram-negative bacilli	Acute onset Fevers, chills, pleuritic chest pain, productive cough	Lobar infiltrate	Sputum Gram stain and culture Blood cultures
M. pneumoniae	Subacute Nonproductive cough Extrapulmonary manifestations Young adults	Interstitial infiltrate Radiographic picture often out of proportion to symptoms and signs	Serology
C. pneumoniae	Subacute Generally mild Persistent, nonproductive cough Pharyngitis, laryngitis common	Patchy, segmental infiltrates	Serology
L. pneumophila	Acute or subactue Cough with scant sputum CNS manifestations common	Patchy infiltrates progressing to consolidation	Serology Urinary antigen Culture (requires special medium)
Influenza	Typical influenza prodrome followed by rapidly progressive pneumonia Occurs during epidemics	Bilateral interstitial infiltrates	Viral culture

who are receiving corticosteroids or who have underlying immuno-globulin defects. The incidence of *Legionella pneumophila* as a cause of pneumonia depends on the geographic area; incidences as high as 25 percent have been reported from some areas. A new species of *Chlamydia* has been identified in recent years as a cause of community-acquired pneumonia (without any history of exposure to birds). This organism, *Chlamydia pneumoniae* (termed TWAR) accounts for 6 to 12 percent of community-acquired pneumonias primarily affecting young adults.

In the elderly, community-acquired pneumonia is often caused by aerobic gram-negative bacilli as well as by *S. aureus*. The frequency of these organisms as etiologic agents in the elderly may be due to increased colonization of the pharynx by gram-negative rods secondary to a serious underlying disease, prior antibiotic therapy, and diminished physical activity. *Influenza A* is the cause of a small, but significant, number of cases of community-acquired pneumonia in the elderly, usually during an epidemic among the elderly in the winter months.

CLINICAL MANIFESTATIONS

The clinical presentation of community-acquired pneumonia varies with the etiologic agent and the condition of the host.

Acute Pyogenic Pneumonia

In an otherwise healthy patient, pneumonia due to pyogenic organisms such as *S. pneumoniae, S. aureus,* or *H. influenzae* typically presents with the acute onset of fever, cough productive of purulent sputum, chest pain, and shortness of breath; the patient is tachypneic and using the accessory muscles of respiration. The clinical syndrome can vary considerably depending on the organism, the immune state, and the age of the host. For example, pneumococcal pneumonia in a young or middle-aged adult characteristically begins with the abrupt onset of rigor, followed quickly by fever, cough productive of blood-tinged sputum, and pleuritic chest pain. However, the elderly patient with the same type of pneumonia may manifest nothing more than deterioration in mental status.

As noted above, the patient with bacterial pneumonia usually manifests respiratory distress. Examination of the affected lung discloses evidence of consolidation, i.e., increased vocal fremitus, dullness to percussion, rales, whispered pectoriloquy, and egophony. Not uncommonly, the patient has abdominal complaints such as pain, nausea and vomiting, and distention.

Atypical Pneumonia

The etiologic agents of the atypical pneumonia syndrome, including *M. pneumoniae, L. pneumophila, Influenza A* virus, and *Chlamydia pneumoniae,* generally evoke a more subacute syndrome, with constitutional complaints, headache, mild fever, and a nonproductive cough. The physical examination in these patients usually does not reveal signs of consolidation.

USUAL DIAGNOSTIC TESTS

Radiology The radiographic manifestations of pneumonia depend on the etiologic agent. In pneumonia due to pyogenic organisms, the chest radiograph usually shows lobar consolidation with homogeneous opacification and air bronchograms. Alternatively, the pattern may be that of a bronchopneumonia, i.e., patchy, inhomogeneous infiltrates; this pattern is common in patients with chronic bronchitis. Certain etiologic agents are likely to cause cavitation or necrosis; in particular, staphylococcal, gram-negative, and anaerobic infections can cause abscesses. Mycoplasmal or viral infections are apt to cause interstitial infiltrates. In pneumonia due to *Legionella* species, the infiltrates may be patchy at the onset but often progress to lobar consolidation, sometimes bilaterally.

Sputum examination Examination of a Gram-stained sputum is an important first step in the evaluation of a patient with pneumonia because it may help to define the etiologic agent responsible for the pneumonia and assist in choosing the initial antibiotic regimen. A first concern in evaluating the specimen is that it really is sputum: > 25 polymorphonuclear leukocytes and < 10 epithelial cells per low power field indicates that the specimen is sputum, uncontaminated by saliva.

In pneumococcal pneumonia, the Gram stain of sputum is apt to be more sensitive than culture, which allows overgrowth of other organisms that comprise the normal flora of the oropharynx. A preponderance of gram-positive, lancet-shaped diplococci *(S. pneumoniae)*, small pleomorphic gram-negative coccobacilli *(H. influenzae)*, or gram-positive cocci in clusters *(Staphylococcus)* provides a presumptive diagnosis. In a patient who has not been receiving antibiotics, a Gram stain of sputum that shows a leukocytosis despite a paucity of organisms suggests either *Legionella, Mycoplasma,* or a virus as the cause of the infection.

There are two important prerequisites in the use of sputum cultures for the diagnosis of pneumonia: (1) adequate samples, as defined above for identifying sputum rather than saliva, and (2) rapid processing of the samples. Even if careful attention is paid to these prerequisites, sputum culture is often nondiagnostic in community-acquired pneumonia. For example, in pneumococcal pneumonia, as many as 50 percent of cultures may be negative. Similarly, in pneumonia caused by *H. influenzae,* about one third to one half the cultures may be negative. Finally, in pneumonia caused by anaerobic organisms, cultures usually yield normal oral flora; however, the Gram stain can be helpful in making the diagnosis of an anaerobic pneumonia by revealing many neutrophils and a mixed oral flora.

Blood cultures Blood cultures are positive in 20 to 30 percent of patients with bacterial pneumonia. Because positive blood cultures provide definitive proof of an etiologic agent, all patients with community-acquired pneumonia should have blood cultures done before starting antibiotic therapy.

Other techniques Serologic tests can be used to diagnose a number of pathogens that have been associated with the atypical pneumonia syndrome, including *Legionella* species, *M. pneumoniae, Chlamydia* species, and *Influenza A* virus. In general, these methods are not useful at the onset of the pneumonia since both acute and convalescent titers are needed. Although cold agglutinins can be determined at the bedside, they are not specific for *M. pneumoniae* and are found only in up to 50 percent of patients with *M. pneumoniae* infection.

NATURAL HISTORY AND PROGNOSIS

Although morbidity and mortality from pneumonia have decreased dramatically since the preantibiotic era, an estimated 50,000 deaths still occur annually from pneumococcal pneumonia alone. Currently, the overall case fatality rate for pneumococcal pneumonia is about 5 percent. If bacteremia is present, the case fatality rate increases to 20 percent; and if central nervous system (CNS) involvement is present, the case fatality rate increases to 60 percent. Other factors which contribute to mortality in patients with pneumococcal pneumonia are the age and underlying condition of the patient, as well as the capsular type of the organism. Increasing age is strongly related to mortality: the case fatality rate for bacteremic pneumococcal pneumonia increases from 20 percent in young adults to 60 percent in patients over age 70. Underlying medical conditions, notably splenectomy or splenic dysfunction, cirrhosis, chronic obstructive pulmonary disease, immunodeficiency syndromes, and malignancies also increase the risk of death from pneumococcal pneumonia. With respect to the capsular type of the organism, type 3 carries a higher risk of mortality than do other capsular types. Finally, certain clinical features of pneumococcal pneumonia carry a poor prognosis: leukopenia, jaundice, extrapulmonary complications, and involvement of three or more lobes of the lung on the chest radiograph.

The mortality from pneumococcal pneumonia deserves special attention because this is the most common type of community-acquired pneumonia. Mortality associated with other pathogens varies; the highest mortality rates are seen in gram-negative infections (30 to 50 percent) whereas pneumonia due to *M. pneumoniae* is rarely lethal.

Much of the morbidity from community-acquired pneumonia is caused by local complications of the infection. At least 10 to 20 percent of patients with pneumococcal pneumonia develop a pleural effusion; the actual number is probably much higher because effusions are easily overlooked unless chest radiographs are also taken in a lateral decubitus position. Most small effusions complicating pneumococcal pneumonia resolve spontaneously. However, if the effusion is large, the patient is severely ill, or clinical recovery is delayed, the effusion should be aspirated to rule out an empyema. The presence of empyema usually mandates the placement of a chest tube for drainage because loculations are apt to form within the pleural cavity. Empyema is more likely to occur in association with anaerobic and gram-negative pneumonias.

Local destruction of lung tissue in community-acquired pneumonia can cause abscess formation. This complication is uncommon in pneumococcal pneumonia, but, as noted above, common in pneumonia due to *S. aureus,* aerobic gram-negative rods and, particularly, to oral anaerobes.

In addition to local complications, hematogenous dissemination of the infection may occur. The most worrisome site of extrapulmonary involvement is the meninges, because meningitis carries a much higher mortality rate and requires higher doses of antibiotics for adequate treatment. The combination of pneumonia, endocarditis, and meningitis in patients with pneumococcal infection carries a particularly high mortality, i.e., about 80 percent. If there is question about meningeal involvement in a patient with community-acquired pneumonia, particularly if the pneumonia is suspected to be due to *S. pneumoniae,* a lumbar puncture must be performed.

In pneumonia due to *M. pneumoniae,* extrapulmonary involvement may help to make the diagnosis. Stevens-Johnson syndrome, Raynaud's phenomenon, and hemolytic anemia are the most common extrapulmonary manifestations. Others include neurologic complications (aseptic meningitis, Guillain-Barré, psychosis), pericarditis, myopericarditis, and arthritis. In *Legionella* infection, nonfocal neurologic abnormalities such as confusion and clumsiness, are related to the severity of metabolic disturbances and fever. Chlamydia infection is often heralded by sore throat and hoarseness, and cough may persist for weeks to months after resolution of the acute pneumonia.

Radiographically, in community-acquired pneumonia, resolution of the infiltrate lags behind clinical recovery. For this reason, the clinical well-being of the patient should always be considered while viewing follow-up radiographs.

TREATMENT AND PREVENTION

If the Gram stain suggests a specific etiology for the community-acquired pneumonia, initial therapy can be tailored to the specific agent. However, if the initial evaluation is nondiagnostic, then a decision has to be made about the empiric use of antibiotics. In young, otherwise healthy adults, empiric therapy, using erythromycin as treatment for pneumococcal infection as well as for an atypical pneumonia, is reasonable. If an atypical pneumonia is not suspected, penicillin or ampicillin is appropriate. In elderly patients or institutionalized individuals in whom Gram-negative or *S. aureus* infections are more common, empiric therapy using broader coverage, i.e., a third-generation cephalosporin or broad-spectrum penicillin, is in order. In situations where aspiration pneumonia is a possibility (alcoholism, impaired mental status), the use of oral clindamycin or high-dose penicillin should be considered to provide proper coverage for oral anaerobes. If suspicion is high for *Influenza A* pneumonia, e.g., as during an epidemic, the use of amantadine within the first 72 h of illness may shorten the severity and duration of infection. Whatever the initial choice of antibiotic regimen, the decision should be continually reassessed based on the cultures, sputum, blood, and clinical response.

Preventive therapy with pneumococcal and influenza vaccines should be used in individuals who are at increased risk of acquiring infection or who would handle infection poorly. These include healthy elderly persons; patients undergoing splenectomy or with splenic dysfunction; adults with chronic liver, renal, cardiac, or pulmonary disease; alcoholics; and patients who are immunosuppressed by virtue of medications, malignancy, or infection by the human immunodeficiency virus.

BIBLIOGRAPHY

For a more detailed discussion, see Hopkins CC: Community-acquired pneumonia, in Fishman AP (ed), *Pulmonary Diseases and Disorders,* 2d ed. New York, McGraw-Hill, 1988, pp 1535–1542.

Falco V, De Sevilla TF, Alegre J, Ferrer A, Vazquez JMM: *Legionella pneumophila.* A cause of severe community-acquired pneumonia. Chest 100:1007–1011, 1991.

Grayston JT: Infections caused by *Chlamydia pneumoniae* strain TWAR. Clin Infect Dis 15:757–763, 1992.

Marrie TJ: *Mycoplasma pneumoniae* pneumonia requiring hospitalization, with emphasis on infection in the elderly. Arch Intern Med 153:488–494, 1993.

Rello J, Quintana E, Ausina V, Net A, Prats G: A three-year study of severe community-acquired pneumonia with emphasis on outcome. Chest 103:232–235, 1993.

Torres A, Serra-Batlles J, Ferrer A, Jimenez P, Celis R, Cobo E, Rodriguez-Roisin R: Severe community-acquired pneumonia. Epidemiologic and prognostic factors. Am Rev Respir Dis 144:312–318, 1991.

Patrick J. Brennan

Nosocomial pneumonia is now the second leading cause of hospital-acquired infection in the United States, having overtaken surgical wound infections and trailing only urinary tract infections. The mortality rate associated with nosocomial pneumonia may be as high as 50 percent and disproportionately affects the elderly, postoperative patients, and those being mechanically ventilated.

DEFINITION

Criteria for the diagnosis of a nosocomial pneumonia by the Centers for Disease Control and Prevention (CDC) are detailed in Table 39-1. The definition relies on airway cultures and radiographic and clinical observations, such as changing sputum character and new auscultatory findings to make the diagnosis. These findings, particularly in the context of persistent fever and failure to wean from ventilatory support, provide strong evidence for the diagnosis of pneumonia.

CLINICAL FEATURES

Nosocomial pneumonia may present with the characteristic findings of an acute bacterial pneumonia such as fever, productive cough, purulent sputum production, and tachypnea. However, in a hospitalized patient, attributing these findings to pneumonia is not always straightforward because of the wide variety of complications that can mimic infection. Among the diseases that may obscure the diagnosis of nosocomial pneumonia are toxic and allergic processes related to drugs and inspired oxygen, atelectasis, pulmonary emboli and infarction, the adult respiratory distress syndrome (ARDS), congestive heart failure, and tracheobronchitis. Moreover, aspiration of gastric or oropharyngeal contents may result in a chemical pneumonitis that is clinically and radiographically indistinguishable from a bacterial pneumonia. Also, ARDS often masks the appearance of a new pneumonia on the chest radiograph.

PATHOGENESIS

In hospitalized patients, infectious agents can be introduced into the lower respiratory tract in three ways: (1) aspiration of gastric or oropharyngeal contents that are colonized with potential pathogens; (2) hematogenous spread of microbial agents to the lungs, e.g., candidal pneumonia; (3) airborne spread via aerosols and droplet nuclei, e.g., *Legionella,* respiratory viruses, tuberculosis.

TABLE 39-1 CDC Criteria for Diagnosis of Nosocomial Pneumonia

One of these four criteria must be met:

1. Rales or dullness to percussion on chest examination. In addition, any of the following:
   a. New onset of purulent sputum or change in sputum character
   b. Organism isolated from blood culture
   c. Pathogen isolated from specimen obtained by transtracheal aspirate, bronchial brush, or biopsy
2. Chest radiograph shows new or progressive infiltrate, consolidation, cavitation, or pleural effusion *and* any of the following: a, b, or c from number 1 above
   d. Isolation of virus or detection of viral antigens from respiratory secretions
   e. Diagnostic single antibody titer (IgM) or 4-fold increase in paired serum samples (IgG) for pathogen
   f. Histopathologic evidence of pneumonia
3. Patient ≤ 12 months of age has two of the following: apnea, tachypnea, bradycardia, wheezing, rhonchi, or cough. In addition, any of the following:
   g. Increased production of respiratory secretions or any of the criteria in number 2 above
4. Patient ≤ 12 months of age shows new or progressive infiltrate, cavitation, consolidation or pleural effusion on chest radiograph. In addition, any of the criteria in number 3 above.

SOURCE: Garner, et al. Am J Infect Control 16(3):128–140, 1988.

Aspiration is the most common of these pathogenetic mechanisms. Aspiration is facilitated by conditions which decrease the gag reflex and cough. The sequence leading to the development of nosocomial aspiration pneumonia is outlined in Table 39-2. Colonization of the oropharynx by hospital flora, usually gram-negative rods, begins within a few days of admission. Colonization is promoted by the use of broad-spectrum antibacterial agents, increased gastric pH, and carriage of organisms from patient to patient on the hands of health care workers.

The risk factors for the development of pneumonia after hospitalization are listed in Table 39-3. Most important is impairment of airway defenses such as a decrease in the gag reflex and the cough mechanism due to general anesthesia, sedatives, and intoxications and the use of respiratory assist devices and feeding tubes. Mechanical ventilators are important portals of entry for large inocula of

TABLE 39-2 Sequence in the Development of Nosocomial Pneumonia

Colonization of the oropharynx with gram-negative rods
Increased gastric pH
Gastric colonization with gram-negative rods
Impaired cellular or barrier defenses of the lung
Reflux and aspiration of gastric/oropharyngeal contents

TABLE 39-3 Risk Factors for Nosocomial Pneumonia

Age > 70 years
Chronic lung disease
Depressed consciousness
Mechanical ventilation
Large volume aspiration
Chest surgery
Intracranial pressure monitoring
Use of histamine type II blockers
Frequent ventilator circuit changes
Fall and winter seasons
Patient position
Devices
In-line medication nebulizers
Humidifiers
Nasogastric feeding
Enteral feeding
Endotracheal tube

bacteria and for enhancing the growth of organisms which contaminate them.

Another factor that has promoted colonization of the gastrointestinal tract and increased the risk of pneumonia in hospitalized patients has been the decrease in gastric acidity that results from blockade of type II histamine receptors. Ability to clear aspirated organisms is also compromised by impaired host defenses, such as the decrease in the immune function that accompanies advanced age, chronic disease of the airways, and massive aspiration.

Airborne spread of pathogens is often unrecognized as a cause of nosocomial pneumonias unless a cluster of infections occurs and reaches epidemic proportions. Recent nosocomial outbreaks of tuberculosis have been recognized because many of the patients involved were infected with human immunodeficiency virus (HIV) and rapidly developed clinically active tuberculosis and died. Immunocompromised hosts may be particularly susceptible to airborne pathogens. Large outbreaks of Legionnaire's disease have occurred in immunocompromised hosts in hospitals in which water systems were contaminated with *Legionella* organisms.

DIAGNOSTIC PROCEDURES

Determining the microbiologic cause of pneumonia is fraught with pitfalls. A Gram stain of respiratory specimens is the first diagnostic test which should be performed. The Gram stain is useful in directing empiric therapy while waiting for the results of culture. The stain must be interpreted in the light of both the adequacy of the sputum sample and the staining technique. Specimens with < 10 epithelial cells and > 25 polymorphonuclear leukocytes per low power field are considered to be adequate. The cytoplasm of leukocytes should stain pink; the nucleus should stain a deeper shade of pink.

Sputum cultures of specimens obtained through the upper airway are frequently contaminated with oropharyngeal flora and are difficult to interpret. Specimens which bypass the upper airway provide more meaningful information. In the past, transtracheal aspiration was the preferred method for obtaining adequate lower respiratory tract specimens. Currently, transtracheal aspiration has been superseded by the use of the sheathed brush technique to obtain specimens during bronchoscopy. The protected brush specimens possess satisfactory sensitivity and specificity for diagnostic purposes. The sheathed brush technique does not eliminate entirely the risk of contamination with oropharyngeal flora, although in some clinics the sensitivity has reached 100 percent and the specificity 80 percent; in others, the sensitivity and the specificity have been as low as 50 percent.

The bronchoscopic approach offers the advantage of permitting tissue biopsy and bronchoalveolar lavage (BAL) in addition to protected brush specimens. BAL has gained widespread acceptance in the diagnosis of pulmonary infections in compromised hosts, particularly in HIV-infected patients where sensitivity and specificity are comparable to tissue biopsy for the diagnosis of pneumocystis. Despite the widespread use of the bronchoscopic technique, a specific microbial etiology is often elusive and the choice of antimicrobial therapy often remains empirical.

The diagnosis of pneumonia in immunocompromised hosts is considered in greater detail elsewhere (see Chapter 46). Compromised hosts suspected of having nosocomial pneumonia should be bronchoscoped early in the course of the illness, and samples obtained for the culture of community respiratory viruses and *Legionella* as well as bacterial and opportunistic pathogens. In addition, blood cultures should be obtained whenever bacterial pneumonia is suspected because they are positive in 5 to 10 percent of patients. If a pleural effusion is present, fluid should be obtained for culture.

MICROBIAL ETIOLOGY

In large, tertiary care hospitals, aerobic gram-negative bacteria have been the most common cause of nosocomial pneumonia. The most common cause of aerobic gram-positive infection has been *Staphylococcus aureus*. Anaerobic flora have been less prevalent in hospitalized patients with nosocomial pneumonias than in those with outpatient pneumonias. However, since the data (Table 39-4) were

TABLE 39-4 Microbial Etiology of Nosocomial Pneumonia

Bacteria*	
Pseudomonas aeruginosa	17%
Stapylococcus aureus	16%
Enterobacter species	11%
Klebsiella pneumoniae	7%
Escherichia coli	6%
Serratia marcescens	4%
Proteus mirabilis	3%
Enterococci	2%
Coagulase-negative staphylococci	2%
Others	
Anaerobes†	35%
Viruses‡	5%
Influenza A/B	
Respiratory syncytial	
Candida species*	5%

*Modified from Schaberg, et al. Am J Med 91(suppl 3B):72S–75S, 1991.
†Craven, et al. Am J Med 91(suppl 3B):44S–53S, 1991.
‡Graham and Hall, Semin Resp Infect 4(4):253–260, 1989.

obtained from large tertiary care hospitals, they may not reflect the frequency of gram-positive and gram-negative nosocomial infections in smaller hospitals.

The prevalence of viral nosocomial pneumonia is probably greatly underestimated due to the limited availability of viral diagnostic methods. Influenza A/B and respiratory syncytial virus are the most common viruses that cause nosocomial infections. In pediatric institutions, respiratory syncytial virus has been responsible for epidemic outbreaks of pulmonary infection. The most contagious of the respiratory viruses, varicella and measles, have caused serious outbreaks of nosocomial infections. In health care settings, cases of measles have occurred in patients and health care workers who were never immunized or had not acquired natural immunity through prior infection.

PREVENTION

Among the risks for nosocomial pneumonia cited in Table 39-3, several important factors such as advanced age and chronic lung disease, cannot be affected. Table 39-5 lists potentially remediable factors. Limiting the use of endotracheal and nasogastric tubes and sedation whenever possible, appropriate positioning of the patient, and the use of cytoprotective agents rather than antacids and H₂-blockers, may minimize the development of nosocomial pneumonia. Such tactics protect natural barriers to colonization and aspiration.

TABLE 39-5 Prevention of Nosocomial Pneumonia

Treatment of underlying disease
Elimination of H_2-blockers and antacids
Elevation of head
Removal of endotracheal and nasogastric tubes
Controlled use of antibiotics
Selective gut decontamination
Infection control
  Surveillance
  Hand washing
  Education
  Proper airway care

THERAPY

The decision to treat a patient for nosocomial pneumonia is made in the face of uncertainty about the diagnosis and the microbial etiology of the disease. Other diagnoses may masquerade as pneumonia and the choice of antimicrobial agents is usually made before sputum culture results are available; moreover, the culture results are often unreliable. Empiric choices must be made among antimicrobials on the basis of the sputum Gram stain, the severity of the patient's illness, and knowledge of local bacterial resistance patterns.

The high mortality rate associated with nosocomial pneumonia and the prevalence of resistant organisms in most hospitals mandates that empiric therapy cover a broad range of organisms until microbial susceptibility tests are complete. Patients who have been hospitalized for more than 3 days and are seriously ill are likely to be colonized with resistant gram-negative rods. *Pseudomonas aeruginosa, Enterobacter* species, as well as other resistant gram-negative rods are frequent causes of pneumonia in patients requiring mechanical ventilation. Therefore, β-lactam agents with reliable activity against these organisms, such as antipseudomonal penicillins and cephalosporins, are the usual drugs of choice for empiric therapy. Empiric combination therapy with an antipseudomonal β-lactam plus an aminoglycoside should be considered if the patient is severely ill, has had prior antimicrobial therapy, or is known to be colonized with a resistant organism. In institutions with a high prevalence of methicillin-resistant *S. aureus,* vancomycin should be used empirically when gram-positive cocci are noted on Gram stain. When mixed gram-positive and gram-negative flora is present on Gram stain, the process may be a polymicrobial anaerobic infection. The broad-spectrum penicillins, e.g., ticarcillin, mezlocillin, piperacillin, and imipenem/cliastatin have excellent activity against the anaerobes, and the use of additional agents with anaerobic activity is usually not necessary when treating these agents. In view of the increasing problems with antimicrobial resistance and drug costs in hospitals, antibiotic therapy for nosocomial pneumonia should be tailored to limit the spectrum of activity and cost as soon as a pathogen and susceptibilities are available.

The emergence of resistance during monotherapy with a β-lactam is a particular problem with *Enterobacter* and *Pseudomonas* species. Multidrug therapy, e.g., antipseudomonal β-lactam plus an aminoglycoside, should be considered when these pathogens have been identified. The addition of an aminoglycoside may result in synergistic killing when used in combination with other agents against gram-negative rods. Trimethoprim-sulfamethoxazole provides excellent activity against most *Enterobacter* species with little risk of resistance emerging during therapy. At this time, aztreonam and the fluoroquinolones are reserved for patients with β-lactam allergies or with organisms not susceptible to the β-lactams. Table 39-6 provides guidance for empiric therapy of nosocomial pneumonia.

TABLE 39-6 Empiric Therapy of Nosocomial Pneumonia*

Therapy	Clinical setting
Monotherapy Options	
β-Lactam*	Not severely ill; only gram-negative flora on Gram stain§
Aztreonam/fluoroquinolones	Not severely ill; only gram-negative flora on Gram stain; patient has β-lactam allergy
Vancomycin	Not severely ill; only gram-positive flora on Gram stain in institution with high prevalence of methicillin-resistant *S. aureus*
Broad-spectrum penicillin	Not severely ill; mixed flora on Gram stain
Imipenem	Severely ill; mixed flora
Combination Therapy	
β-Lactam† + anaerobic coverage‖	Nonintubated; severely ill; mixed flora
β-Lactam‡ + aminoglycoside	Intubated; severely ill; gram-negative flora severely ill
Aztreonam + aminoglycoside	Severely ill; gram-negative flora; β-lactam allergic patient
Vancomycin/aztreonam/ metronidazole	Severely ill; mixed flora; β-lactam allergic patient

*Antimicrobial choices for specific pathogens are considered in Chapter 37. Decisions regarding empiric therapy should always be made with the knowledge of local susceptibility patterns.
†Third-generation +/– antipseudomonal activity.
‡Third-generation with antipseudomonal activity.
§Consider combination therapy if *Pseudomonas* sp. and *Enterobacter* sp. are suspected.
‖ Anaerobic coverage (e.g., metronidazole or clindamycin) should be added if a cephalosporin with limited anaerobic spectrum is chosen (e.g., ceftazidime, cefoperazone, ceftriaxone).

BIBLIOGRAPHY

For a more detailed discussion, see Counts GW, Stamm WE: Nosocomial pneumonias, in Fishman AP (ed), *Pulmonary Diseases and Disorders,* 2d ed. New York, McGraw-Hill, 1988, pp 1431–1440.

Cohn DL: Bacterial pneumonia in the HIV-infected patient. Infect Dis Clin North Am 5:485–507, 1991.

Edlin BR, Tokars JI, Grieco MH, Crawford JT, Williams J, Sordillo EM, et al: An outbreak of multidrug-resistant tuberculosis among hospitalized patients with the acquired immunodeficiency syndrome. N Engl J Med 326:1514–1521, 1993.

Lowry PW, Tompkins LS: Nosocomial legionellosis: A review of pulmonary and extrapulmonary syndromes. Am J Infect Control 21:21–27, 1993.

McCabe RE: Diagnosis of pulmonary infections in immunocompromised patients. Med Clin North Am 72:1067–1089, 1988.

1993 Revised Classification System for HIV Infection. MMWR 41:17, 1992.

Rossman MD: The resurgence of tuberculosis and non-tuberculosis mycobacteria, in Fishman AP (ed), *Update: Pulmonary Diseases and Disorders.* New York, McGraw-Hill, 1992, pp 287–297.

Rubin RH: Pneumonia in the immunocompromised host, in Fishman AP (ed), *Pulmonary Diseases and Disorders,* 2d ed. New York, McGraw-Hill, 1988, pp 1745–1760.

Shelhamer JH, Toews GB, Masur H, Suffredini AF, Pizzo PA, Walsh TJ, et al: Respiratory disease in the immunosuppressed patient. Ann Intern Med 117:415–431, 1992.

Mindy G. Schuster

The spectrum of anaerobic lung infections includes lung abscess, necrotizing pneumonia, and empyema.

Lung abscess is defined as a suppurative process with a single or dominant cavity of at least 2 cm, usually with an air-fluid level on chest radiograph.

Necrotizing pneumonia represents an analogous but more diffuse process with multiple small cavities < 2 cm in size.

Pulmonary gangrene is a term used to describe tissue destruction that is often the consequence of necrotizing pneumonia.

Empyema is a suppurative infection of the pleural space which is most often the result of contiguous spread from a necrotizing pneumonia.

ETIOLOGY AND MICROBIOLOGY

Anaerobic pulmonary infection is almost always the result of aspiration of oropharyngeal secretions which typically contain anaerobes and aerobes in a ratio of 3 to 5:1. Rarely is embolization from septic thrombophlebitis or spread from a subdiaphragmatic collection the inciting event. Most of the available information about the etiology of anaerobic lung infection comes from studies which used transthoracic and transtracheal needle aspiration. Anaerobes can be isolated in this manner in 60 to 100 percent of cases of lung abscesses and necrotizing pneumonia and 75 percent of empyemas.

Anaerobes alone are isolated in approximately 60 percent of cases of lung abscess, especially if aspiration occurs out of hospital and involves community-acquired organisms. In aspiration that occurs in hospital, mixed infections with anaerobes and aerobes (often *Staphylococcus aureus, Klebsiella* species, and *Pseudomonas*) predominate, reflecting the change in oropharyngeal flora in hospitalized patients.

The most frequently recovered anaerobes are peptostreptococci, *Bacteroides melaninogenicus,* and *Fusobacterium nucleatum. Bacteroides fragilis* is seen in < 10 percent of cases. Other anaerobes that have been described in anaerobic lung infection are listed in Table 40-1.

PATHOGENESIS

About 50 percent of healthy subjects have been demonstrated to aspirate during sleep. However, most instances of anaerobic lung infection are associated with a predisposing condition (Table 40-2) in which impaired consciousness leads to aspiration. Predisposing

TABLE 40-1 Bacteriology of Aspiration Pneumonia in 70 Patients—
Specific Data

Bacteriologic results	No. of patients	
Anaerobic Isolates		
Bacteroides melaninogenicus group	27	(1)*
B. fragilis group	10	
Other bacteroides (*B. oralis, B. corrodens* or *B. gracilis, B. pneumosintes*)	12	
Fusobacterium nucleatum	19	
F. necrophorum	1	
Unidentified anaerobic gram-negative rods	4	(1)
Peptostreptococcus species	34	(6)
Microaerophilic streptococcus	9	(1)
Veillonella	4	
Gram-positive non–spore-forming rods (*Eubacterium, Propionibacterium, Bifidobacterium* species)	14	
Clostridium species	2	
Aerobic and Facultative Isolates		
Staphylococcus aureus	11	(2)
Streptococcus pneumoniae	11	(2)
Other streptococci	5	
Enterobacteriaceae	19	(2)
Pseudomonas (*P. aeruginosa* and *P. maltophilia*)	8	

*Parentheses indicate number of organisms recovered in pure culture.
SOURCE: Based on data in Bartlett, Gorbach, Finegold, 1974.

TABLE 40-2 Predisposing Conditions for
Anaerobic Lung Infections

Altered Consciousness
  Periodontal disease/gingivitis
  Alcoholism
  Cerebrovascular accident
  Seizure disorder
  Diabetic coma
Dysphagia
  Esophageal disease
  Neurologic disease
  Intestinal obstruction
Other
  Bronchiectasis
  Bronchial obstruction
Risks for Gram-negative Rod Involvement
  Alcoholism
  Chronic illness
  Inpatient aspiration
  Endotracheal intubation
  H_2-antagonists and antacids

conditions include alcoholism, neurologic disorders, and dysphagia. In contrast, chronic obstructive pulmonary disease is not, per se, a predisposing condition. Because oropharyngeal anaerobes colonize the gingival crevice, lung abscess is extremely rare in edentulous patients.

Pulmonary segments that are dependent while the patient is supine are most frequently involved in aspiration. The most common site is the posterior segment of the right upper lobe (because of the direct take-off of the right main-stem bronchus), followed by the apical-posterio-segment on the left and the superior segments of the lower lobes. When aspiration occurs in the sitting position, the basal segments of the lower lobes may be involved.

The earliest expression of infection is pneumonia without cavity formation. Inflammation and necrosis then lead to abscess formation. Subsequently, bronchopleural fistulae may develop, leading to empyema.

CLINICAL MANIFESTATIONS

History Symptoms may be subacute or acute. Most often, patients present with malaise, low-grade fever, and productive cough. Approximately 40 to 50 percent of patients have a history of weight loss. The median duration of symptoms before hospitalization is about 2 weeks. There is little in the clinical presentation to distinguish anaerobic pulmonary infections from other bacterial lung infections. Subacute, indolent presentations may mimic pulmonary tuberculosis, and acute presentations may resemble pneumococcal pneumonia. Putrid sputum, considered the hallmark of anaerobic lung infection, is seen in 40 to 60 percent of cases.

Physical examination The physical signs of an anaerobic pulmonary infection depend on its stage of evolution and duration. A fever spike is common early, e.g., in necrotizing pneumonia, but less prominent when a lung abscess has formed. The signs of a necrotizing pneumonia do not differ from those of other types of pneumonia. A lung abscess before drainage is manifested by localized dullness to percussion and decreased breath sounds. Once drainage (of foul-smelling sputum) occurs, fever drops; bronchial breathing can then be heard over the affected area because of improved transmission of breath sounds by consolidated tissue surrounding the abscess cavity. By the time that an empyema develops, the patient is often debilitated and dyspneic and presents signs of a pleural effusion.

DIAGNOSTIC TESTS

Microbiological diagnosis Because the normal oropharyngeal flora includes anaerobic bacteria, expectorated sputum specimens are unreliable. Ideal specimens include transthoracic or transtracheal aspirates (often difficult to obtain), blood cultures (associated with a yield of < 5 percent), and pleural fluid. Specimens obtained during fiberoptic bronchoscopy with use of a protected brush are acceptable when combined with quantitative cultures and transported quickly. Anaerobic specimens should be sent in a syringe after expelling as much air as possible. Often many of these techniques are unavailable or too cumbersome. Consequently, diagnosis depends on the presence of putrid sputum along with the appropriate history and chest radiograph. In these cases in which a microbiologic diagnosis is often not achieved, the patient is treated empirically.

Chest radiography The earliest chest radiograph finding after aspiration is a parenchymal infiltrate consistent with pneumonia. Progression to cavity formation with air-fluid level is unusual within the first week after aspiration and takes an average of 12 days to occur. Necrotizing anaerobic pneumonias are often confined to one lobe, but spread can occur rapidly to involve both lungs. Chest radiography reveals evidence of pneumonitis with multiple small cavities. A pleural effusion raises the suspicion of empyema.

DIFFERENTIAL DIAGNOSIS

Organisms other than anaerobic bacteria may cause cavitary pneumonia and lung abscess. Tuberculosis cavities are usually thinner and often lack surrounding infiltrate; nonetheless, sputum smears for acid-fast bacilli may be necessary to distinguish the two entities. Many aerobic bacteria can also cause necrotizing pneumonia, including *S. aureus, Klebsiella pneumoniae,* and *Pseudomonas aeruginosa.* Less commonly, *Pneumococcus, E. coli,* and *Proteus* are the etiologic agents. Additionally, *Legionella, Nocardia,* and *Actinomycosis,* and some fungi may cause cavitation.

In patients who lack the usual predisposing conditions for aspiration or do not respond appropriately to antibiotic therapy, the diagnosis of cavitating lung carcinoma should be considered. Fiberoptic bronchoscopy, with biopsy or transthoracic needle biopsy, may be necessary to exclude this possibility. Other noninfectious causes of cavitary disease in the lungs include vasculitis, e.g., Wegener's granulomatosis or pulmonary infarction.

NATURAL HISTORY AND PROGNOSIS

Patients with anaerobic lung abscess may not become afebrile for 5 to 7 days, even with appropriate antibiotic therapy. Chest radiography often worsens during this period of time as well. The apparent lack of response to therapy during the first week does not require that antibiotics be changed or added. By the end of the first week of treatment, most patients start to feel better. This improved sense of well-being is accompanied by a decrease in sputum production and the disappearance of fever. Continuing fever after a week of therapy is unusual and prompts consideration of fiberoptic bronchoscopy to establish a diagnosis and evaluate the possibility of bronchial obstruction. Full recovery may require several months. Because cavitary lesions do not close for an average of 65 days, the chest radiograph is an insensitive measure of response to therapy.

One half the patients with necrotizing pneumonia become afebrile by the second day of therapy; 80 percent become afebrile after 5 days. Patients with empyema often demonstrate recurrent fever and may not become afebrile for several weeks despite drainage.

Complications Approximately one third of patients with lung abscess, and one half of patients with necrotizing pneumonia, develop empyema. On rare occasion, hematologic dissemination occurs via the vertebral arteries resulting in brain abscess, which is usually solitary. Dissemination to other organs does occur but is exceedingly rare.

Prognosis The prognosis for anaerobic lung abscess is genreally good; infection is the cause of death in 4 percent of patients. The mortality rate is higher in necrotizing pneumonia, i.e., it may approach 25 percent, probably because of the propensity of infection to spread rapidly to adjacent lobes. Mortality is about as high in nosocomial anaerobic pulmonary infections because of the general debilitation of the patients and the virulence of gram-negative rods which are often part of a mixed anaerobic/aerobic infection. Poor prognostic indicators include a large abscess cavity > 6 cm in diameter, necrotizing pneumonia, > 8 weeks of symptoms before diagnosis, bronchial obstruction, and the underlying diseases associated with debilitation.

TREATMENT

Traditionally, the mainstay of treatment for anaerobic lung infections has been penicillin. However, increasing numbers of oropharyngeal anaerobes are now β-lactamase producers, i.e., in 15 to 25 percent of patients, leading to treatment failures. Some studies favor clindamycin over penicillin because fever generally lasts longer with penicillin and the incidence of treatment failures is higher with penicillin. However, this preference is debatable because the likelihood of side effects with clindamycin is greater and the cost is higher. Some clinicians use penicillin alone if the patient is mildly or moderately ill. In the seriously ill patient, they either add metronidazole or resort to clindamycin.

Metronidazole is active against all gram-negative anaerobes but ineffective against most microaerophilic streptococci. Therefore, metronidazole is used only in conjunction with penicillin. Other antibiotics that are active against a wide variety of anaerobes but have not been well studied include ticarcillin/clavulanate, amoxicillin/clavulanate, ampicillin/sulbactam, chloramphenicol, and imipenem. Third-generation cephalosporins have less activity against anaerobes than do cefoxitin or penicillins. A significant percentage of anaerobes are resistant to tetracycline. Quinolones and aztreonam have little activity against anaerobes.

Penicillin is given in doses of 12 to 18 million units per day. Some studies suggest that oral penicillin may be effective, but most experts start with intravenous therapy. After clinical improvement occurs, treatment can be changed to oral penicillin at 750 mg every 6 h or clindamycin, 300 mg every 6 h. Therapy may need to be continued for 2 to 4 months.

Postural drainage is an important component of treatment. Bronchoscopy is indicated in treatment failure or when a foreign body is suspected. Surgical resection is rarely necessary. Indeed, it is usually contraindicated because of the risk of spillage to adjacent lung tissue. Indications for surgical resection include failure of medical therapy, hemorrhage, and suspected neoplasm. Drainage is the mainstay of therapy for empyema, and failure to establish drainage promptly may result in rapid clinical deterioration. Although antibiotics do play a major role in treatment, they are ineffective when used without proper drainage.

BIBLIOGRAPHY

For a more detailed discussion, see Finegold SM: Anaerobic infections of lungs and pleura, in Fishman AP (ed), *Pulmonary Diseases and Disorders,* 2d ed. New York, McGraw-Hill, 1988, pp 1505–1516.

Bartlett JG: Antibiotics in lung abscess. Semin Respir Infect 6:103–111, 1991.

Gary JJ, Johnson AC, Garner FT: The role of the prosthodontist regarding aspirative dysphagia. J Prosthet Dent 67:101–106, 1992.

Hill MK, Sanders CV: Anaerobic disease of the lung. Infect Dis Clin North Am 5:453–466, 1991.

Khawaja IT, Buffa SD, Brandstetter RD: Aspiration pneumonia. A threat when deglutition is compromised. Postgrad Med 92:165–168, 173–177, 1992.

Abby Huang

The term *atypical pneumonia* is used to differentiate between those pneumonias which present in the traditional clinical fashion and those which do not. Typical (classical) bacterial pneumonias present with rigors, fever, a productive cough, pleuritic chest pain, and lobar infiltrates. Atypical pneumonias usually present in a more insidious fashion with malaise, headache, fever, nonproductive cough, and nonlobar infiltrates. The common etiologic agents involved in atypical pneumonia include *Mycoplasma pneumoniae, Chlamydia pneumoniae, Chlamydia psittaci, Coxiella burnetii, Legionella pneumophila,* and a number of viruses, such as influenza A and B, adenovirus, and respiratory syncytial virus.

Mycoplasma pneumoniae PNEUMONIA

Epidemiology

M. pneumoniae, which is the primary cause of atypical pneumonia, is the etiologic agent in approximately 20 percent of all cases of pneumonia in the general population. Infection occurs throughout the year, but the incidence appears to increase during the late summer and fall. The incidence is highest in children and young adults (ages 5 to 20). Horizontal spread is common and enclosed populations, e.g., college students, military recruits, or families, appear to be particularly prone to *M. pneumoniae* infection.

Pathogenesis

M. pneumoniae is the smallest free-living organism and, unlike true bacteria, it lacks a cell wall. Infection appears to occur by inhalation of infected respiratory material during close contact with an acutely ill individual. Following attachment of the organism to respiratory tract epithelial cells, *M. pneumoniae* produces hydrogen peroxide and superoxide, causing injury to the epithelial cells with resultant stasis of cilia. Aside from the direct effect of the organism on respiratory epithelial cells, immune-mediated mechanisms probably play a role in the development of clinically evident pneumonia and some of the extrapulmonary complications.

Clinical Manifestations

The incubation period after exposure is 14 to 21 days. Most patients develop pharyngitis or tracheobronchitis. Pneumonia occurs in only 10 percent of patients and usually is mild. The onset of illness is gradual, usually beginning with fever, malaise, and headache. An intractable, nonproductive cough occurs in almost all patients. In up to 50 percent of patients with pneumonia, upper respiratory tract signs and symptoms such as sore throat, rhinorrhea, and earache are present. Musculoskeletal and gastrointestinal symptoms are common but minor. Other less common findings include cervical lymphadenopathy, conjunctivitis, skin rashes, sinusitis, and pulse-temperature dissociation. Pleuritic chest pain is uncommon.

Physical examination of the chest often reveals rales and rhonchi. Signs of pulmonary consolidation are uncommon.

Extrapulmonary Manifestations

The most characteristic extrapulmonary manifestation of infection with *M. pneumoniae* is autoimmune hemolytic anemia which results from the production of cold hemagglutinins. Nervous system manifestations occur in approximately 7 percent of infected patients; they include aseptic meningitis, encephalitis, transverse myelitis, neuropathies, Guillain-Barré syndrome, and sensorineural hearing loss. Dermatologic manifestations usually consist of macular, pete-chial, or morbilliform eruptions. However, erythema nodosum, urticaria, erythema multiforme, and Stevens-Johnson syndrome have been reported. Cardiac involvement is infrequent (7.5 percent in one series) but may be manifested as myocarditis, pericarditis, congestive heart failure, and conduction disturbances.

Laboratory Findings

Except for occasional increases in the hepatic transaminases, routine blood studies are typically normal. The white blood cell count may be elevated but uncommonly exceeds 15,000 per cubic millimeter. Band forms may be found not in excess of 10 percent. Gram stain of the sputum usually reveals polymorphonuclear leukocytes, but no predominant bacterial organism is seen. Routine sputum cultures typically grow only normal oral flora.

The chest radiograph usually reveals a unilateral patchy segmen-tal infiltrate that in 75 to 90 percent of patients involves the lower lobes. However, a wide variety of radiographic abnormalities have been reported, including lobar consolidation involving upper lobes, multilobe infiltrates, pleural effusion, lung abscess, pneumatocele formation, and hilar adenopathy.

Diagnosis

M. pneumoniae infection is diagnosed by culturing the organism or by detecting an increase in the titer of specific antibodies. The organism can be isolated from throat washings, sputum, or throat swabs using specialized culture medium, e.g., SP-4; growth takes 2 to 3 weeks. The most commonly used serologic test is complement fixation (CF); a 4-fold rise in specific antibody in paired sera is diagnostic of recent infection. Specific antibody begins to increase 1 week after illness and peaks at 3 to 4 weeks. If the first serologic sample is drawn late in the illness, then a 4-fold decrease in titer is diagnostic. Cold agglutinin antibodies, which are not specific to *M. pneumoniae* infections, also begin to increase 1 week after illness and peak at 4 weeks. A cold agglutinin titer of 1:64 or higher, in combination with an increase in CF antibody titer (1:64 or greater) is diagnostic. Other diagnostic tests are under development. These include detecting specific IgM antibody by enzyme-linked immunosorbent assay (ELISA), demonstrating antigen in respiratory secretions by ELISA or DNA probes, and detecting *M. pneumoniae* by the polymerase chain reaction.

Treatment

M. pneumoniae pneumonia usually resolves without treatment, but symptoms may last from 2 to 6 weeks. Tetracycline and erythromycin (2 g per day) are equally effective, and both reduce the duration of respiratory symptoms; 10 to 14 days of treatment are often needed. Antibiotic therapy does not eliminate the carrier state and generally cannot stop the spread of infection. Despite appropriate drug therapy and prompt clinical response, *M. pneumoniae* often persists in respiratory tract secretions for up to 6 to 13 weeks after completion of treatment.

Chlamydia psittaci PNEUMONIA

Epidemiology

Psittacosis (parrot fever) is a worldwide zoonosis caused by *C. psittaci*. It is an infection of birds that is transmissible to human beings. Parrots are the main reservoir, but almost any bird species can host the organism. Psittacosis in people is usually a sporadic disease; 40 to 60 cases are reported annually in the United States. It is an important occupational hazard to people in the poultry business, as well as pet shop employees, zoo workers, pigeon fanciers, bird owners, and veterinarians. Approximately 20 percent of patients who have psittacosis deny previous contact with birds. Human infection may be in the form of either a respiratory or a systemic illness.

Pathogenesis

C. psittaci is an obligate intracellular parasite present in the blood, tissues (especially the liver, spleen, and kidneys), excreta, and feathers of infected birds. Human infection follows inhalation of dried bird excreta, but it may also be acquired by handling contaminated feathers or tissues or, rarely, from bites. Human-to-human transmission and transmission by other animals, including cattle, sheep, and cats, is rare. From the lungs, *C. psittaci* is carried by the blood to the reticuloendothelial cells of the liver and spleen and then is spread hematogenously to the lungs and other organs. In the lungs, *C. psittaci* produces a lymphocytic inflammatory reaction in both alveolar and interstitial spaces. The lower lobes are most often involved. These areas become edematous, thickened, and necrotic.

Clinical Manifestations

Psittacosis can present as a mild flulike syndrome or as a severe systemic illness. The incubation period is usually 7 to 15 days, but can be as long as 30 to 39 days. The onset is sudden with chills and high fever; rarely it develops insidiously over 2 to 4 days. Severe headache, arthralgias, myalgias (particularly in the back and neck), pharyngitis, and malaise are common. Respiratory symptoms often predominate, usually with a persistent, hacking cough that is sometimes productive of scant mucoid sputum. Less common respiratory manifestations include tachypnea, dyspnea, hemoptysis, and pleuritic chest pain.

The physical examination usually underestimates the extent of pulmonary involvement. Rales may be heard over localized areas of the lower lung fields. Signs of consolidation are unusual, but do occur occasionally. Nontender hepatomegaly is common. Ten to 70 percent of patients have palpable splenomegaly which, when found in association with an atypical pneumonia, should suggest the diagnosis of psittacosis. As is seen in certain other intracellular infections, e.g., brucellosis, typhoid, a pulse-temperature dissociation may occasionally be present.

Extrapulmonary Manifestations

Nervous system findings include delirium, lethargy, and transient meningeal or focal neurologic signs which can progress to coma. Cardiac involvement is unusual but may present as myocarditis, pericarditis, or culture-negative endocarditis. Dermatologic manifestations include a rash resembling the rose spots of typhoid fever (Horder's spots), a measleslike eruption, erythema nodosum, and vasculitic lesions. Other manifestations of psittacosis include anemia, hepatitis, pancreatitis, acute renal failure, and reactive arthritis.

Laboratory Findings

Routine laboratory tests are typically nonspecific. The leukocyte count is usually normal, but leukopenia and leukocytosis can occur.

Other abnormalities include increased liver transaminases and muscle enzymes, an increase in serum bilirubin level, and proteinuria.

Radiographic findings are varied and are often more extensive than the physical examination suggests. The most common finding is a patchy infiltrate that extends from the hilar area and involves the lower lobes. Infiltrates are usually unilateral but may be bilateral. Consolidation and, rarely, pleural effusions, may be seen.

Diagnosis

Exposure to birds provides an important clue for the diagnosis of psittacosis. The diagnosis is confirmed by culture or a 4-fold increase in acute and convalescent serum antibody to *C. psittaci*. Although isolation of Chlamydiae can be done from tissue culture, this procedure is hazardous to laboratory personnel. The diagnostic method of choice is serologic testing by CF. Antibodies usually appear by the end of the second week of illness; early treatment with tetracycline can delay the appearance of antibody for several weeks. A single titer of 1:32 in a patient with a compatible illness is presumptive evidence of psittacosis. Cross-reactions with Brucella, *C. burnetii*, and *L. pneumophila* may occur and give false-positive CF tests.

Treatment

Tetracycline (2 to 3 g per day) is the mainstay of treatment. Because the response may be slow, a therapeutic trial with tetracycline cannot be relied on as a diagnostic maneuver. Relapses are common and therapy should be continued for 10 to 14 days after defervescence to minimize recurrence.

The use of tetracycline-laced poultry feed, a 30-day quarantine for imported birds, and an increase of domestically produced parakeets have decreased the incidence of psittacosis.

Chlamydia pneumoniae PNEUMONIA

Epidemiology

C. pneumoniae (TWAR) is a recently described respiratory pathogen which causes approximately 10 percent of adult cases of pneumonia. The first strain (TW-183) was isolated from a Taiwanese child's eye in 1965, whereas a second isolate (AR-39) came from the throat swab of a University of Washington student in 1983. The name TWAR was derived from these two isolates and is used interchangeably with *C. pneumoniae*. All evidence suggests that *C. pneumoniae* is primarily or exclusively a human pathogen with no known animal reservoir. The TWAR antibody has been found in up to 50 percent of adult populations; this high incidence exceeds the frequency of antibodies to all other chlamydia strains. Antibody prevalence is low in children but increases during adolescence, reaching a plateau around 30 to 40 years of age. In teenagers and young adults, TWAR infection is usually mild; the illness is often more severe in older adults.

Pathogenesis

C. pneumoniae is an obligate intracellular bacterium. The organism's primary mode of transmission seems to be from person to person. Although the method of spread is unknown, it probably occurs via respiratory secretions or aerosols, as is the case for many other respiratory pathogens. Suitable animal models have not been developed. Because of the usual benign course of illness, specimens for pathologic examination are not widely available.

Clinical Manifestations

Pulmonary infections caused by *C. pneumoniae* range from mild illness (pharyngitis, bronchitis) to severe disease (pneumonia). The incubation period is unknown, but available data suggest that TWAR has a relatively long incubation period. Compared to other common respiratory pathogens, it is not highly infectious and symptoms are more gradual in onset, the patients often complaining of fever, sore throat, and laryngitis. Cough, often hacking, may not begin for several days to a week, giving the appearance of a biphasic illness.

On chest examination, rales are almost always present even in patients with relatively mild symptoms. Pharyngeal erythema, usually without exudate, is a common finding, and sinus tenderness is present in about one third of patients with TWAR pneumonia.

Extrapulmonary Manifestations

Very few extrapulmonary manifestations have been seen with *C. pneumoniae* infections. Myocarditis and endocarditis, which have been associated with other chlamydia species, also have been associated with *C. pneumoniae,* both with and without pneumonia.

Laboratory Findings

Routine laboratory tests are of little help in establishing a diagnosis. The leukocyte count is increased in only 15 to 28 percent of individuals with TWAR pneumonia.

Chest radiographs usually reveal single, subsegmental infiltrates. However, more diffuse changes, including consolidation, pleural effusion, and bilateral infiltrates have been reported.

Diagnosis

Definitive diagnosis of *C. pneumoniae* infection requires isolation of the organism or demonstration of an appropriate antibody response. Although culture of the organism is difficult, the development of a TWAR-specific fluorescein-conjugated monoclonal antibody has greatly increased the detection of the organism in cell culture. Recently, the isolation of TWAR has been improved with the use of HL cells, a human cell line used to isolate respiratory syncytial virus. This new development will make the diagnosis of TWAR infections more widely available because any laboratory capable of cell culture should be able to isolate *C. pneumoniae* using this cell line.

The two primary serologic tests for *C. pneumoniae* are CF and microimmunofluorescence (MIF). The CF test is widely available and has been used to diagnose psittacosis for many years. Unfortunately, the test is not species specific; it cannot distinguish between antibody to *C. trachomatis, C. psittaci,* and *C. pneumoniae.* The MIF test is specific for *C. pneumoniae* and can distinguish between IgM and IgG antibody to TWAR. In acute primary TWAR infection, an increase in IgM antibody occurs 3 weeks after the onset of illness, and the level remains high for 2 to 6 months. The IgG antibody appears 6 to 8 weeks after the onset of primary infection and can persist for years. In reinfection, the IgM antibody titer remains low, but the IgG antibody may show a rise within 1 to 2 weeks, reaching a very high titer. The criteria for diagnosing acute infection using MIF consists of demonstrating a 4-fold rise in specific antibody in paired sera or detecting an IgM antibody titer $\geq 1:16$ or an IgG $\geq 1:512$. The convalescent titer should not be obtained before the third week of illness because the MIF antibody may be slow to rise during the first infection.

Treatment

Tetracycline (2 g per day) is the therapy of choice, but erythromycin is also effective. Because patients often respond slowly and incompletely to antibiotic therapy, treatment should be continued for at least 14 days. Recently, ciprofloxacin has been found to show in vitro activity against TWAR. However, no clinical studies of efficacy have been performed.

Q FEVER PNEUMONIA

Epidemiology

Q (query) fever is caused by *C. burnetii,* a rickettsia that is highly resistant to desiccation. The organism exists in two forms—phase I and phase II—with the phase II variant being less virulent. A spore stage probably explains the organism's ability to withstand harsh conditions. Human infection is rare in the United States; approximately 20 to 60 cases of Q fever are reported each year. The disease is usually maintained by animal-to-animal spread via ticks, and the most common reservoirs are sheep, goats, cattle, and ticks. Q fever is an important occupational hazard for abattoir workers and veterinarians. Epidemics have occurred in medical research facilities, particularly among those using sheep and goats for experimental purposes. Recent outbreaks have occurred in parturient cats.

Pathogenesis

C. burnetii is a highly contagious obligate intracellular organism that does not need an arthropod vector to maintain itself in nature. The milk, feces, urine, and parturient material of infected animals are the major sources of infection for human beings. Infection usually occurs by inhalation of aerosol particles that contain *C. burnetii*. Other modes of transmission include ingesting contaminated raw milk, person-to-person spread via droplets, penetration of the organism through skin abrasions, and blood transfusion. After inhalation, organisms multiply in the lung (or other sites of entry) and then spread hematogenously to other organs. The alveolar walls of the lungs become thickened by a mononuclear infiltrate composed mostly of macrophages and the bronchiolar mucosa may become necrotic.

Clinical Manifestations

The incubation period of Q fever is 20 days, with a range of 2 to 5 weeks. The illness often begins abruptly. The most common syndrome is a self-limited, flulike illness that consists of high fevers, severe headache, malaise, and myalgias. Although the development of pneumonia is variable, three distinct pulmonary syndromes can be seen—atypical pneumonia, rapidly progressive pneumonia, and most commonly, an asymptomatic infiltrate in a febrile patient. A nonproductive cough is present in over 50 percent of patients. Headache is common and pleuritic chest pain occurs infrequently. A pulse-temperature dissociation may be seen.

Examination of the chest usually reveals rales; occasionally, signs of consolidation are present. The physical examination typically underestimates the extensive infiltrates seen on the chest radiograph.

Extrapulmonary Manifestations

Gastrointestinal manifestations usually consist of hepatitis with hepatomegaly and marked increase in the transaminases. Encephalitis, focal neurologic signs, and neuropathy are rare. Other complications of Q fever include hemolytic anemia, optic neuritis, uveitis, iritis, osteomyelitis, and glomerular nephropathy. The most devastating, and often fatal, complication is endocarditis, which is common in chronic Q fever.

Laboratory Findings

Routine laboratory tests yield little helpful information. The white blood cell count is usually normal or mildly increased with a slight shift to the left. The serum transaminases and alkaline phosphatase levels may be increased.

The chest radiograph usually shows single or multiple alveolar infiltrates involving the lower lobes. Lobar consolidation is found in up to 25 percent of patients. Coin lesions, platelike linear atelectasis, pleural effusions, and inflammatory pseudotumors of the lung have also been seen.

Diagnosis

Q fever is diagnosed by isolating *C. burnetii* or by finding an increase in the titer of specific antibodies. Culture of the organism is hazardous to laboratory personnel and is not done routinely. Electron microscopy can detect intracytoplasmic organisms in macrophages, and fluorescent antibody can identify *C. burnetii* in tissue. Diagnosis is usually made by a 4-fold rise in specific antibody titer in paired sera; the level of specific antibodies is determined by CF, microagglutination, indirect immunofluorescence (IFA), or ELISA. The IFA titers peak before the CF titers (4 to 8 weeks versus 12 weeks). The IFA is particularly useful if only one serum specimen is available because it can detect both IgM and IgG antibodies. In contrast, IgM antibodies may persist for up to 2 years.

Phase I and phase II antibodies can also be detected, but their clinical significance is not fully understood. Phase II antibodies increase in acute infection, whereas a high titer of phase I antibody suggests chronic disease, such as endocarditis.

Treatment

Tetracycline (2 g per day) is the drug of choice for Q fever pneumonia. Doxycycline and chloramphenicol are effective alternatives and erythromycin has also been used successfully. Rifampin, in combination with doxycycline, trimethoprim-sulfamethoxazole, and certain of the quinolones also have antirickettsial activity. Treatment should be continued for 2 weeks.

LEGIONNAIRES' DISEASE

Epidemiology

There are over 30 species in the Legionellaceae family. At least 19 cause pneumonia, but L. *pneumophila* is the most common species implicated in human disease. Natural and artificial aquatic habitats, such as freshwater lakes, ponds, stagnant rainwater, hot water heaters, air conditioning cooling towers, and tap water serve as reservoirs for the organism. Besides being the cause of Legionnaires' disease, *L. pneumophila* is also the cause of Pontiac fever.

Legionnaires' disease is often associated with point-source epidemics, such as outbreaks in hotels or hospitals. However, sporadic cases probably outnumber the cases involved in outbreaks. In prospective studies of community-acquired and nosocomial pneumonia, the incidence of Legionnaires' disease has ranged from 1 to 15 percent and 1 to 40 percent, respectively. Predisposing risk factors include chronic obstructive pulmonary disease, cigarette smoking, age > 50 years, malignancy such as hairy cell leukemia and immunosuppression, e.g., in patients receiving corticosteroids and in the transplant recipient.

Pathogenesis

L. pneumophila is an intracellular, gram-negative bacilli found in water. The mechanism by which it is transmitted to human beings is not entirely clear, but three ways by which the organisms have been introduced into the lungs have been identified—aerosolization via respiratory equipment, humidifiers, or air conditioning systems; aspiration of contaminated water; or direct instillation into the lung during respiratory tract manipulation. Person-to-person spread does not seem to occur.

Once the organisms reach the lung, alveolar macrophages phagocytize but do not kill them. *L. pneumophila* replicates within the macrophages until the cells rupture, thereby releasing the bacteria; the cycle is then repeated. Microscopically, acute purulent pneumonia is seen.

Clinical Manifestations

L. pneumophila can cause two different illnesses, namely, Pontiac fever and Legionnaires' disease. Pontiac fever is an acute self-limiting illness. The incubation period is 48 h and the exposure attack rate is high (up to 95 percent). The major symptoms are high fever, myalgias, malaise, and headache. Pneumonia does not occur but a nonproductive cough may be present. Patients usually recover within 1 week without antibiotic treatment or sequelae.

The major manifestation of Legionnaires' disease is pneumonia. The incubation period is 2 to 10 days. In the first 48 h, there is usually a gradual onset of nonspecific symptoms, such as anorexia, malaise, headache, and myalgia. Almost all patients develop fever which tends to increase and become sustained. A dry, nonproductive cough occurs after 1 or 2 days of illness and may be accompanied by pleuritic chest pain. Gastrointestinal symptoms such as nausea, vomiting, diarrhea, and abdominal pain are often prominent features. Change in mental status, ranging from confusion to coma or a grand mal seizure, is a common neurologic finding.

On physical examination, a pulse-temperature dissociation is sometimes found. Early in the course of the disease, the lung examination usually reveals only scattered rales or rhonchi. However, after the illness progresses, signs of consolidation are almost always present. The findings in the chest typically correlate with the changes seen on chest radiograph.

Extrapulmonary Manifestations

The extrapulmonary manifestations usually occur from local infection or bacteremic dissemination. They may not become apparent until weeks to months after resolution of the pneumonia. The abnormalities in other organ systems include sinusitis, perirectal abscess, pericarditis, endocarditis, pyelonephritis, peritonitis, and pancreatitis. Neurologic manifestations include brain abscess, tremors, ataxia, peripheral neuropathies, and global dysfunction. Wound infections have occurred from contact with water colonized with *Legionella* organisms.

Laboratory Findings

Several nonspecific laboratory findings have been associated with *Legionella* infections. The leukocyte count is frequently elevated with a shift to the left in 50 to 75 percent of cases. However, leukopenia and thrombocytopenia sometimes occur in severe disease. Abnormalities in the liver function tests, hypophosphatemia, hematuria, and increased creatinine phosphokinase also occur. Hyponatremia occurs in about 50 percent of patients, probably due to salt and water loss from diarrhea rather than from the syndrome of inappropriate antidiuretic hormone secretion. Gram stain of the sputum shows numerous white blood cells with few or no visible organisms.

No radiographic findings are pathognomonic for *Legionella* infection. A unilateral alveolar infiltrate at the onset is typical. In 70 percent of the patients, the infiltrate progresses to consolidation. Lower lobe involvement is common. Spread can be ipsilateral or, less commonly, contralateral, the latter leading to noncontiguous involvement of pulmonary lobes. Pleural effusions can be seen. Cavitation occasionally occurs in immunosuppressed patients.

Diagnosis

Specialized laboratory tests are needed to make the diagnosis of Legionnaires' disease (Table 41-1). Culture of respiratory tract specimens on selective media is the best method of confirming the diagnosis. Legionellae are nutritionally fastidious and will not grow on standard bacteriologic media. Buffered charcoal yeast extract agar containing L-cysteine is commonly used to isolate *Legionella* organisms. Three to 5 days are required for detection of growth.

Direct or indirect fluorescent antibody staining of clinical specimens is a rapid method for the detection of legionellae. The test is highly specific but its sensitivity is variable (25 to 80 percent); a negative test does not rule out the disease.

L. pneumophila antigen can be detected in the urine by radioimmunoassay. The test can remain positive for weeks after the episode of pneumonia. The principal drawback of the test is that it only detects *L. pneumophila* serogroup 1. However, because this species causes 80 to 90 percent of the clinically apparent infections, this shortcoming is relatively minor.

Measuring the serum antibody titer by ELISA or IFA is probably the least helpful test for the diagnosis of *Legionella* infection. A 4-fold or greater rise in paired sera is required. The antibody response appears 4 to 8 weeks after the onset of illness. Because the antibody can persist for months after the development of Legionnaires' disease, it may be difficult to distinguish past from present infection. Other drawbacks to serologic testing include cross-reactivity to other gram-negative bacteria, such as *Pseudomonas* species, and the failure of antibody titer to increase in 30 percent of patients with Legionnaires' disease.

Treatment

Erythromycin (2 to 4 g per day) is the drug treatment of choice for these infections. Tetracyclines probably are as effective. Doxycycline (200 mg per day) is the preferred agent if erythromycin cannot be given. Trimethoprim-sulfamethoxazole (20 mg/kg per day trimethoprim component) also has been used successfully in patients with Legionnaires' disease. In seriously ill patients, rifampin (600 mg every 12 h) should be added to erythromycin. However, rifampin should not be given alone because of the possibility of the emergence of resistance. The quinolones, i.e., ciprofloxacin 750 mg every 12 h, have excellent potential as treatment for Legionnaires' disease and patients unresponsive to erythromycin have been treated successfully with ciprofloxacin.

Antibiotics should be given intravenously for the first 5 to 7 days until the patient has shown objective clinical improvement. The clinical response to erythromycin is usually prompt and many patients begin to feel better within the fi rst 2 days of therapy. Treatment should be given for at least 3 weeks to prevent relapse.

TABLE 41-1 Laboratory Diagnostic Tests for Legionnaires' Disease

Method	Suitable specimens	Advantages	Disadvantages	Turnaround time	Sensitivity	Specificity	Chances of false-positive/false-negative results*
Culture	All lower respiratory tract sections/tissues including sputum; blood, pleural fluid, abscesses; must be fresh; avoid collection in saline solutions	Independent of species or serogroup	Requires use of selective media and freshly collected, non-fixed specimens	2–7 days mean 3 days	? 80–90% for sputum. TTA† >95% for lung tissue.	100%	0% 10–20%
Immunofluorescent detection of bacteria	Same as for culture except for blood; can be fixed, although non-fixed specimens are best	Rapid	Technically demanding, serogroup specific; polyvalent antisera required	1–3 h	25–75% for sputum (mean 60%). >95% for lung tissue.	95–99.9%‡	4–60%/17–35

Antibody determination	Serum	Samples easy to obtain	Time-consuming, requires use of multiple antigens and paired sera	Weeks§	60–70%	95–99%‡	25–60%/25–30
Urinary antigen detection	Urine	Samples easy to obtain	Serogroup-specific, requires use of multiple antisera; unable to distinguish between acute and chronic (relapsing) disease; not available commercially	1–6 h	60–80%	98–99.9%	4–40%/17–30

*With disease prevalence equal to 5%. Lowest estimate of false-positive rate is for highest estimated specificity, and lowest estimate of false-negative rate is for highest estimated sensitivity.
†Transtracheal aspirate.
‡Higher specificity estimate is for *L. pneumophila*, and lower one is for other *Legionella* species.
§Long turnaround time because of the need to test paired sera collected 2–6 weeks apart. The test itself takes less than 4–6 h to perform.
SOURCE: Table 102-2 from Meyer RD, Edelstein PH: Legionnaires' disease, in Fishman AP (ed). *Pulmonary Diseases and Disorders*, 2d ed., New York, McGraw-Hill, 1988, p 1635.

BIBLIOGRAPHY

For a more detailed discussion, see Nash TW, Murray HW: The atypical pneumonias, in Fishman AP (ed), *Pulmonary Diseases and Disorders,* 2d ed. New York, McGraw-Hill, 1988, pp 1613–1628.

LaForce FM: Antibacterial therapy for lower respiratory infections in adults: A review. Clin Infect Dis 14:S233–237, S244–245, 1992.

Mandell GL, Douglas RG, Bennett JM (eds): *Principles and Practice of Infectious Disease,* 3d ed. New York, Churchill Livingstone, 1990, pp 1440–1444, 1446–1455, 1472–1475, 1764–1772.

Martin RE, Bates JH: Atypical pneumonia. Infect Dis Clin N Am 5:585–601, 1991.

Meyer RD, Edelstein PH: Legionnaires' disease, in Fishman AP (ed), *Pulmonary Diseases and Disorders,* 2d ed. New York, McGraw-Hill, 1988, pp 1629–1638.

Rello J, Quintana E, Ausina V, Net A, Prats G: A three-year study of severe community-acquired pneumonia with emphasis on outcome. Chest 103:232–235, 1993.

Infection Due to Mycobacterium Tuberculosis

Randi Silibovsky

DEFINITION

The term *tuberculosis* (TB) refers to disease caused by *Mycobacterium tuberculosis* or rarely, in the United States, by *Mycobacterium bovis*. *M. bovis*, once an important human pathogen causing infections clinically identical to that of *M. tuberculosis*, has become rare in the United States due to the slaughter of tuberculin-positive cattle and the pasteurization of milk. The spectrum of disease produced by these organisms ranges from subclinical to lethal, and the clinical manifestations are determined by the balance struck between the defenses of the host and the virulence of the organism.

Infection may be held in check for years only to reactivate as concomitant medical conditions cause host immunity to wane. Although the lung is the initial and principle site of infection, extrapulmonary sites may also be involved. Without therapy, a chronic wasting course is common, often culminating in death. This chapter is confined to infection caused by *M. tuberculosis*.

ETIOLOGY

M. tuberculosis is a nonmotile and nonsporulating bacillus, 0.2×5.0 μm in size, with several clinically important biologic properties. First, it is an obligate aerobe that grows best in human tissues in which the P_{O_2} is highest, such as the lung apices. Second, the lipid content of its cell wall is high and, as a result, is acid fast, i.e., it is resistant to decolorization with acid alcohol after staining with carbolfuchsin. Third, it is slow growing. As a result, tuberculous lesions typically evolve in a subacute to chronic course, and 3 to 8 weeks is required for primary isolation by culture. Finally, mycobacterial cell walls and cytoplasm contain many antigens; development of hypersensitivity to these antigens is important in the pathogenesis of TB.

EPIDEMIOLOGY

Tuberculosis is a major world health problem with an estimated 8 million new cases and 3 million deaths each year. It is estimated that there are 1 billion infected persons worldwide, making TB one of the most prevalent infections in the world. In the United States and other developed countries, the incidence of TB declined progressively after 1900. However, in 1985, the incidence of the disease leveled off and subsequently has increased. It is estimated that there have been 27,000 "excess" cases of TB between 1985 and 1990, above that predicted by previous trends. The disease is most prevalent in urban areas. Populations with a disproportionately high incidence of TB include Hispanics, African-Americans, immigrants (especially Asian), alcoholics, drug-dependent individuals, the homeless, prison inmates, persons in residential care facilities and other closed institutions, and human immunodeficiency virus (HIV)-infected individuals. Among African-Americans and Hispanics, the disease is increasing in younger age groups while the elderly form an ever-increasing risk group in the caucasian population.

Infection with the HIV is contributing significantly to both the increasing incidence and changing epidemiologic trends. This presumption is supported by several lines of evidence: (1) the sharpest rises in reported cases of TB have occurred in regions, e.g., New York City, and in demographic groups, e.g., Hispanics, African-Americans, with the highest prevalence of HIV infection; (2) the incidence of TB in HIV-infected patients is increased 500-fold over that of the general population; and (3) the risk of active TB in HIV-infected patients with a positive purified protein derivative (PPD) has been demonstrated to be 8 percent per year, far in excess of the estimated lifetime risk of reactivation in PPD-positive individuals in the general population. Infection in HIV-positive individuals may occur either by primary acquisition or by reactivation. Because of the intrinsic virulence of the organism, TB typically occurs early in the course of HIV infection at a time when host immunity is only mildly to moderately impaired.

Mode of Transmission

Infection occurs primarily by inhalation of droplet nuclei, i.e., respiratory secretions aerosolized by coughing, sneezing, or talking. They are sufficiently small to dry while airborne, to remain suspended for long periods, and to reach the alveoli where infection begins. Large drops of respiratory secretions are of no real concern because they drop to the floor or, if inhaled, are trapped and removed by mucociliary action and coughing. Prolonged exposure to an infectious environment is usually required for infection to occur and brief contact is of little risk. However, patients with laryngeal tuberculosis and extensive cavitary pulmonary disease are often highly contagious. Mycobacteria are susceptible to ultraviolet irradiation, and transmission of infection rarely occurs in daylight. Most patients become noninfectious within 2 weeks after the institution of appropriate chemotherapy because of a decrease in the number of organisms excreted and a decrease in cough. Fomites are not important in the transmission of tuberculosis.

PATHOGENESIS AND PATHOLOGY

Primary Infection

It is estimated that only a few bacilli have to reach the alveoli to establish an infection. Initial infection usually occurs in the lower lung fields due to the greater distribution of ventilation to the lung bases. In the first few weeks following infection, host defenses are nonspecific and relatively ineffective; the bacilli multiply in the alveolar spaces and within alveolar macrophages after ingestion. Concurrent with the initial pulmonary site of infection, hematogenous seeding of distant sites occurs. Bacterial multiplication proceeds slowly, both in the initial focus and in metastatic foci. Although any tissue can be seeded hematogenously, organs with the higher blood flows tend to receive the most bacilli, and tissues with the highest P_{O_2} provide the most favorable environment for multiplication. Thus, frequently infected areas include the lung apices, renal cortex, vertebral column, and metaphyseal ends of long bones. Approximately 6 to 8 weeks after initial infection, specific cell-mediated immunity develops, providing effective killing of most organisms within macrophages and containment of infection by the formation of granulomas. The tuberculin skin test becomes positive at this time.

Several characteristic pathologic features occur at the site of initial infection: caseating necrosis, granulomas, and Langhans' giant cells (fused macrophages with the nuclei in a peripheral position). In time, healing ensues leading to fibrosis and calcification of the granulomas. The combination of a calcified lesion in the periphery of a lower lobe and an ipsilateral calcified hilar lymph node is known as a *Ghon complex*. In the United States, the primary lesion of tuberculosis seems to heal completely in 95 percent of individuals, leaving no residual evidence of disease.

Postprimary (Reactivation) Infection

The apparently healed lesions of primary infection contain small numbers of dormant, but viable, tubercle bacilli; these lesions can break down and lead to reactivation infection. Reactivation is most apt to occur within 2 years after the initial infection, or at times of decreased host resistance such as occurs with aging or systemic illness; it may even occur many decades after the initial infection. Reactivation tuberculosis has been estimated to occur in up to 10 percent of infected individuals. When reactivation occurs, it most commonly takes place in the apical posterior segments of the upper lobes of the lungs, which are rarely the site of primary infection. Reactivation may also occur at extrapulmonary sites to which organisms have been disseminated.

Reinfection

Previously infected individuals are typically resistant to exogenous reinfection by inhaled bacilli; in these patients, cellular immune mechanisms are primed to neutralize invading mycobacterial organisms in an efficient and expeditious manner. However, protection against reinfection is not absolute and, although rarely, exogenous reinfection can occur in response to a particularly heavy exposure or in a patient with compromised immune function.

CLINICAL MANIFESTATIONS

Primary Tuberculosis

Once predominantly a pediatric disease, primary TB is increasingly a disease of adults. It is usually asymptomatic. In patients who are symptomatic, the most common syndrome is a pneumonic process with fever and nonproductive cough. In most patients with this form, the process is self-limited and will resolve without specific antituberculous therapy.

A second form of primary TB is tuberculous pleurisy with effusion that is caused by rupture of a subpleural focus into the pleural space. Affected individuals often have high fever, cough, and pleuritic chest pain and may be dyspneic. Although primary tuberculous pleuritis resolves spontaneously in most cases, up to 60 percent of untreated patients will develop reactivation tuberculosis within 5 years of the initial infection.

Reactivation Tuberculosis

In adults, reactivation (postprimary) tuberculosis is the most common clinical form of tuberculosis. Symptoms usually begin insidiously and progress over a period of many weeks or months before the diagnosis is made. Although a subacute to chronic presentation is the more common, rapidly progressive disease can occur in the immunocompromised patient. Constitutional symptoms, including anorexia, weight loss, and night sweats, are often prominent. In most patients, fevers are low grade, but, when the disease progresses rapidly, temperatures are often higher, sometimes accompanied by chills.

Pulmonary symptoms are common; they include cough and sputum production. Sputum may be scanty at first, but typically increases if the disease is progressive. Dyspnea is uncommon unless underlying chronic lung disease is present. Hemoptysis is common, the result of bleeding from tortuous, dilated bronchial vessels that feed affected areas of lung. In some patients, hemoptysis is massive and life threatening.

Physical findings in the lung in patients with pulmonary TB are generally nonspecific and few, and can be appreciated when the disease is extensive. Rales may be heard, typically during an inspiratory effort after a short cough (posttussive rales). This is characteristic of apical disease. Dullness with decreased fremitus may indicate pleural thickening or fluid. When the lesions are extensive, signs of consolidation (whispered pectoriloquy, tubular breath sounds) can be heard. Distant hollow breath sounds may be heard over cavities.

Extrapulmonary Tuberculosis

Approximately 15 percent of all newly recognized cases of TB in the United States are extrapulmonary. The incidence of extrapulmonary TB is particularly high in patients infected with HIV: extrapulmonary involvement occurs in two thirds of such patients, most often in patients with profound HIV-induced immunosuppression.

Although the clinical features of extrapulmonary TB vary widely, certain generalizations can be made. Only about 25 percent of patients have a past history of tuberculosis, and virtually all of these have received inadequate treatment. Typically, except in children, the latent period between the first episode of infection and the extrapulmonary presentation is long. In approximately 50 percent of patients with extrapulmonary TB, the chest radiographs are normal; most others have evidence of old inactive pulmonary disease. Although all organ systems can be involved, the most common are the genitourinary tract, the musculoskeletal system, and the lymph nodes.

The clinical course of extrapulmonary TB depends on the site that is involved. Certain forms are particularly fulminant: miliary TB, tuberculous meningitis, and TB of the pericardium. These patients are usually febrile and have prominent constitutional symptoms suggestive of infection. Without therapy, the course is progressively downhill, and the mortality rate is extremely high, death often occurring within weeks. Patients with TB of the peritoneum or pleura also have prominent constitutional symptoms, including fever, but their course is more indolent. Indeed, spontaneous resolution of pleural TB is common without treatment even though, as noted above, the high incidence of subsequent pulmonary or extrapulmonary reactivation is high. Finally, focal involvement of the genitourinary tract, lymph nodes, bones, or joints leads to site-specific symptoms and signs, but fever and other constitutional complaints are uncommon. Although these forms of extrapulmonary TB are focally destructive, they are rarely lethal.

DIAGNOSIS

A presumptive diagnosis of tuberculosis is usually based on clinical suspicion, chest radiography, skin test, examination of sputum or other body fluids for acid-fast bacilli (AFB) and, possibly, histologic findings in a biopsy of infected tissue. A definitive diagnosis requires isolation of *M. tuberculosis* on culture.

Chest radiography Chest radiographic findings vary according to the type of disease. In patients with primary pulmonary infection, unilateral patchy parenchymal infiltrates in the lower lobe, paratracheal or hilar adenopathy, or pleural effusion may be present. In patients with reactivation TB, typical features include unilateral or bilateral infiltrates in the apical/posterior pulmonary segments which often progress to cavitation. Apical lordotic views, chest tomograms, and computed tomography scans may be helpful in documenting cavitary disease. The radiographic features of reactivation TB in HIV-positive patients are often atypical, and include lower lobe noncavitary infiltrates, hilar adenopathy, and pleural effusion.

Microbiologic studies Collection of sputum or other body fluid for AFB stain and culture is essential for establishing the diagnosis of TB. In pulmonary disease, an early morning sputum collection is optimal; multiple specimens maximize the yield. If patients are unable to produce sputum spontaneously, attempts should be made to induce sputum using nebulized hypertonic saline. Alternatively, sputum swallowed during the night may be obtained by aspirating gastric contents immediately after the patient awakens in the morning; this procedure is used more often in children than in adults. Fiberoptic bronchoscopy, in conjunction with lavage and transbronchial biopsy, has become the procedure of choice for collection of respiratory specimens when sputum is unavailable or unrevealing. The yield from culture of respiratory secretions (sputum, bronchial washings) is significantly higher than that of AFB stain, particularly for noncavitary disease where the mycobacterial load is lower. Thus, negative smears alone do not exclude the diagnosis of TB; it is imperative that culture results be checked. It is important to bear in mind that it may take up to 6 weeks to grow and identify *M. tuberculosis* in culture and, therefore, that the definitive diagnosis of infection may be delayed.

Body fluids, such as pleural fluid, cerebrospinal fluid, urine, or joint fluid should be sent for AFB stain and culture when tuberculosis involvement of the related organs or structures is suspected.

Tissue biopsy The demonstration of caseating granulomas or AFB in tissue specimens provides strong but presumptive evidence for TB; once again, cultures of tissue specimens are essential to make a definitive microbiologic diagnosis. Tissues that are frequently examined histologically include the lung, pleura, liver, and bone marrow.

Skin testing The tuberculin skin test is an important adjunct to diagnosis. Infection with *M. tuberculosis* usually results in development of skin hypersensitivity within 2 to 10 weeks. Tuberculin PPD is the preferred reagent. A 5-tuberculin unit (TU) dose of PPD (intermediate strength) should be used routinely. One tenth of 1 cc is applied (Mantoux text) via an intracutaneous injection on the volar aspect of the forearm. Precise intracutaneous injection producing a raised, blanched wheal is necessary. The reaction is read in 48 to 72 h; a positive test usually is defined as > 10 mm of induration (NOT erythema). False-positive reactions, usually indurations of < 10 mm, sometimes occur due to cross-sensitization with other nonpathogenic mycobacteria. In high-risk individuals, such as contacts of active cases and in HIV-positive patients, indurations to 5 to 10 mm should be considered positive. Overall, in up to 20 percent of newly diagnosed cases of TB, the initial 5 TU PPD may be falsely negative. The incidence of a negative test is particularly high in miliary TB (up to 50 percent) and pleural TB (up to 33 percent).

Tuberculin PPD is also available in a second strength dose (250 TU). Because this strength elicits nonspecific reactivity, a false-positive reaction is frequent. Additionally, 25 percent of those who are nonreactive to 5 TU will also be nonreactive to 250 TU. Therefore, the frequency of both false-positive and false-negative reactions to 250 TU limits its usefulness. The 1-TU dose has not been adequately standardized for clinical use.

Routine laboratory studies Laboratory findings in patients with TB include a normocytic, normochromic anemia, as well as a low serum albumin and a high serum globulin. The white blood cell count is usually normal, but ranges between 10,000 to 15,000 in some patients. Monocytosis, often said to be characteristic of TB, actually occurs in < 10 percent of patients. Hematuria or pyuria may indicate coexisting renal tuberculosis. Marked albuminuria is uncommon; when present, it usually indicates associated amyloidosis. Hyponatremia due to inappropriate secretion of antidiuretic hormone may accompany tuberculosis meningitis as well as pulmonary disease. Hyponatremia should also suggest the possibility of adrenal insufficiency. Hypercalcemia is observed early in the course of some patients with pulmonary TB and is usually mild. An elevated erythrocyte sedimentation rate is common but nonspecific.

DIFFERENTIAL DIAGNOSIS

Tuberculosis may be confused with several other infectious and noninfectious diseases. Chronic pulmonary infections due to anaerobic bacteria, nocardia, actinomycosis, atypical mycobacteria, and fungi, e.g., histoplasmosis, share many of the clinical, radiographic, and, in some instances, the histologic features of tuberculous disease. The noninfectious diseases most often confused with TB are sarcoidosis and bronchogenic carcinoma. One helpful, albeit not infallible, radiographic clue to distinguishing between TB and carcinoma of the lung is the proclivity of TB to affect the apical and posterior segments of the upper lobes. Isolated involvement of the anterior segment of the upper lobe, therefore, is more suggestive of cancer of the lung than of TB.

MANAGEMENT

The chemotherapy of active tuberculosis is based on five basic principles:

1. Multiple drugs should be used to prevent the emergence of drug-resistant organisms.
2. In the event of treatment failure, drugs should be changed in combination rather than singly; in these cases, testing for drug sensitivity is mandatory.
3. Single daily dosages of drugs are preferred.
4. Prolonged chemotherapy is necessary.
5. No matter what regimen is chosen, it is important to follow patients closely to ensure compliance and to monitor drug effectiveness and toxicity.

Most patients with TB should be hospitalized and kept in respiratory isolation for the initial phase of therapy. Two weeks of therapy will greatly decrease the infectiousness of patients with pulmonary TB, although a few mycobacteria may still be present on sputum smears or cultures. Beyond this time period, respiratory isolation and, indeed, continued hospitalization, are usually unnecessary. Patients with extrapulmonary tuberculosis are much less infectious and can sometimes be managed entirely as outpatients if their clinical state permits.

Treatment of Active Pulmonary Tuberculosis

There are a large number of possible combinations of drugs and durations of administration. Table 42-1 lists the agents effective against TB along with appropriate dosing and side effects. Table 42-2 summarizes the acceptable drug regimens for initial treatment of pulmonary TB. The current minimal acceptable duration of therapy is 6 months. HIV-infected patients with TB should be treated for a minimum of 9 months and at least 6 months after obtaining a negative culture. In the case of INH resistance, therapy should be continued for a total duration of 12 months.

Particularly alarming is the increase in the number of persons with multi-drug-resistant TB (MDR-TB) caused by strains resistant to two or more drugs. Treatment for MDR-TB often requires the use of second line TB drugs. Therapy for 18 months to 2 years may

TABLE 42-1 Treatment of Tuberculosis in Adults and Children

	Dosage		Most common side effects*	Tests for side effects*	Drug interactions†
	Daily dose	Twice weekly dosage			
			Commonly used agents		
Isoniazid	5–10 mg/kg up to 300 mg PO or IM	15 mg/kg PO or IM	Peripheral neuritis, hepatitis, hypersensitivity	SGOT/SGPT (not as a routine)	Phenytoin—synergistic Antabuse
Rifampin	10 mg/kp up to 600 mg PO	10 mg/kg up to 600 mg PO	Hepatitis, febrile reaction, purpura (rare)	SGOT/SGPT (not as a routine)	Rifampin inhibits the effect of oral contraceptives, quinidine, corticosteroids, coumarin drugs and methadone, digoxin, oral hypoglycemics; PAS may interfere with absorption of rifampin.
Streptomycin	15–20 mg/kg up to 1 g IM	25–30 mg/kg	8th nerve damage, nephrotoxicity	Vestibular function, audiograms‡; BUN and creatinine	Neuromuscular blocking agents—may be potentiated to cause prolonged paralysis
Pyrazinamide	15–30 mg/kg up to 2 g PO	50–70 mg/kg	Hyperuricemia, hepatotoxicity	Uric acid, SGOT/SGPT	
Ethambutol	15–25 mg/kg	50 mg/kg PO	Optic neuritis (reversible with discontinuation of drug; very rare at 15 mg/kg), skin rash	Red-green color discrimination and visual acuity.‡ Difficult to test in a child under 3 years.	

TABLE 42-1 Treatment of Tuberculosis in Adults and Children *(Continued)*

	Dosage		Most common side effects*	Tests for side effects*	Drug interactions†
	Daily dose	Twice weekly dosage			
				Less commonly used agents		
Capreomycin	15–30 mg/kg up to 1 g IM		8th nerve damage, nephrotoxicity	Vestibular function, audiograms‡; BUN and creatinine	Neuromuscular blocking agents—may be potentiated to cause prolonged paralysis
Kanamycin	15–30 mg/kg up to 1 g IM		Auditory toxicity, nephrotoxicity, vestibular toxicity (rare)	Vestibular function, audiograms‡; BUN and creatinine	Neuromuscular blocking agents—may be potentiated to cause prolonged paralysis
Ethionamide	15–30 mg/kg up to 1 g PO		GI disturbance, hepatotoxicity, hypersensitivity	SGOT/SGPT	
p-Aminosalicylic acid (aminosalicylic acid)	150 mg/kg up to 12 g PO		GI disturbance, hypersensitivity hepatotoxicity, sodium load	SGOT/SGPT	
Cycloserine	10–20 mg/kg up to 1 g PO		Psychosis, personality changes, convulsions, rash	Psychological testing	Alcohol—may aggravate or precipitate psychiatric problems

*Check product labeling for detailed information on dose, contraindications, drug interaction, adverse reactions, and monitoring.
†Reference should be made to current literature, particularly on rifampin, because it induces hepatic microenzymes and therefore interacts with many drugs.
‡Initial examination should be done at start of treatment.
BUN = blood urea nitrogen; SGOT = serum glutamic-oxaloacetic transaminase; SGPT = serum glutamic-pyruvic transaminase.
SOURCE: From Davidson PT. Treatment of mycobacterial disease of the lungs caused by *Mycobacterium tuberculosis*, in Fishman AP (ed), *Pulmonary Diseases and Disorders*, 2d ed., New York, McGraw-Hill, 1988, p 1870.

TABLE 42-2 Acceptable Drug Regimens for First Treatment of
Pulmonary Tuberculosis

I. 6-month duration*		
INH 300 mg		
Rifampin 600 mg		Daily for 2 months
Pyrazinamide 25–30 mg/kg		
	THEN	
INH 300 mg		Daily for 4 months
Rifampin 600 mg		
II. 9-month duration*		
INH 300 mg		
Rifampin 600 mg		Daily for 9 months
	OR	
INH 300 mg		
Rifampin 600 mg		Daily for 1 month
	THEN	
INH 900 mg		
Rifampin 600 mg		Twice weekly for 8 months
III. Regimen for HIV-positive patients*		
INH 300 mg		
Rifampin 600 mg		Daily for 2 months
Pyrazinamide 25–30 mg/kg		
	THEN	
INH 300 mg		Daily for 7 months or for 6
Rifampin 600 mg		months after cultures negative (whichever is longer).

*Ethambutol (15–25 mg/kg) is added to the initial regimen if INH-resistant
organisms are suspected.
SOURCE: Modified from MacGregor RR. Treatment of mycobacterial disease
of the lungs caused by *Mycobacterium tuberculosis,* in Fishman AP (ed),
Pulmonary Diseases and Disorders, 2d ed. New York, McGraw Hill, 1988,
p 1878.

be necessary, and patients often receive three drugs, one as an
injection, after drug susceptibility testing. Even with treatment, the
death rate from MDR-TB is 40 to 60 percent, the same as for TB
patients who receive no treatment. For persons coinfected with HIV
and MDR-TB, the death rate may be as high as 80 percent.

Treatment of Extrapulmonary Tuberculosis

The basic principles that underlie the treatment of pulmonary TB
also apply to extrapulmonary forms of the disease. While prospective, randomized trials of treatment regimens for extrapulmonary
TB are few, clinical experience has indicated that 9-month regimens
are effective. Regimens of 6 months are probably as effective in
extrapulmonary as in pulmonary disease, but in some instances such
as lymphadenitis and bone and joint tuberculosis, longer therapy
may be necessary.

The use of adjunctive therapies such as surgery and corticosteroids are more commonly required in extrapulmonary TB than in pulmonary disease. Surgery may be necessary to obtain specimens for diagnosis and to treat such processes as constrictive pericarditis and spinal cord compression. Corticosteroids may be of benefit in preventing cardiac constriction from TB pericarditis and in decreasing the neurologic sequelae of tuberculous meningitis.

Chemoprophylaxis

Chemoprophylaxis is intended to prevent the development of clinical disease in infected patients at increased risk for reactivation (Table 42-3). Isoniazid (INH) is the only drug shown to be effective

TABLE 42-3 High-Risk Groups Recommended for Preventive Therapy

1. Persons with < 5 mm of induration to PPD
    a. Children and adolescents who have been close contacts of infectious persons within the past 3 months are candidates for preventive therapy until a repeat tuberculin skin test is done 12 weeks after the last contact with an infectious source.
2. Persons with ≥ 5 mm of induration to PPD
    a. HIV-positive patients or persons with risk factors for HIV infection and suspected of having HIV infection but whose HIV status is unknown.
    b. Close contacts of persons with newly diagnosed infectious tuberculosis.
    c. Persons with abnormal chest radiographs that show fibrotic lesions likely to represent old, healed tuberculosis.
3. Persons with ≥ 10 mm induration to PPD
    a. Recent converters (< 35 years old) as indicated by PPD testing that demonstrated a ≥ 10 mm increase in induration within a 2-year period.
    b. HIV-positive intravenous drug users.
    c. Persons with medical conditions that have been reported to increase the risk of tuberculosis.
    d. Persons < 35 years old who are
        (1) Foreign-born from high-prevalence countries.
        (2) Members of medically underserved low-income populations, including high-risk racial or ethnic minority populations, especially blacks, Hispanics, and Native Americans.
        (3) Residents of facilities for long-term care (e.g., correctional institutions, nursing homes, and mental institutions).
4. Persons with > 15 mm induration to PPD
    a. All persons < 35 years of age with no risk factors.
    b. Recent converters (≥ 35 years of age) as indicated by PPD testing that demonstrated a ≥ 15 mm increase in induration within a 2-year period.

SOURCE: From Rossman MD. The resurgency of tuberculous and non-tuberculous mycobacteria, in Fishman AP (ed), *Update: Pulmonary Diseases and Disorders,* New York, McGraw Hill, 1992, p 291.

in chemoprophylaxis. Caution must be exercised in using INH prophylaxis in the elderly because of an increased risk of INH-induced hepatitis. When isoniazid-resistant organisms are suspected or when isoniazid cannot be tolerated, rifampin therapy has been suggested, but its efficacy as a prophylactic agent has not been documented in large scale trials. The suggested duration of INH therapy ranges from 6 to 12 months. Results with 6 months of treatment are nearly as effective as 12 months (65 percent versus 75 percent reduction in disease). The American Thoracic Society recommends 6 months of preventive therapy only if the chest radiograph is normal; otherwise a full 12-month course should be administered. Additionally, HIV-positive patients who fulfill criteria for prophylaxis should receive a minimum of 12 months of preventive therapy.

BIBLIOGRAPHY

For a more detailed discussion, see Stead WW, Bates JH: Epidemiology and prevention of tuberculosis, in Fishman AP (ed), *Pulmonary Diseases and Disorders,* 2d ed. New York, McGraw-Hill, 1988, pp 1795–1810.

Des Prez RM, Heim CR: Mycobacterium tuberculosis, in Mandell GL, Douglas RG, Bennett JM (eds), *Principles and Practice of Infectious Diseases,* 3d ed. New York, Churchill Livingstone, 1990, pp 1877–1906.

Pearson ML, Jereb JA, Frieden TR, Crawford JT, Davis BJ, Dooley SW, et al: Nosocomial transmission of multidrug-resistant *Mycobacterium tuberculosis.* A risk to patients and health care workers. Ann Intern Med 117:191–196, 1992.

Rossman M: The resurgence of tuberculosis and nontuberculosis mycobacteria, in Fishman AP (ed), *Update: Pulmonary Diseases and Disorders.* New York, McGraw-Hill, 1992, pp 287–297.

Weissler JC: Tuberculosis—immunopathogenesis and therapy. Am J Med Sci 305:52–65, 1993.

Jerry M. Zuckerman   Patrick J. Brennan

The nontuberculous mycobacteria (NTM) are ubiquitous microorganisms commonly found in soil and water. Generally, they are nonpathogenic for human beings. Isolation of NTM from a human specimen in the microbiology laboratory may represent either colonization or environmental contamination or infection.

Beginning in the 1950s, NTM were recognized as a cause of human disease. Since then, NTM have been implicated in pulmonary disease, lymphadenitis, skin and soft tissue infections, catheter-associated infections, surgical wound infections, and disseminated disease (especially in patients with human immunodeficiency virus [HIV] infection). This chapter focuses primarily on the NTM responsible for pulmonary disease: *Mycobacterium avium-intracellulare* (MAI), *Mycobacterium kansasii*, *Mycobacterium fortuitum*, and *Mycobacterium chelonae*.

CLASSIFICATION AND MICROBIOLOGY

The NTM are acid-fast, aerobic, non–spore-forming nonmotile bacteria that are easily cultured in the microbiology laboratory. These organisms generally grow slowly and require 2 to 8 weeks for detection on culture media. In the microbiology laboratory, the sputum specimen or sample obtained during bronchoscopy should be processed to promote the recovery of mycobacteria. The sample is liquefied by a mucolytic agent, usually *N*-acetyl-L-cysteine, thereby decreasing its mucin content, and then decontaminated, usually with NaOH, to eliminate other bacterial flora. The sample is then concentrated by centrifugation. Finally, it is plated on appropriate culture media that are maintained at different temperatures and at different exposures to light. Other samples suitable for culture include tissue specimens, body fluids, e.g., cerebrospinal fluid, pleural fluid, urine, and blood. Swabs of body fluid and tissue are not suitable for recovery of mycobacteria.

All mycobacterial isolates should be identified with respect to species as an aid in determining the clinical significance of the organism and the therapeutic options available for dealing with it. NTM are indistinguishable from *Mycobacterium tuberculosis* (MTB) with respect to acid-fast staining and histologic appearance.

In the 1950s, Runyon developed a classification system based on the growth rates, pigment production, and colonial morphology of the mycobacterial isolates. Runyon's classification (Table 43-1) divides the mycobacteria into four groups: photochromogens (group

TABLE 43-1 Classification (Runyon) on Nontuberculous Mycobacteria*

Class	Organism	Site of clinical infection[†]
Group I: Photochromogens	M. kansasii	Pulmonary
	M. simiae	Pulmonary
	M. marinum	Skin, soft tissue
Group II: Scotochromogens	M. scrofulaceum	Lymphadenitis
	M. szulgai	Pulmonary
Group III: Nonchromogens	M. avium-intracellulare	Pulmonary, lymphadenitis
	M. xenopi	Pulmonary
	M. ulcerans	Skin, soft tissue
Group IV: Rapid growers	M. fortuitum	Skin, soft tissue
	M. chelonae sp. abscessus	Skin, soft tissue
	M. chelonae sp. chelonae	Skin, soft tissue

*Nonpathogenic NTM are not included.
[†]The site of infection listed is the one with which a particular mycobacterium is most often associated.

I), scotochromogens (group II), nonchromogens (group III), and rapid growers (group IV). Final identification of the organism is determined by the optimal temperature for growth and a battery of biochemical tests, e.g., niacin accumulation test, nitrate reduction, iron uptake, and others. Newer methods for the more rapid and reliable speciation of mycobacterial isolates are being developed. Among these are nucleic acid probes and gas liquid chromatography. Nucleic acid probes for the identification of MTB, MAI and *M. gordonae* are now commercially available.

EPIDEMIOLOGY AND PATHOGENESIS

The primary reservoirs for NTM are in the environment. Pulmonary disease arises from the inhalation of aerosolized organisms. Soft tissue infection follows direct inoculation of NTM from a contaminated source. Disseminated disease in immunocompromised patients can occur after ingestion of organisms which subsequently traverse the intestinal mucosa. Animal-human or human-human transmission does not appear to be an important mechanism for transmission of the disease.

Because NTM infections are not reportable to the Centers for Disease Control and Prevention (CDC), the exact incidence and prevalence of these infections are unknown. However, two national surveys performed by the CDC in the early 1980s indicate that the prevalence of NTM disease in the United States is about 1.8 cases per 100,000. MAI was the most common isolate reported; prevalence of disease due to MAI was estimated to be 1.1 cases per 100,000. The CDC surveys found some geographic variability in the mycobacterial isolates: *M. kansasii* was more commonly isolated from the midwestern and southern states and MAI from the southeastern states.

Pulmonary infections due to *M. kansasii* and MAI generally occur in individuals who are in their fifth decade or older. Most of these individuals have underlying lung disease, such as chronic obstructive pulmonary disease, pneumoconiosis, bronchiectasis, or a history of tuberculosis. However, recent reports have highlighted the ability of MAI to infect patients without predisposing conditions.

Infections due to *M. kansasii* occur approximately three times more frequently in men than women. In contrast, MAI infections affect men and women equally, although women predominate in the group of patients without predisposing risk factors. Pulmonary infections due to *M. fortuitum* and *M. chelonae* occur more often in female patients who are nonsmokers and who have no underlying lung disease. Other species of mycobacteria, e.g., *M. szulgai*, *M. xenopi*, *M. simiae*, and *M. malmoense* are less common causes of pulmonary infection.

MAI has recently emerged as an important pathogen in patients with acquired immunodeficiency syndrome (AIDS). MAI infection is identified ante mortem in as many as one quarter of AIDS patients; at autopsy up to 50 percent of AIDS patients have MAI infection. MAI infection is typically a late manifestation of AIDS, usually appearing when CD4 counts drop below $100/mm^3$.

CLINICAL MANIFESTATIONS

The symptoms of patients with NTM pulmonary disease are similar to those of pulmonary tuberculosis. These symptoms are variable and nonspecific: productive cough, dyspnea, malaise, fatigue, and infrequently, hemoptysis. Constitutional symptoms such as fever, night sweats, and weight loss are generally less pronounced than in tuberculosis infections. Most cases are indolent. Frequently, patients with NTM pulmonary disease are treated for exacerbations of their underlying lung disease and weeks to months often elapse before the NTM infection is diagnosed.

The physical examination and laboratory findings of patients with NTM pulmonary disease are also nonspecific. Frequently the abnormalities on physical examination are attributed to the underlying lung disorder. The radiographic studies are also nonspecific. The chest radiographs commonly demonstrate thin-walled cavities that resemble those of pulmonary tuberculosis. In other instances, the radiographs show a diffuse, nodular process without cavitation. The disease is often bilateral and affects multiple lobes. In contrast to tuberculosis, mediastinal and hilar adenopathy and pleural effusions are rare.

The clinical presentation of MAI infection in patients with AIDS differs from that seen in the non-AIDS population. MAI infection in patients with AIDS is invariably widely disseminated, and pulmonary disease usually does not dominate the clinical picture. Intra-abdominal lymph nodes, liver, spleen, bone marrow, and gastrointestinal tract are among the most common sites of infection. Although the organism is often recovered from the respiratory tract, pulmonary parenchymal involvement is not usually extensive or clinically significant. Constitutional symptoms predominate, with fever, anorexia, and weight loss. Because of the propensity to involve the gastrointestinal tract and intra-abdominal lymph nodes, patients commonly present with abdominal pain and diarrhea. Respiratory symptoms are uncommon.

The chest radiograph in AIDS patients with disseminated MAI is commonly normal, even though organisms are recovered from the respiratory tract. When abnormal, a variety of radiographic patterns may be seen, including interstitial and nodular infiltrates and focal areas of consolidation. Mediastinal and hilar adenopathy may occur in isolation or in association with parenchymal infiltrates.

DIAGNOSTIC CONSIDERATIONS

Because of the lack of specificity of the history, physical examination, and chest radiographs, isolation of NTM in culture is essential for diagnosis. Skin testing using protein purified derivatives from NTM is not useful because of low specificity due to cross reactivity among mycobacterial species. In patients in whom the acid-fast bacilli (AFB) smear is positive, it is imperative that they initially be treated as if they have tuberculosis until the organism is finally identified.

Regardless of whether the AFB smear is positive or negative, once NTM grow in culture, their clinical importance must be determined. Unlike MTB, where isolation of even a single colony is always clinically significant, positive cultures of NTM are not always meaningful. When NTM are isolated from sputum, a major clinical issue arises: does this represent true disease, colonization, or contamination? Factors in favor of disease include an illness consistent with a mycobacterial infection, compatible radiographic findings, exclusion of other causes of infection, e.g., MTB and fungi, repeated isolation of the same species, and moderate or heavy growth in cultures.

In 1990, the American Thoracic Society published its diagnostic criteria for NTM infections (Table 43-2). The recommendations distinguish between cavitary and noncavitary forms of lung disease. For patients with cavitary lung disease, two or more sputums (or bronchial washings and sputum) should be AFB smear positive or have moderate-to-heavy growth of NTM on culture. For patients

TABLE 43-2 Diagnostic Criteria for Pulmonary Disease Caused by Nontuberculous Mycobacteria

I. For patients with cavitary lung disease
  1. Presence of two or more sputum specimens (or sputum and a bronchial washing) that are acid-fast bacilli smear positive and/or result in moderate-to-heavy growth of NTM on culture.
  2. Other reasonable causes for the disease process have been excluded, e.g., tuberculosis, fungal disease, etc.

II. For patients with noncavitary lung disease
  1. Presence of two or more sputum specimens (or sputum and a bronchial washing) that are acid-fast bacilli smear positive and/or produce moderate-to-heavy growth of NTM on culture.
  2. If the isolate is *M. kansasii* or *M. avium* complex, failure of the sputum cultures to clear with bronchial toilet or within 2 weeks of institution of specific mycobacterial drug therapy (although only studied for these two species, this criterion is probably valid for other species of NTM).
  3. Other reasonable causes for the disease process have been excluded.

III. For patients with cavitary or noncavitary lung disease whose sputum evaluation is nondiagnostic or another disease cannot be excluded
  1. A transbronchial or open lung biopsy yields the organism and shows mycobacterial histopathologic features, i.e., granulomatous inflammation, with or without acid-fast bacilli.
  2. A transbronchial or open lung biopsy that fails to yield the organism but shows mycobacterial histopathologic features in the absence of a prior history of other granulomatous or mycobacterial disease plus (1) presence of two or more positive cultures of sputum or bronchial washings; (2) other reasonable causes for granulomatous disease have been excluded.

SOURCE: Reprinted with permission from American Thoracic Society. Am Rev Resp Dis 14:940–953, 1990.

with noncavitary lung disease, in addition to satisfying the same criteria, they must remain culture positive after a trial of bronchial hygiene or a 2-week course of specific antimycobacterial therapy. Moreover, other disease processes should be excluded in both groups. Finally, in patients from whom tissue specimens are obtained, invasive disease is considered to be present if the sample shows the histologic changes of mycobacterial disease and if the organism is grown on culture.

Diagnosis of MAI infection in the AIDS patient is less problematic. Recovery of MAI from blood is a simple and highly sensitive means of establishing the diagnosis. The yield of blood cultures approaches 100 percent when either the lysis-centrifugation technique (DuPont isolators) or radiospirometric system (BACTEC) is used. Biopsies of liver, lymph nodes, or bone marrow also provide a high diagnostic yield. Specimens from the respiratory tract (sputum, lavage fluid) are frequently positive but are more useful as markers of disseminated disease than as indicators of parenchymal lung infection.

TREATMENT

There have been no controlled clinical trials evaluating the efficacy of various treatment regimens for pulmonary disease due to NTM. If the disease is asymptomatic or stable clinically, the decision can be made to withhold specific antimycobacterial therapy and treat only the underlying pulmonary disorder. However, if the disease is progressive or the patient is very symptomatic, a trial of antimicrobial therapy is indicated.

Drug susceptibility testing for NTM is not standardized. In vitro, the NTM, except for *M. kansasii*, are usually resistant to most of the antituberculous drugs tested at concentrations effective against MTB (Table 43-3). However, in vitro susceptibility patterns do not predict clinical response to therapy for the NTM. For several reasons, patients may respond favorably to multiple drug regimens despite in vitro resistance of isolates to individual drugs. First, susceptibility testing currently relies on the same techniques and drug combinations that are effective for MTB; the possibility exists that NTM might be sensitive in vitro to higher drug concentrations. Second, in vitro susceptibility patterns are difficult to relate to in vivo effectiveness because the organism multiplies primarily within phagocytic cells and it is the concentration of the drug in tissue, rather than in serum, that may be of major importance in determining therapeutic efficacy. Third, antimycobacterial agents are tested individually against the isolate, whereas combination therapy may have additive or synergistic therapeutic effects. Therefore, except for *M. fortuitum* and *M. chelonae* (see below), susceptibility patterns should not guide selection of antimicrobial agents. In general, treatment requires multiple drugs for synergy and to prevent the emergence of resistant organisms.

TABLE 43-3 Usual Susceptibility Patterns of Nontuberculous Mycobacteria to Various Antibiotics

	Species		
Antibiotic	M. kansasii	M. avium-intracellulare	M. fortuitum/chelonae
Isoniazid	I	R	R
Rifampin	S	R	R
Streptomycin	I	R	R
Pyrazinamide	R	R	R
Ethambutol	S	I	R

S = susceptible; R = resistant; I = intermediate

Mycobacterium kansasii *M. kansasii* is one of the more commonly isolated NTM. It is sensitive in vitro to most of the antimycobacterial agents. Drug regimens that contain rifampin seem to be more effective than those that exclude it; when rifampin is included, the conversion rate of sputum at 4 months is almost 100 percent. However, no controlled clinical trials of the best regimen have yet been done. In 1990, the American Thoracic Society recommended the following for *M. kansasii* pulmonary disease: isoniazid (300 mg), rifampin (600 mg), and ethambutol (15 mg/kg) given daily for 18 months. For patients unable to tolerate isoniazid, streptomycin can be given with rifampin and ethambutol for the first 3 months. The efficacy of a shortened course of therapy or intermittent therapy for *M. kansasii* pulmonary infection has not yet been adequately studied. For organisms resistant to rifampin, a clinical trial is currently under way evaluating the following regimen: daily isoniazid in high dosage (900 mg), ethambutol in high dosage (25 mg/kg), and sulfamethoxazole (3.0 g); treatment with these agents is continued for 18 to 24 months; during the first 6 months, streptomycin or amikacin is added to the regimen.

Mycobacterium avium-intracellulare *M. avium-intracellulare* is another commonly isolated NTM. Antimycobacterial drugs are 10 to 100 times less active in vitro against MAI than against MTB. Nonetheless, most patients with MAI respond clinically when the antimycobacterial drugs are used in combination. For patients with progressive symptoms or extensive disease, the American Thoracic Society recommends an initial four-drug regimen: isoniazid (300 mg), rifampin (600 mg), and ethambutol (25 mg/kg for the first 2 months; thereafter, 15 mg/kg) daily with streptomycin added for the initial 3 to 6 months of therapy. Treatment is continued for 18 to 24 months or for a minimum of 12 months after sputum cultures become negative. The success rate for this regimen is 50 to 80 percent but up to 20 percent of patients experience a relapse. If the sputum fails to convert, additional drugs such as cycloserine or ethionamide are sometimes helpful.

In patients with AIDS who have disseminated MAI infections, new treatment protocols have recently been explored. Included in these regimens have been various combinations of clofazimine (an antileprosy drug), ciprofloxacin, amikacin, rifabutin, ethambutol, rifampin, and isoniazid; they have been successful in clearing bacteremia and in leading to the abatement of symptoms. Two new macrolide antibiotics, clarithromycin and azithromycin, also appear to have excellent activity, both in vitro and in vivo, against MAI (as well as *M. fortuitum* and *M. chelonae*). The effectiveness of these macrolide antibiotics seems to be related to their high degree of penetration into tissue and macrophages. Although these new treatment regimens appear useful for disseminated MAI in the AIDS patient, it is unknown how effective they will be for pulmonary MAI disease in the non-AIDS population.

When MAI is limited to a solitary pulmonary nodule, surgical resection is curative. Furthermore, if a patient has progressive disease despite chemotherapy, surgical excision of diseased lung becomes an option if the disease is localized and the patient is able to tolerate surgery. After surgery, these patients should receive a course of drug therapy.

Mycobacterium fortuitum and Mycobacterium chelonae M. *fortuitum* and *M. chelonae* are rapidly growing mycobacteria that are resistant to all standard antituberculosis drugs. *M. fortuitum* is usually sensitive to amikacin, ciprofloxacin, cefoxitin, imipenem, sulfonamides, and doxycycline. *M. chelonae* subspecies *abscessus* is sensitive only to amikacin, cefoxitin, and, in about 30 percent of patients, to erythromycin. *M. chelonae* subspecies *chelonae* is more sensitive to erythromycin and occasionally responds to doxycycline. As noted above, in contrast to other NTM where in vitro testing for drug susceptibility may not be helpful, in pulmonary infections with *M. fortuitum* and *M. chelonae*, susceptibility testing of the various agents should be performed on isolates from all patients with clinically active disease. Because 90 percent of the isolates will be susceptible to amikacin and cefoxitin, patients with pulmonary disease caused by rapidly growing mycobacteria should initially be treated with high dose cefoxitin (12 g/day) and amikacin (serum levels of approximately 20 µg/ml). The final therapeutic regimen should be based on in vitro susceptibility results. In general, combination therapy is preferable. The intravenous route should be used for the first 4 to 8 weeks, followed by an oral regimen administered for an additional 6 months. If the isolate is not susceptible to any oral antibiotics, therapy should be reserved for clinically or radiographically significant exacerbations; antibiotics are then administered exclusively by the intravenous route.

The risks and benefits of drug administration must be weighed against the potential risks of not treating the patient. All patients, particularly the elderly, must be monitored closely for drug toxicity during the course of any therapeutic regimen. Ethambutol may cause an optic neuritis with loss of visual acuity and red-green color discrimination. Isoniazid and rifampin may cause a drug-induced hepatitis. Streptomycin and amikacin can lead to renal toxicity as well as auditory and vestibular dysfunction. If toxicity develops, the treatment regimen should be reevaluated based on the patient's clinical status, long-term prognosis, and the availability of effective alternative antimicrobial agents.

BIBLIOGRAPHY

For a more detailed discussion, see Davidson PT: Diseases caused by mycobacteria other than mycobacterium tuberculosis, in Fishman AP (ed), *Pulmonary Diseases and Disorders,* 2d ed. New York, McGraw-Hill, 1988, pp 1863–1868.

American Thoracic Society: Diagnosis and treatment of disease caused by non-tuberculosis mycobacteria. Am Rev Respir Dis 142:940–953, 1990.

Hopewell P, Cynamon M, Starke J, Iseman M, O'Brien R: Evaluation of new anti-infective drugs for the treatment of disease caused by *Mycobacterium kansasii* and other mycobacteria. Infectious Diseases Society of America and the Food and Drug Administration. Clin Infect Dis 15 (Suppl 1):S307–312, 1992.

Kirschner RA Jr, Parker BC, Falkinham JO III: Epidemiology of infection by nontuberculous mycobacteria. *Mycobacterium avium, Mycobacterium intracellulare,* and *Mycobacterium scrofulaceum* in acid, brown-water swamps of the southeastern United States and their association with environmental variables. Am Rev Respir Dis 145(2 Pt 1):271–275, 1992.

Rossman MD: The resurgence of tuberculosis and non-tuberculous mycobacteria, in Fishman AP (ed), *Update: Pulmonary Disease and Disorders.* New York, McGraw-Hill, 1992, pp 287–297.

Shafer RW, Sierra MF: *Mycobacterium xenopi, Mycobacterium fortuitum, Mycobacterium kansasii,* and other nontuberculous mycobacteria in an area of endemicity for AIDS. Clin Infect Dis 15:161–162, 1992.

Wolinsky E: Mycobacterial diseases other than tuberculosis. Clin Infect Dis 15:1–10, 1992.

Neil O. Fishman

The causative organisms of the endemic mycoses, *Histoplasma capsulatum, Blastomyces dermatitidis,* and *Coccidioides immitis,* share several environmental and pathophysiologic characteristics. They are all found in the soil and their reproductive cycles require heat and moisture. The organisms grow as molds in the soil, and their spores are the infective agents. These spores are inhaled and lodge in the alveoli when soil containing the organisms is disturbed. In general, the severity of symptoms in community-acquired fungal pneumonias depends on the size of the inoculum and the immune status of the host. This chapter focuses on endemic fungal pneumonias in the normal host; disease in immunocompromised individuals is discussed in Chapter 46.

HISTOPLASMOSIS

Epidemiology

Histoplasmosis is the most common and most extensively studied systemic fungal infection in the United States. The most significant endemic area surrounds the Ohio and Mississippi River valleys, and extends into the neighboring states of Texas, Oklahoma, Kansas, Pennsylvania, Maryland, and Virginia; it is estimated that 80 percent of the population has been infected with *H. capsulatum* in this region. The majority of cases are asymptomatic and of no clinical consequence.

The organism is much more prevalent at sites where avian or bat excrement have collected for several years. Birds appear to be resistant to histoplasma infection due to high body temperature. Bats, however, may be infected, have yeast forms in their feces, and can spread the organism to new habitats. Bird roosts, chicken houses, and sites frequented by bats such as caves, attics, and hollow trees are most likely to be point sources in endemic areas. Any disturbance at these sites markedly increases the number of infectious airborne spores.

Pathogenesis

Spores are inhaled, settle in the alveoli, and germinate in 2 to 3 days to release yeast forms that are phagocytized by macrophages. The yeast multiplies intracellularly in the nonimmune host and more macrophages are recruited to the region, resulting in small areas of pneumonitis at each infected site. Infected macrophages migrate to the mediastinal lymph nodes and subsequently gain access to the fixed reticuloendothelial system, producing new focal infiltrates in the liver and spleen. Both animal and clinical studies have shown that this process continues for 14 days, at which time the onset of acquired immunity results in tissue necrosis and caseation. The lesions eventually calcify and are readily apparent on chest radiographs. Viable organisms are trapped in the necrotic tissue and persist despite calcification; however, it is not clear whether they can reactivate.

In the vast majority of cases, the inoculum is small and the disease is asymptomatic. Infected individuals may eventually exhibit a few small calcifications in the lung, mediastinal lymph nodes, liver, and spleen. However, larger inocula usually result in a more severe illness, particularly in the nonimmune host.

Clinical Presentation

Acute symptomatic pulmonary histoplasmosis is characterized by a nonspecific influenza-like illness, with fever, chills, arthralgias, myalgias, headache, and nonproductive cough. Chest pain varies from vague to prominent and may be more severe on deep inspiration. This finding is probably attributable to enlarged mediastinal lymph nodes and can be diagnostically helpful when present. Nausea, vomiting, and diarrhea occur occasionally, and dyspnea has been reported following heavy inhalations. The duration of illness is related to the severity of symptoms, i.e., mild disease resolves quickly, whereas more advanced presentations persist for prolonged periods.

There is a paucity of physical findings in acute disease, but hepatosplenomegaly may be present with heavy infections. Erythema nodosum or erythema multiforme may occur in either symptomatic or asymptomatic disease and is seen more frequently in young women. These findings are often accompanied by arthralgias or frank arthritis. Routine laboratory studies are usually within normal limits.

Radiographic Findings

Visible infiltrates occur only in 25 percent of individuals with acute pulmonary histoplasmosis resulting from a small or modest inhalation inoculum. Similarly, calcifications develop in just one fourth of these patients. Heavy exposures result in many small scattered infiltrates, often with ipsilateral mediastinal or hilar adenopathy. When the fungus infects individuals with abnormal pulmonary architecture, such as smokers with centrilobular emphysema, the infection primarily involves the apices rather than the lower lung fields, as seen in normal individuals. The inflammatory infiltrate surrounds and outlines the abnormal air spaces, mimicking the cavitary lesions of reactivation tuberculosis.

Diagnosis

This is largely a clinical diagnosis in the appropriate epidemiologic setting with characteristic radiographic findings. Serologic data can provide strong confirmatory evidence, but culture or histologic proof is rarely obtained. The histoplasmin skin test is an important epidemiologic tool, but is not useful diagnostically.

Complement fixation (CF) is the most reliable test for the detection of serum antibody to *H. capsulatum.* A CF titer to the yeast-phase antigens of 1:32 or greater, or an appropriately timed 4-fold increase in titer is evidence of active or recent infection. Unfortunately, up to 30 percent of lifelong residents in endemic areas have persistent elevations of their CF titers. Of note, cross reactivity with *Blastomyces* is a documented problem with this study. Currently available immunodiffusion tests are more specific but lack the sensitivity of CF.

Treatment

Patients with acute pulmonary histoplasmosis seldom require antifungal therapy. Short-course amphotericin B is recommended for prolonged or severe infections with progressive ventilatory failure; the dose in adults is 0.5 mg/kg daily intravenously for 2 to 3 weeks. Ketoconazole has not been investigated in acute histoplasmosis but is probably an appropriate alternative given its efficacy in other clinical syndromes. Itraconazole, a new triazole antifungal agent, was recently approved for the treatment of histoplasmosis. The drug has excellent in vitro activity against *H. capsulatum,* and clinical studies have shown it to be an effective alternative to amphotericin B. The dose is 200 to 400 mg orally per day in single or divided doses.

Complications

Complications of acute pulmonary histoplasmosis are attributable to the healing of the disease in immunocompetent patients. Large calcified hilar and mediastinal lymph nodes may erode into adjacent structures, leading to cough, expectoration of broncholiths, and formation of tracheoesophageal fistulae. In rare instances, massive fibrosis surrounds the healing of mediastinal disease; the resultant mediastinal fibrosis may cause bronchial stenosis or occlusion of pulmonary arteries, veins, or the superior vena cava. Finally, caseous lymph nodes can erode into the pericardial or pleural spaces causing pericarditis or pleural effusion, respectively.

BLASTOMYCOSIS

Blastomycosis is a systemic pyogranulomatous disease caused by the dimorphic fungus *Blastomyces dermatitidis.* Initial infection occurs via the lungs and is usually followed by hematogenous dissemination. This is a multisystem disease that can involve the lungs, skin, bone, genitourinary system, and central nervous system (CNS).

Epidemiology

Detailed epidemiologic studies have been hampered by the lack of sensitive, specific skin test reagents. Current knowledge regarding blastomycosis has been derived from reports describing sporadic disease in both dogs and human beings, as well as from a limited number of small epidemics. The endemic area of blastomycosis appears to overlap the endemic region of histoplasmosis, but the blastomycosis belt extends further north into northern Wisconsin and Minnesota, as well as to the Canadian provinces of Ontario and Manitoba.

B. dermatitidis is also a soil-dwelling organism that lives in very specific and well-circumscribed areas. Most epidemics have been associated with waterways and soil that has been amply enriched by organic nitrogen through the droppings of various animal and bird species; decaying vegetation and wood have also been commonplace during recent outbreaks.

Pathogenesis

The portal of entry for blastomycosis in human beings appears to be the lung. Therefore, the manifestations of disease at the body sites result after dissemination from a primary pulmonary infection, although this is frequently not evident clinically. As with histoplasmosis, pulmonary infection occurs after inhalation of spores, which then convert to the yeast phase in the lung. The initial inflammatory response consists of clusters of neutrophils, and then progresses to noncaseating granulomas with epithelioid and giant cells. The response in cutaneous disease is unique and consists of prominent pseudoepitheliomatous hyperplasia with microabscess formation. The immunologic responses in blastomycosis are not well defined due to the lack of appropriate antigens for study. However, both cellular and humoral immunity appear to contribute in this infection.

Clinical Presentation

Blastomycosis is a systemic disease with a wide spectrum of pulmonary and extrapulmonary manifestations. Pulmonary disease may be acute or chronic and can mimic infection with a variety of other organisms, including bacteria, tuberculosis, and other fungi. *B. dermatitidis* infection can involve almost every body organ, with skin, bone, and the genitourinary tract being the most common to manifest clinically. Approximately 60 to 70 percent of infected individuals will present with extrapulmonary disease during the chronic phase of illness.

Acute pulmonary infection is frequently unrecognized. Symptoms are nonspecific and include an influenza-like syndrome with abrupt onset of fever, chills, arthralgias, and myalgias. Cough is initially nonproductive, but can become mucopurulent. The chest radiograph usually demonstrates lobar or segmental consolidation during the acute illness; pleural effusion and hilar adenopathy are uncommon.

Chronic blastomycosis is a progressive disease with a subacute indolent onset. As noted above, the clinical manifestations are protean and the first evidence of blastomycosis is commonly the appearance of disseminated disease. Pulmonary disease presents as a chronic pneumonia with productive cough, hemoptysis, weight loss, and pleuritic chest pain. The radiographic appearance is variable, but upper lobe fibronodular disease, with or without cavitation, is common and may be confused with tuberculosis. Large mass lesions, miliary disease, pleural effusions, and pneumothorax have all been described. Miliary disease carries a 50 percent mortality rate, and pleural disease does not respond well to therapy. Skin disease is the most common extrapulmonary manifestation of blastomycosis, followed by bone, genitourinary tract, and CNS disease.

Diagnosis

No pathognomonic syndrome points toward a diagnosis of blastomycosis. Serologic studies are neither sensitive nor specific. Therefore, definitive diagnosis requires culture of the organism from clinical specimens. However, a presumptive diagnosis can be made by visualization of the characteristic yeast in pus, sputum, secretions, or histologic specimens. Sputum and pus can be examined by wet preparation, with or without potassium hydroxide treatment; the yeast has a large refractile cell wall with single broad-based buds.

Treatment

Many patients with acute primary pulmonary blastomycosis will have self-limited disease, but there is no way of determining which patients will later present with extrapulmonary disease. Therefore, all patients with blastomycosis should receive antifungal therapy, whether they are presenting with acute or chronic disseminated manifestations of the disease. Amphotericin B was previously the treatment of choice for blastomycosis. However, ketoconazole is an effective alternative in immunocompetent patients with mild to moderate disease; the dose is 400 to 800 mg daily and should be continued for a minimum of 6 months. Ketoconazole does not cross the blood-brain barrier and, therefore, should not be used in patients with central nervous system disease. Itraconazole was recently approved for the management of blastomycosis and may be effective in CNS infections. The dose is 200 to 400 mg daily.

Amphotericin B is now reserved for those with life-threatening disease or for individuals who fail oral therapy. Although the exact dose and duration of therapy are uncertain, most studies recommend 1.5 to 2.5 g of amphotericin B at a dose of 0.3 to 0.6 mg/kg daily.

COCCIDIOIDOMYCOSIS

Epidemiology

Approximately 100,000 people are infected with *Coccidioides immitis* in the United States annually. The majority of these infections occur in the lower Sonoran Desert and the central valley of California and the adjacent areas of northern Mexico. The characteristic climate conditions are a semiarid desert with short intense periods of rain followed by rapidly rising temperatures, which favor sporulation of the fungus. Following sporulation, the fragile arthroconidia break off and become airborne, giving rise to the infecting aerosol. Once the arthroconidia reach the alveolar spaces following inhalation, they convert to the tissue phase of the organism, resulting in the production of the pathognomonic giant spherule. The spherule enlarges, septations develop, and endospores are produced. On maturation, the spherule ruptures, releasing large numbers of endospores which can then repeat the cycle.

Clinical Presentation

Sixty percent of infected individuals have asymptomatic infections, identifiable only by skin testing. Approximately 40 percent develop symptoms of primary infection 1 to 3 weeks following exposure. Symptoms include a nonproductive cough, fever, and pleuritic chest pain, which is seen more frequently in coccidioidomycosis than in the other endemic mycoses. In addition to nonspecific influenza-like complaints, many patients develop an erythematous rash over the trunk early in the course of the disease, but this usually resolves quickly. Erythema nodosum and erythema multiforme occur with increased frequency during the course of the disease, and are usually associated with an arthralgia-myalgia complex; this constellation of signs and symptoms is known as "valley fever," and it occurs much more frequently in young women.

Radiographic presentations vary significantly in coccidioidomy-

cosis and range from infiltrates to frank pneumonia. Hilar adenopathy may occur in a substantial number of patients, usually
ipsilateral to the infiltrate. In most cases, these manifestations
resolve spontaneously, but about 5 percent of those infected have
pulmonary residua, most commonly a pulmonary nodule or thin-
walled cavity. Pleural disease is also common and many patients
will have small pleural effusions during the acute phase of their
illness; secondary pleural involvement may occur with the rupture
of the classic thin-walled cavities. Rarely, widespread rapid dissemination may occur with a miliary and usually fatal picture. Common
sites for dissemination include the musculoskeletal system, the CNS,
and skin. This phenomenon is much more common in men, pregnant
women, immunocompromised hosts, and dark-skinned races.

In some patients, the acute pneumonia does not resolve, but
progresses to chronic pulmonary disease with low-grade fever,
anorexia, cough, weight loss, and chest pain. Cavitary lesions are
usually a part of this syndrome. Most cavities are < 2 cm in diameter
and are asymptomatic; however, they can be associated with fever
and hemoptysis. Long-term follow-up reveals that most small
cavities stabilize and regress in size without therapy. A small
proportion will continue to enlarge and approach the pleural
surface; this is an indication for antifungal therapy and possibly
surgical intervention.

Diagnosis

Serodiagnosis is highly developed and very useful in coccidioidomycosis. IgM antibodies appear early in infection and can be measured
by either the tube precipitin test or latex agglutination. The
antibodies appear in the second or third week of infection, reach
their peak at 1 month, and are usually gone by 6 months. Although
they are highly specific, the test is not very sensitive, with only 50
percent of patients demonstrating an IgM titer during acute pulmonary coccidioidomycosis. The CF test is well standardized in this
disease. A 4-fold titer rise is diagnostic, and a rising titer is cause
for concern. Titers of 1:16 or greater are frequently seen in
disseminated disease. When rising titers are observed, the risk for
dissemination is high and the patient should be carefully reassessed.

Culture of the fungus is not difficult but is extremely hazardous
to laboratory personnel. The mycelial phase grows readily under
standard lab conditions, but the arthroconidia are extremely fragile
and can break off with even the simplest of maneuvers; opening the
Petri dish might produce sufficient air currents to aerosolize the
infecting particles. Therefore, the clinician must notify the laboratory when a diagnosis of coccidioidomycosis is suspected so that
appropriate precautions may be taken.

Skin testing in coccidioidomycosis is also well developed. There are two available antigens: coccidioidin, made from mycelial filtrates, and the more recently developed spherulin, made from the tissue phase of the organism. Both preparations are equally effective in documenting previous infection. Skin testing is particularly useful when the previous test status of the individual is known. Conversion of the test to positive in the presence of a compatible acute illness is diagnostic. When a previously positive skin test becomes negative in the setting of progressive disease, this is indicative of the development of selective anergy and correlates well with dissemination.

Treatment

Most patients with primary pulmonary coccidioidomycosis do not require treatment; the usual course is spontaneous resolution in immunocompetent patients. Antifungal therapy is indicated for those with persistent symptoms beyond 6 to 8 weeks and for individuals at high risk for dissemination, i.e., immunosuppressed patients, diabetics, and members of dark-skinned races. The drug of choice is amphotericin B; the exact dose and duration of therapy are not known, but a total dose of 1.0 to 1.5 g appears reasonable during the acute phase of the illness. Ketoconazole appears to be an effective alternative for all but CNS disease at doses of 200 to 400 mg daily. Disseminated disease, however, requires amphotericin B in larger doses, usually greater than 2.5 g. Meningeal involvement necessitates both intrathecal and intravenous amphotericin B.

BIBLIOGRAPHY

For a more detailed discussion, see Rubin RH: Fungal infections in the immunocompromised host, in Fishman AP (ed), *Pulmonary Diseases and Disorders,* 2d ed. New York, McGraw-Hill, 1988, pp 1761–1774.

Daar ES, Meyer RD: Medical management of AIDS patients. Bacterial and fungal infections. Med Clin North Am 76:173–203, 1992.

Dismukes WE, Bradsher RW Jr, Cloud GC, Kauffman CA, Chapman SW, George RB, et al: Itraconazole therapy for blastomycosis and histoplasmosis. Am J Med 93:489–497, 1992.

Loyd JE, Tillman BF, Atkinson JB, Des Prez RM: Mediastinal fibrosis complicating histoplasmosis. Medicine 67:295–310, 1988.

Medoff G, Kobayashi GS: Systemic fungal infections: An overview. Hosp Pract (Off Ed) 26:41–52, 1991.

Milatovic D, Voss A: Efficacy of fluconazole in the treatment of systemic fungal infections. Eur J Clin Microbiol Infect Dis 11:395–402, 1992.

Sarosi GA, Bates JH, Bradsher RW, et al: Chemotherapy of the pulmonary mycoces: Official statement of the American Thoracic Society. Am Rev Respir Dis 138:1078–1081, 1988.

Sarosi GA, Davies SF (eds): *Fungal Diseases of the Lung,* 2d ed New York: Raven Press, 1993, p 352.

Neil O. Fishman

Viruses are the most common causes of pneumonia in infants and children, but, in general, are less common causes of pulmonary disease in adults. Viruses of six major families cause acute respiratory disease, but the RNA viruses account for the greatest number of cases. Although respiratory viruses vary significantly with respect to the composition and organization of their genomes, their pathophysiology and resultant clinical syndromes are relatively similar from virus to virus. Therefore, clinical signs and symptoms are not sufficient criteria on which to base an etiologic diagnosis.

EPIDEMIOLOGY

The true incidence and prevalence of viral pneumonias are difficult to estimate inasmuch as most published series deal only with hospitalized patients. There is an increased incidence of disease reported in the young, in closed populations (such as nursing homes and military recruits), and in individuals who have underlying cardiac and pulmonary diseases. Death rates from viral pneumonia vary with respect to the causative virus and host immune factors; the highest mortality rates have been reported during epidemics and pandemics of influenza A. Additionally, long-term pulmonary sequelae have been described in infants, young children, and some adults.

Certain epidemiologic and clinical clues can assist in the diagnosis of viral respiratory disease. First, viral pneumonias are seen most commonly during the winter months. Second, a few clinical syndromes, such as croup or bronchiolitis, are pathognomonic for just one or two viruses. Finally, many agents have distinctive epidemiologic patterns that can help narrow the etiologic spectrum. For example, adenoviruses are an important cause of pneumonia in military recruits but are predominantly a pediatric pathogen in the civilian population. "Winter infantile wheezing" syndrome is most likely attributable to infection with either respiratory syncytial virus (RSV) or parainfluenza virus, type III; the common cold is usually due to rhinovirus and typically exhibits a bimodal distribution, with peaks in the early fall and late winter or early spring.

Ultimately, the diagnosis of viral pneumonia can be difficult, particularly if the patient is coinfected with a bacterial pathogen at the time of presentation. There are few radiographic clues that help distinguish bacterial from viral pneumonia or one virus from another. However, it is now possible to establish a laboratory identification of certain common viral respiratory pathogens within several hours through the use of new immunofluorescent techniques.

Pathophysiology

The majority of viral respiratory pathogens are transmitted from person to person via small droplet aerosols. These small particles can spread across considerable distances and are able to inoculate the lower respiratory tract epithelium directly. Rhinoviruses and RSV are frequently transmitted by hand-to-hand or hand-to-fomite-to-hand inoculation of conjunctival or nasal membranes. Finally, cytomegalovirus, and possibly other herpesviruses, reach the lung by hematogenous spread. The route of entry and site of inoculation can often explain the development of prodromal symptoms during a viral syndrome. Therefore, RSV causes a localized upper respiratory prodrome before the development of pneumonia, whereas influenza virus initially manifests with pulmonary and systemic symptoms because it inoculates the lower respiratory tract directly.

The signs and symptoms of viral respiratory infections are produced by the interplay of viral cytopathic effect and the resultant inflammatory response; the pathologic changes that result from these processes are similar irrespective of the etiologic viral agent. Necrosis and sloughing of respiratory epithelium results in increased mucous production and bronchiolar plugging. A mononuclear inflammatory infiltrate develops within a week, and intranuclear inclusion bodies can be detected during the latter stages of infection. Parainfluenza virus and measles pneumonia are characterized by multinucleated giant cells.

Humoral and cell-mediated responses and nonspecific host defenses are activated to control progression of and to clear the viral infection. For example, high concentrations of interferon, which inhibits the cell-to-cell spread of virus, are found in the lung. Both specific antiviral antibody and cytotoxic T lymphocytes are found approximately 3 days following infection, but the relative contribution of each arm of the immune system to final recovery is not yet clear. Of note, extrarespiratory spread of virus is rare. The systemic and constitutional signs of viral infection are attributable to soluble inflammatory mediators, such as interferon. Secondary bacterial infection of the lung occurs after viral infection of the lower respiratory tract; increased bacterial adherence and colonization is due to viral damage of the mucociliary escalator and alterations of alveolar macrophage and neutrophil phagocytic function.

Laboratory Diagnosis

The "gold standard" of laboratory diagnosis of viral infections is isolation and identification of the virus in cell culture. As noted, the presentations of viral pneumonias are sufficiently homogeneous to warrant obtaining viral cultures for specific diagnosis. Nasal washes, nasopharyngeal swabs, throat swabs, tracheal aspirates (if the patient is intubated), bronchoalveolar lavage, and transbronchial biopsies are all suitable specimens. The specimen should be placed in a protein-containing carrier medium and transported promptly to the laboratory. The sample is then inoculated onto several tissue culture cell lines and observed for cytopathic effect over several weeks. Some viruses, e.g., influenza virus, rhinovirus, and herpes simplex virus, will grow within 74 h, whereas others, e.g., cytomegalovirus and varicella zoster virus, take several weeks to produce cytopathic changes. Nonrespiratory specimens such as stool, urine, and blood, can also be cultured for viruses.

Rapid immunofluorescence techniques are available to assist in the identification of many respiratory viruses within just a few hours. Commercial kits are available for the rapid detection of influenza virus A and B; parainfluenza virus types I, II, and III; respiratory syncytial virus; and adenovirus. Serologic studies currently play a small role in the routine diagnosis of viral respiratory diseases.

INFLUENZA VIRUSES

Epidemiology

Influenza is the most common cause of lower respiratory tract infections in the United States. The most demonstrative figures on the impact of influenza are the 20,000 deaths that occur annually and the 3.9 million hospitalizations necessitated by the disease. Children younger than 5 years and persons 65 years and older have significantly greater complication rates than individuals between these extremes of age. Additionally, people with cardiac or pulmonary disease, diabetes, asthma, and immunosuppressed systems are also at greater risk for severe influenza and resultant complications.

Influenza A virus causes the most severe and widespread disease; influenza B virus causes more localized outbreaks. Infection with influenza C virus is common, but rarely causes detectable disease. Influenza virus is a negative-strand RNA virus with a segmented genome; it has a lipid envelope with surface hemagglutinin and neuraminidase glycoprotein projections. Two types of antigenic changes occur among influenza viruses. Minor changes (antigenic drifts) occur in the hemagglutinins and neuraminidases of both influenza A and B and are due to spontaneous point mutations. This process is thought to account for influenza epidemics which occur every few years. Major changes (antigenic shifts) occur only in influenza A and are caused by reassortment of genomic segments between viral strains. This process results in a new viral subtype and is responsible for pandemic outbreaks.

Clinical Presentations and Complications

The onset of influenza is usually abrupt and is commonly associated with extrapulmonary and systemic symptoms such as fever, headache (frequently retrobulbar), arthralgias, myalgias, and muscle tenderness. Patients may also present with conjunctivitis or complain of photophobia, anorexia, or nausea. Respiratory symptoms include dry cough, sore throat and coryza; these usually resolve in 3 to 5 days, followed by defervescence 1 to 2 days later. However, total recovery may take up to several weeks and can be complicated by hyperreactive airway disease, tracheobronchitis, primary influenza pneumonia, and secondary bacterial pneumonia. The wheezing (or occasionally cough-equivalent bronchospasm) and tracheobronchitis are self-limited and resolve with symptomatic therapy, but the other two entities carry a more significant morbidity and mortality.

Primary influenza pneumonia is the least common and most serious complication of influenza and is believed to represent widespread infection of the lung with the virus. Individuals with elevated left atrial pressures, such as those with mitral valve stenosis, appear to be at greatest risk for this complication. Pregnant women have also been at increased risk during some outbreaks; this is not directly related to the altered mechanics of breathing characteristic of late pregnancy, inasmuch as there is no correlation with stage of pregnancy. Clinically, patients with primary pneumonia give a history of an acute influenza-like illness that does not resolve, but progresses steadily over 24 to 48 h to frank pneumonia. They appear seriously ill with marked dyspnea and cyanosis. Auscultation does not reveal evidence of consolidation, and the chest film demonstrates diffuse involvement of the lungs with interstitial or patchy infiltrates. The white blood cell count may be elevated with a left shift; leukopenia can be seen, however, and is a poor prognostic sign. The sputum Gram stain should have few neutrophils and no predominant organisms. Mortality is high and most patients die with a picture of adult respiratory distress syndrome.

Secondary bacterial pneumonia occurs far more frequently than primary influenza pneumonia. Patients often note a period of improvement of their acute influenza-like illness for 1 to 4 days, after which they develop signs and symptoms of bacterial pneumonia. The most common organisms associated with secondary pneumonia are *Streptococcus pneumoniae, Staphylococcus aureus,* and *Haemophilus influenza,* although gram-negative bacilli should be considered in residents of nursing homes and in patients in intensive-care units. Once again, the sputum Gram stain can be helpful in identifying likely pathogens and in assisting with empirical antimicrobial therapy.

Extrapulmonary complications of influenza are rare but include myocarditis and various neurologic entities such as encephalitis, transverse myelitis, and Guillain-Barré syndrome. Rye's syndrome is a complication of influenza B infection and is increased in frequency with concomitant use of aspirin. Therefore, children should receive aspirin-free antipyretics such as acetaminophen or ibuprofen during influenza season.

Treatment and Prophylaxis

Uncomplicated influenza is generally treated symptomatically with hydration, analgesics, antipyretics, and rest. Specific antiviral therapy is available only for influenza A infections; both amantadine and the closely related analogue rimantadine (which is not yet licensed in the United States) demonstrate excellent in vitro activity against influenza A and can reduce the severity and duration of fever and systemic symptoms if initiated during the first 72 h of illness. The dosage is 200 mg orally initially, followed by 100 mg once or twice daily for the duration of fever; dosage must be adjusted for individuals with renal insufficiency. Amantadine causes neurologic side effects such as dizziness, insomnia, and extrapyramidal symptoms with increased frequency in the elderly population. Rimantadine has poorer penetration into the central nervous system and thus has a decreased incidence of neurologic side effects.

The major public health measure for the prevention of influenza A and B infections has been the use of trivalent inactivated influenza vaccines. Efficacy rates for the vaccine have been reported to be between 67 and 92 percent. The only contraindication to the vaccine is allergy to eggs, because the vaccine viruses are grown in embryonated eggs. The vaccine must be reformulated and administered annually due to the changing antigenic patterns of influenza A and B. The vaccine is recommended for use in (1) adults or children with cardiac or pulmonary disorders; (2) residents of nursing homes or other chronic care facilities; (3) health care workers; (4) any individual over the age of 65; (5) adults or children with chronic diseases such as diabetes mellitus or renal disease; and (6) all immunosuppressed patients.

The vaccine is not contraindicated in pregnancy but is generally administered during the second or third trimesters. Amantadine may also be used for prophylaxis and is particularly useful during severe epidemic outbreaks as an adjunct to protect individuals during the 10 to 14 days necessary for antibodies to develop following immunization.

RESPIRATORY SYNCYTIAL VIRUS

Epidemiology

Respiratory syncytial virus is the most common cause of pneumonia in children under 3 years of age. Approximately 50 percent of all pneumonias in this age group are caused by RSV, and approximately 50 percent of all RSV pneumonias occur before 2 years of age. Because RSV infection does not produce absolute immunity, individuals continue to have mildly symptomatic or asymptomatic infections through adulthood. However, lower respiratory tract involvement is confined to children under the age of 2, the elderly, and the immunosuppressed host. Local epidemics during the winter and spring are an annual occurrence, although RSV disease abates during influenza outbreaks; this is known as viral interference. Infection within families and infections in day care centers are the major routes of transmission. However, several nonsocial outbreaks of RSV infections have been reported.

Clinical Presentations

Bronchiolitis characterized by airway hyperreactivity is the most characteristic presentation of RSV infection, but more children actually have pneumonia without clinically evident bronchospasm. The most important difference between these two presentations is that bronchiolitis is typically seen in the infant, whereas pneumonia is more common in the toddler. RSV pneumonia is associated with hypoxia and apneic spells in infants and can also present as a "viral sepsis" syndrome; this latter complication is more common in premature infants. Mechanical ventilation may be required in hospitalized infants with severe pneumonia. Children may also develop a rash several days into RSV infection, ranging from mild erythema to a confluent maculopapular eruption. Fever is uncommon beyond the first day of infection, as are conjunctivitis and otitis media. Radiographic diagnosis is suggested by air trapping and multilobar patchy infiltrates, but no pattern is pathognomonic. Additionally, right upper lobe collapse or consolidation has been reported in a high percentage of patients with RSV pneumonia.

Treatment

The majority of children with RSV infection can be managed at home with symptomatic care and humidification. Approximately 1 percent of cases, primarily infants under 6 months of age, require hospitalization. The keystone of management here is supplemental oxygen therapy. The role of bronchodilators in treating RSV pneumonia is controversial. The most significant advance in the management of RSV infection has been the introduction of ribavirin, a synthetic nucleoside analogue of guanosine that has broad antiviral activity. It is administered as an aerosol and has been shown to be effective in the treatment of RSV pneumonia and bronchiolitis. Ribavirin limits the severity of symptoms and shortens the duration of illness, although viral shedding does not differ from that in controls. The Committee on Infectious Diseases for the American Academy of Pediatrics currently recommends that ribavirin be considered for infants at risk or for those suffering complicated RSV infection. Ribavirin aerosol, at a concentration of 20 mg/ml of water, must be delivered 12 to 18 h per day for 3 to 7 days to achieve the desired dosage. The aerosol is sticky and can precipitate within any ventilator apparatus.

PARAINFLUENZA VIRUSES

The second most common cause of lower respiratory tract infections leading to hospitalization in infants is parainfluenza virus. Although there is not a strict relationship between specific viral types and particular clinical syndromes, infection with parainfluenza virus types I and II typically manifests as croup, whereas parainfluenza virus type III more commonly causes laryngotracheobronchitis and pneumonia. When pneumonia occurs, it is usually mild with few reported fatalities. Parainfluenza virus type III causes infection in early childhood; parainfluenza virus types I and II are seen during later childhood. Epidemics caused by parainfluenza types I and II usually occur in the fall, whereas parainfluenza type III infections occur in sporadic endemic outbreaks. Type II virus is isolated less commonly than either types I or III and is usually associated with more mild upper respiratory infections. Patterns of transmission for the parainfluenza viruses are similar to those discussed for RSV. Reinfection with all the parainfluenza viruses is common in children.

Laryngotracheobronchitis and croup represent different ends of a single clinical spectrum. The onset of illness is usually characterized by cough, hoarseness, and fever, which may persist for 2 to 3 days. Lower respiratory tract disease with wheezing, air trapping, and hypoxemia will predominate the clinical presentation in some patients; others will develop the brassy, barklike cough and inspiratory stridor characteristic of croup. It is not difficult to recognize and diagnose these syndromes during epidemic periods. Patients are usually not severely ill. However, it is imperative to distinguish croup from acute bacterial epiglottitis, which can rapidly progress to airway obstruction within a period of several hours. A lateral neck film can be helpful in this regard, but the patient should not be removed from medical observation and resuscitative equipment for an extended period of time. Optimally, the diagnosis of epiglottitis should be made in a controlled setting with direct laryngoscopy. Radiographic studies are of limited value in the diagnosis of parainfluenza virus infections.

Symptomatic therapy with supplemental oxygen, humidification, antipyretics, and occasionally cough suppressants is the mainstay of therapy for both croup and laryngotracheobronchitis. However, racemic epinephrine administered via aerosol has been shown to provide prompt symptomatic relief in double-blind placebo-controlled studies of more severely ill patients, although this therapy has no effect on the pace of the illness or on arterial oxygen tension. Ribavirin has in vitro activity against parainfluenza virus types I, II, and III, but clinical efficacy has not yet been studied effectively.

OTHER VIRAL PNEUMONIAS SEEN IN ADULTS

There are 41 adenovirus serotypes that cause disease in normal adults. Acute respiratory disease in military recruits is associated with types IV, VII, and XXI; lower respiratory disease, including pneumonia and bronchiolitis, is associated with types III, VII, and XXI. Sporadic cases of adenoviral pneumonia in adults are still reported, and immunocompromised patients are susceptible to severe and occasionally fatal adenoviral pneumonias. A wide range of radiographic findings are described, including feathery irregular infiltrates, indistinct segmental margins, and a predilection for the lower lobes. Diagnosis rests on viral isolation. No effective antiviral agents are active against adenovirus, but a vaccine is available for prophylaxis and is currently being used in military recruits.

Both measles and varicella zoster virus infection can be complicated by pneumonia at the time of acute exanthem. Radiographic evidence of pneumonia is seen commonly in uncomplicated cases of measles. Individuals born after 1956 who received the killed measles vaccine (prior to 1969) can develop an atypical measles syndrome characterized by an atypical rash that begins peripherally and progresses centripetally, high fever, and interstitial pulmonary infiltrates.

When varicella develops in adulthood, 16 percent of patients will develop radiographic evidence of pneumonia; the pneumonia can be severe with mortality rates of 13.5 to 45 percent reported in the literature. Radiographic features can include nodular or reticular densities bilaterally, as well as extensive interstitial infiltrates. As the pneumonia resolves, the lesions may calcify and leave multiple calcifications scattered throughout all lung fields. Intravenous acyclovir appears to be an effective therapy for varicella pneumonia in both normal and immunocompromised hosts, although published clinical data are limited. The dose of acyclovir is 12.4 mg/kg administered every 8 h for 7 days. Acyclovir has been used to treat varicella pneumonia successfully during pregnancy and has been recommended for use in children with varicella complicating leukemia. Varicella hyperimmune globulin is effective as prophylactic therapy if given within 72 h of the onset of lesions.

The other common respiratory viruses—rhinoviruses, coronaviruses, and enteroviruses—rarely cause pneumonia in normal adults. Similarly, herpes simplex virus, cytomegalovirus, and Epstein-Barr virus, are more frequent cases of pneumonias in immunocompromised patients, although sporadic cases of pneumonia caused by these viruses have been reported in previously healthy adults. It is interesting to note that herpes simplex virus typically infects squamous epithelium; therefore, factors that cause squamous metaplasia of the tracheobronchial tree such as traumatic endotracheal intubation, burns, radiation therapy, cytotoxic chemotherapy, and smoking, predispose individuals to lower respiratory tract infection with this virus.

BIBLIOGRAPHY

For a more detailed discussion, see Douglas RG Jr, Edelson PJ: Respiratory viral infections, in Fishman AP (ed), *Pulmonary Diseases and Disorders,* 2d ed. New York, McGraw-Hill, 1988, pp 1583–1596.

Anderson DJ, Jordan MC: Viral pneumonia in recipients of solid organ transplants. Semin Respir Infect 5:38–39, 1990.

Bender BS, Small PA: Influenza: Pathogenesis and host defense. Semin Respir Infect 7:38–45, 1992.

Greenberg SB: Viral pneumonia. Infect Dis Clin North Am 5:603–621, 1991.

Whimbey E, Bodey GP: Viral pneumonia in the immunocompromised adult with neoplastic disease: The role of common community respiratory viruses. Semin Respir Infect 7:122–131, 1992.

Patrick J. Brennan

The number of individuals in the United States with immunocompromising conditions has increased dramatically since the beginning of the 1980s due largely to the spread of the human immunodeficiency virus (HIV) pandemic. Prior to the revision of the Acquired Immunodeficiency Syndrome (AIDS) surveillance definition by Centers for Disease Control and Prevention, > 250,000 individuals in the United States met the definition of AIDS. The new case definition recognizes the profound susceptibility of HIV-infected persons to *Mycobacterium tuberculosis* and includes pulmonary tuberculosis among AIDS-defining illnesses. Despite significant advances in the treatment and prophylaxis of opportunistic infections in patients infected with HIV, pulmonary complications continue to be important causes of morbidity and mortality in this population.

The maturation of solid organ and bone marrow transplantation into accepted therapeutic modalities for the treatment of a variety of end-organ diseases and hematologic malignancies has further expanded the pool of compromised patients. Recipient and graft survival now exceeds 80 percent for some transplant groups. More than 100,000 solid organ transplant operations were performed between 1980 and 1990, and in the case of renal transplantation, has become the preferred treatment modality for end-stage renal disease. Advances in transplant biology and pharmacology have established a pool of patients with long-term survival and susceptibility to infection. Congenital defects in immunity constitute a relatively small proportion of the population of compromised hosts.

PATHOGENESIS OF PNEUMONIA IN THE COMPROMISED HOST

Susceptibility to opportunistic pulmonary pathogens is a function of the specific immune defect, as well as the duration and severity of the defect. Table 46-1 relates immune deficiency to the susceptibility to pulmonary pathogens. HIV infection is currently the most prevalent immunocompromising condition in the world with more than one million infected Americans and tens of millions carrying the virus in Africa and Asia. The progressive loss of CD4 cells, T-helper lymphocytes, results in progressive and profound susceptibility to infection when the CD4 count drops below 200 mm^3. Susceptibility to protozoans, mycobacteria, and cytomegalovirus (CMV) infection in HIV-infected individuals is mediated by loss of

TABLE 46-1 Relationship Between Types of Pulmonary Infection and Defects in Host Defenses in the Immunocompromised Patient

Host defense defect	Conditions commonly associated	Pulmonary infection to which patient is predisposed
Impaired antibody formation	Congenital and acquired hypoglobulinemias, chronic lymphocytic leukemia, multiple myeloma, B cell lymphoma, AIDS	*Streptococcus pneumoniae, Hemophilus influenzae* type B
Depressed cell-mediated	Lymphoma, AIDS, transplantation, prolonged corticosteroid therapy	Typical and atypical mycobacteria, *Nocardia asteroides,* fungi, herpes group viruses, measles virus, *Pneumocystis carinii, Toxoplasma gondii, Strongyloides stercoralis*
Decrease in the number of fully functional granulocytes	Myeloproliferative disorders, cytotoxic chemotherapy, congenital defects	Oral bacterial flora, *Staphylococcus aureus,* Enterobacteriaceae, *Pseudomonas aeruginosa, Acinetobacter, Aspergillus* species
Defects in complement	Congenital and acquired hypocomplementemic states, hypocomplementemic vasculitis	*Streptococcus pneumoniae, Haemophilus influenzae* type B
Oral and tracheobronchial ulcerations and/or obstructions	Tumors of respiratory tract, cytotoxic chemotherapy	Oral bacterial flora, Enterobacteriaceae

CD4 cells. Virtually all cases of *Pneumocystis carinii* pneumonia (PCP) in HIV occur in individuals with CD4 counts below 200. It is not always possible to quantify the immune defect with such precision. The duration of the defect is important in the development of infection, particularly in neutropenic hosts. Normal hosts who develop transient neutropenia related to antimicrobial therapy are at little increased risk for infection, whereas leukemics undergoing cytotoxic chemotherapy with a 2 to 3 week neutropenic nadir are very susceptible to nosocomial gram-negative bacteria, *Straphylococcus aureus,* and fungi.

The widespread use of chemoprophylaxis in preventing PCP and the development of antiretroviral agents has drastically reduced the number of cases of PCP in HIV-infected patients. Nonetheless, pneumonia remains a leading cause of HIV-related mortality and morbidity. Recurrent bacterial pneumonia is now recognized as an AIDS-defining condition in the CDC's *1993 Revised Classification for HIV Infection.* Progression to symptomatic HIV disease is often manifested by pulmonary infection such as bacterial pneumonias, including *Legionella,* and tuberculosis when CD4 counts fall below 500/mm³. The exact incidence of bacterial pneumonia in HIV-infected persons is not known. The rate for pneumococcal pneumonia among HIV-infected persons is estimated to be approximately 100-fold greater than for immunologically normal persons. B cell dysfunction seen in patients with HIV infection is responsible for their increased rate of bacterial pneumonia. Neutrophil defects and cytotoxic chemotherapy are usually associated with gram-negative bacterial pneumonias, nocardiosis and invasive pulmonary aspergillosis. These diseases are now being seen increasingly in the latter stages of HIV infection.

Tuberculosis has emerged as a major pulmonary pathogen in HIV-infected persons. Susceptibility to *M. tuberculosis* varies in degree depending on the cause of the cell-mediated immune defect. HIV-infected persons possess a 200-fold greater risk than the population at large of developing active tuberculosis. The increasing prevalence of tuberculosis in society places at jeopardy all patients with defects in cell-mediated immunity, whether congenital or acquired through pharmacologic or infectious processes. HIV-infected persons with undiagnosed pulmonary conditions should be evaluated for tuberculosis infection and isolated until proven not to have tuberculosis. This approach has placed a tremendous burden on hospital isolation facilities in the areas of high prevalence of tuberculosis and HIV. Outbreaks of multidrug resistant (MDR) tuberculosis have exacted a heavy toll among HIV-infected patients and health care workers. Among HIV-infected patients developing MDR-tuberculosis, the mortality rate has ranged from 72 to 89 percent in various outbreaks with death occurring between 4 and 16 weeks after diagnosis. Six health care workers have acquired MDR-tuberculosis occupationally and died. Four of the deaths occurred among HIV-infected persons.

Other patient populations possess characteristic susceptibilities to infection based on their immune defect. The pharmacologic agents used to prevent allograft rejection are, for the most part, broadly immunosuppressive, but exert their most important effects on cell-mediated immunity leaving the host vulnerable to protozoan, mycobacterial, and viral infections. Infections in solid organ transplant recipients predominate in the body cavity in which the organ is implanted. Thus, pneumonia is a relatively infrequent complication of renal transplantation occurring in approximately 1 percent, whereas 5 percent of heart and heart-lung transplant recipients may develop pneumonia. As in HIV infection, PCP in allograft recipients has been well controlled by the use of co-trimoxazole. The most serious pulmonary complications of transplantation are latent viral infections, most often caused by CMV, which occur through transmissions from the donor organ or reactivation of a prior infection. The intensity of immunosuppression plays an important role in the development of posttransplant infection with the largest proportion of serious infections occurring in the first 6 months after the transplant. Episodes of allograft rejection treated with more intensive immunosuppression potentiate the development of infectious processes. The murine monoclonal antibody, OKT3, an anti-CD3 antibody, has been associated with life-threatening CMV infections. The highest mortality associated with CMV pneumonia occurs following bone marrow transplantation when graft-versus-host disease appears to play a role that is absent in solid organ recipients.

Individuals with neutrophil defects or prolonged neutropenia are likely to develop infection with filamentous fungi, such as aspergillus, or bacterial pathogens.

MANIFESTATIONS OF PNEUMONIA IN THE COMPROMISED HOST

The clinical manifestations of pulmonary infection in the compromised host may be obscured by the underlying host defense defect. Neutropenic hosts may have minimal pulmonary infiltrates with invasive pulmonary aspergillus infection until neutrophil recovery occurs. Following marrow recovery in these patients, pulmonary infiltrates may become more apparent and progress to cavitation. Pharmacologic immunosuppression with corticosteroids may ablate the febrile response. HIV-infected patients often have atypical presentations of tuberculosis compared to non-HIV patients with earlier progression to active disease following infection and more frequent appearance of disease in the lower lobes. CMV infection typically has an insidious onset in all groups of compromised patients. Fever, mild dyspnea, and subtle pulmonary infiltrates may progress within a few days to arterial oxygen desaturation, hypoxemia, and respiratory failure. The absence of the usual signs of pulmonary infection in compromised hosts mandates the early and aggressive use of pulmonary diagnostic studies when infection is suspected. The initial pulmonary findings may be so subtle that pulmonary infection may not be suspected until a routine chest radiograph is obtained as part of a fever work-up. Noninfectious processes may complicate the diagnostic work-up in the compromised host. Disease entities, such as pulmonary embolus, cardiogenic and noncardiogenic pulmonary edema, and allergic and toxic pulmonary reactions, may obscure an infectious process. When pulmonary infection occurs in a compromised host, the outcome is death in 15 to 40 percent of patients.

MICROBIAL AGENTS OF PNEUMONIA IN COMPROMISED HOSTS

The opportunistic agents causing pulmonary infection in compromised hosts are usually not pathogens for immunocompetent individuals. Conditions such as HIV infection may leave the host susceptible to different agents at different stages of disease. As the loss of CD4 cells progresses, the patient with HIV infection will progress from normal immunity to susceptibility, to a succession of opportunists as immunity wanes. When the CD4 count falls below 500 cells/mm^3, bacterial pneumonias (pneumococcus and *Legionella*) and *M. tuberculosis* increase in frequency. Fungi and protozoal infections increase as the CD4 count falls below 200 cells. In the terminal phases of disease infection with *Mycobacterium avium* complex, higher bacteria and aspergillus become more common. Other conditions, such as congenital immune globulin deficiency states, cause more circumscribed defects with susceptibility to a single class of pathogen such as bacteria.

Bacteria

Bacterial pneumonias are most common in individuals with neutrophil defects such as patients with leukemia. In this setting, gram-negative organisms such as *Enterobacter* species and *Pseudomonas* are most prevalent. A broad range of bacterial pathogens have been reported in patients with HIV infection. *Pneumococcus, S. aureus, Streptococcus* species, higher bacteria, and *Rhodococcus equi* are among the gram-positive organisms causing bacterial pneumonia in HIV-infected patients. *Haemophilus influenzae* is the most common gram-negative bacterial pneumonia agent associated with HIV. Legionnaire's disease, a bacterial process requiring intact cell-mediated immunity for immune defense, has been implicated in nosocomial outbreaks among solid organ transplant recipients.

Viruses

The most important viral pulmonary pathogen in all compromised patient populations due to its prevalence and virulence is CMV. Mortality among allogeneic bone marrow transplant recipients is 90 percent despite antiviral therapy. CMV may be transferred from donor to recipient with solid organ allografts and through blood transfusion. Community acquired viral infections such as influenza, respiratory syncytial virus, and adenovirus are also important causes of morbidity. Defective cell-mediated immunity is essential to reactivation of latent herpesvirus infections such as CMV.

Fungi

The most common fungal infection in patients with defective cell-mediated immunity is *Cryptococcus neoformans.* Invasive pulmonary aspergillosis plagues neutropenic patients and is sometimes seen in patients with impaired cellular immunity as well. In geographic regions such as the southwestern United States and the Midwest, the regional mycoses *Histoplasma capsulatum* and *Coccidioides immitis* are prevalent among organ transplant recipients and HIV-infected persons. Histoplasmosis, coccidioidomycosis, and cryptococcosis are inhaled and may establish a subclinical pulmonary infection before disseminating. Clinical pulmonary disease may occur as well.

Protozoa

The natural reservoir of *P. carinii* is not known. Impairment of T-cell function and pharmacologic steroid doses are two important factors in the development of pneumonia with this agent, which is considered by some to be a fungal organism. Childhood leukemics, HIV-infected patients, patients on corticosteroids, and solid organ transplant recipients are more often affected by this agent. Toxoplasmosis is rarely implicated in pulmonary infection. When it does occur, it is seen in patients with T-lymphocyte dysfunction such as heart transplant recipients.

Mycobacteria

Impaired cell-mediated immunity greatly increases the risk for mycobacterial infection. The resurgent epidemic of tuberculosis is fueled by conditions such as poverty, homelessness, and HIV infection. The largest numbers of new cases of tuberculosis are occurring in regions of high HIV prevalence. Nontuberculosis mycobacterial infections (*Mycobacterium avium* complex, rapid growers, and others) may disseminate in patients with impaired cellular immunity.

DIAGNOSIS

Relying on a clinical impression when pulmonary infection occurs in the immunocompromised patient is treacherous due to the variety of intercurrent illnesses and infectious and noninfectious processes, which can obscure the true diagnosis. Diagnostic material obtained from deep in the respiratory tract must be obtained expeditiously in most cases to secure the diagnosis. The simultaneous occurrence of more than one disease process in the same organ system, often times duel infections, is commonplace among compromised hosts.

The most readily available tool for diagnosis of pulmonary infection is the microscopic examination of expectorated sputum. Sputum Gram stain and culture lack specificity in all hosts as collection through the colonized upper airway may contaminate the specimen. The presence of > 25 neutrophils per high powered microscope field or < 10 epithelial cells per field indicates a satisfactory specimen. Sputum examination is most useful for the diagnosis of bacterial processes and PCP in HIV-infected individuals. Evidence of tissue invasion is required for the diagnosis of pulmonary fungal infections; therefore, microscopic examination of sputum is of little utility. Sputum cultures from a compromised host which repeatedly yield a fungal organism should be strongly suspected to represent evidence of an invasive fungal infection. Similarly, direct sputum examination is of little use in the diagnosis of respiratory viral infection. Viral cultures and immunofluorescence staining of nasopharyngeal aspirates obtained early in the course of an illness are sensitive and specific for the diagnosis of community-acquired viral infections (Influenza A and B, respiratory syncytial virus, parainfluenza, adenovirus).

In the setting of HIV infection, induced sputum examination with methenamine silver staining has a sensitivity of > 80 percent, a rate comparable to bronchoscopy with bronchoalveolar lavage. Sputum induction and staining for pneumocystis and acid-fast organisms is well established as the initial diagnostic step in mild to moderately ill HIV-infected patients. The utility of sputum induction to diagnose PCP in non–HIV-infected patients is unknown.

Severity of disease, availability of sputum, pace of the pneumonia, and knowledge of the host's immune defect will guide the clinician in judging the need for more invasive diagnostic studies. Transtracheal aspirates (TTA) effectively bypass the colonized upper airway and yield reliable deep respiratory cultures free of upper airway contamination. TTA is rarely considered a diagnostic option with the widespread availability of bronchoscopy. In experienced hands, TTA has a complication rate lower than that of bronchoscopy with biopsy. Skinny needle biopsy of peripheral pulmonary lesions under fluoroscopic guidance is an acceptable alternative to open lung biopsy in nonemergent situations. Bronchoscopy with alveolar lavage has supplanted TTA as a diagnostic intervention because of the low risk associated with the procedure and comparable diagnostic yields. TTA and skinny needle procedures are less useful than bronchoscopy for the diagnosis of diffuse pulmonary processes. In the setting of diffuse infiltrates, the diagnostic yield of bronchoscopy is 80 to 95 percent. Bronchoscopy is less effective as a diagnostic tool in the evaluation of bacterial pneumonia because of contamination of the bronchoscope in the upper airway. Protected brush specimens obtained through the bronchoscope are now achieving diagnostic yields for bacterial pneumonia similar to those of TTA.

The traditional "gold standard" for the diagnosis of pulmonary infiltrates in compromised patients has been open lung biopsy because of its utility in obtaining large pieces of tissue and the potential for control of complications such as bleeding. In experienced hands, thoracoscopic biopsy can serve the same function with much less morbidity. Open lung biopsy and thoracoscopic biopsy are particularly rewarding in diffuse processes where bronchoscopy with lavage has not been diagnostic. Mortality related to open lung biopsy and thoracoscopy are virtually zero in clinics which perform these procedures routinely, i.e., when local experience is high. In most instances, bronchoscopy is undertaken as an intermediate diagnostic step before moving to open lung biopsy or thoracoscopic biopsy.

The radiographic appearance of pneumonia is considered in detail elsewhere. Diffuse infiltrates are more likely to be caused by protozoal or viral infections, whereas patchy may be mycobacterial or fungal. Radiographic appearance is not a specific diagnostic tool in this setting, and should be used to direct further diagnostic studies.

PREVENTION OF PNEUMONIA

Table 46-2 lists methods used to prevent pneumonia. Immunization with pneumococcal and influenza vaccine should be standard practice for compromised hosts. Family members as well as the immunodeficient patient should be encouraged to receive influenza vaccine. The use of chemoprophylaxis with co-trimoxazole for the prevention of PCP is well established among children with leukemia, solid organ transplant recipients, and HIV-infected persons, as is the use of immune globulin infusions for hypogammaglobulinemics.

ANTIMICROBIAL THERAPY

The choice of agents for initial antimicrobial therapy for pneumonia in the compromised host is made after examination of the patient, chest radiograph, and sputum Gram stain, and with the knowledge

TABLE 46-2 Measures to Prevent Pneumonia in Compromised Host

Hand washing
Reverse isolation
Protected environments
Antibacterial prophylaxis for neutropenic patients
Prophylaxis against *Pneumocystis carinii* pneumonia for patients with
cell-mediated immune defects
Vaccination
  Influenza
  Pneumococcal vaccine

SOURCE: Adapted from Henderson DK: Prevention of respiratory infection in immunocompromised patients, pp 428–429, in Shelhamer JH, Moderator, Respiratory disease in the immunocompromised patient. Ann Intern Med 117:415–431, 1992.

of the defect in host immunity. Antimicrobials should be initiated while decisions about diagnostic studies are being formulated. The pace of the illness should be considered when determining the span of initial therapy. The sudden onset of respiratory symptoms is more suggestive of a bacterial process, particularly when the chest radiograph reveals a lobar or segmental infiltrate. Neutropenic hosts warrant empirical therapy using agents with broad coverage for gram-positive and gram-negative organisms. A broad-spectrum β-lactam, in combination with an aminoglycoside, is appropriate therapy for the neutropenic patient. Patients with cell-mediated immune defects, such as organ transplant recipients, can be managed effectively at the outset using co-trimoxazole while undergoing further diagnostic studies. Fulminant disease or associated findings suggestive of CMV infection (recent seroconversion, relative neutropenia, or thrombocytopenia) necessitates empirical antifungal and antiviral therapy. Table 46-3 offers guidelines for initial therapy of pneumonia in the compromised host while diagnostic studies are being performed.

SUMMARY

Pneumonia is a common cause of morbidity and mortality in immunocompromised patients. More than one pathogen per episode is not uncommon. Among HIV-infected persons, bacterial pneumonias are now being seen commonly, whereas pneumocystis is readily prevented by chemoprophylaxis. Aggressive diagnostic evaluation is imperative to limit the toxicity of empirical antimicrobial therapy and tailor the regimen to the specific pathogen. A knowledge of the host's immune defect is important in directing the work-up and choice of initial therapy.

TABLE 46-3 Initial Therapy of Pneumonia in Immunocompromised Host

Clinical Setting	Antimicrobial Agent
A. Febrile Neutropenic (gram-negative, staphylococcus fungi)	β-Lactam + Aminoglycoside*
— No response	Add amphotericin
— Patchy/diffuse infiltrate	β-Lactam + Aminoglycoside + Add amphotericin B
B. Solid Organ Transplant Interstitial process (PCP, CMV)	Co-trimoxazole + Ganciclovir
Lobar infiltrate (Pneumococcus, *H. influenzae,* staphylococcus)	Co-trimoxazole
Diffuse process (PCP, viruses, fungi)	Co-trimoxazole + Ganciclovir + Amphotericin B
C. Hypogammaglobulinemic (Bacterial processes)	Erythromycin or β-Lactam
D. HIV Infection Interstitial process (PCP, virus)	Co-trimoxazole or Pentamidine
Lobar infiltrate —Purulent sputum (Bacterial)	Erythromycin or Co-trimoxazole
Nosocomial pneumonia (Resistant gram-neg., staph)	β-Lactam + Aminoglycoside*
E. Bone Marrow Transplant	
Allogeneic Interstitial process	Ganciclovir + Immune globulin (IVIG)
Patchy/diffuse	Ganciclovir + IVIG + Amphotericin B + β-Lactam + Aminoglycoside

* Choice of β-lactam and aminoglycoside should be based on institutional susceptibility profiles.

BIBLIOGRAPHY

For a more detailed discussion, see Rubin RH: Pneumonia in the immuno-compromised host, in Fishman AP (ed), *Pulmonary Diseases and Disorders,* 2d ed. New York, McGraw-Hill, 1988, pp 1745–1760.

Cohn DL: Bacterial pneumonia in the HIV infected patient. Infect Dis Clin North Am 5:485–507, 1991.

Fishman JA: *Pneumocystis carinii* pneumonia, in Fishman AP (ed), *Update: Pulmonary Diseases and Disorders.* New York, McGraw-Hill, 1992, pp 263–286.

Janzen DL, Adler BD, Padley SP, Muller NL: Diagnostic success of bronchoscopic biopsy in immunocompromised patients with acute pulmonary disease: Predictive value of disease distribution as shown on CT. Am J Roentgenol 160:21–24, 1993.

McCabe RE: Diagnosis of pulmonary infections in immunocompromised patients. Med North Am 72:1067–1089, 1988.

1993 Revised Classification System for HIV Infection. MMWR 41:17, 1992.

Rossman MD: The resurgence of tuberculosis and nontuberculosis mycobacteria, in Fishman AP (ed), *Update: Pulmonary Diseases and Disorders.* New York, McGraw-Hill, 1992, pp 287–297.

Shelhamer JH, Toews GB, Masur H, Suffredini AF, Pizzo PA, Walsh TJ, et al: Respiratory disease in the immunosuppressed patient. Ann Intern Med 117:415–431, 1992.

Jay Kostman

This chapter focuses on several microorganisms which are unusual, but important, causes of pneumonia.

NEISSERIA MENINGITIDIS

The meningococcus is a gram-negative diplococcus surrounded by a polysaccharide capsule, the basis for the system used for typing the organism. It is a fastidious organism, requiring enriched media, an atmosphere of 5% to 10% carbon dioxide, a moist environment, and temperatures of 35°C to 37°C for optimal growth.

Epidemiology

In nonepidemic periods, 10 to 20 percent of the population may be nasopharyngeal carriers of the organism at one time or another. The organism is probably transmitted from carrier to carrier by the respiratory route. Close contact, as in the case of military service or boarding schools, can cause rapid development of new carriers.

Meningococcal pneumonia was common during the influenza pandemic of 1918–1919. In more recent times, serogroups Y and W-135 have been associated with both outbreaks and nosocomial disease. *N. meningitidis* is the responsible pathogen in 3 to 5 percent of all community-acquired pneumonias.

Clinical Manifestations

Little distinguishes the presentation of meningococcal pneumonia from that of pneumococcal pneumonia. Pharyngitis is often an early complaint with meningococcus. Fever, chills, and a productive cough with pleuritic chest pain are common complaints. Systemic complications, such as sepsis, meningitis, and diffuse intravascular coagulation, are unusual. Local pulmonary complications, such as abscess formation and necrosis, occasionally occur. A large number of cases of pneumonia in a closed setting should raise suspicion of meningococcal pneumonia.

The radiologic findings in meningococcal pneumonia are also nonspecific. However, more than one lobe is involved in 40 percent of the cases, particularly the right middle and lower lobes.

Diagnosis and Treatment

Gram stain of a sputum specimen is the initial step in diagnosis of meningococcal pneumonia. A predominance of the characteristic gram-negative diplococci should prompt culture on an enriched medium, e.g., Thayer-Martin agar. Blood and cerebrospinal fluid cultures are rarely positive in meningococcal pneumonia.

Penicillin, in doses of 2 to 4 million units per day, is effective therapy for most patients with meningococcal pneumonia. In the penicillin-allergic patient, a third-generation cephalosporin or chloramphenicol can be substituted.

Because the spread of meningococci is primarily via the respiratory route, patients suspected of having meningococcal pneumonia should be placed in respiratory isolation. In general, isolation precautions suffice to protect hospital personnel unless exposure is heavy or intimate, e.g., mouth-to-mouth resuscitation. In the case of heavy or intimate exposure, personnel should receive chemoprophylaxis with rifampin, 600 mg every 12 h for 2 days.

PASTEURELLA MULTOCIDA

Epidemiology

P. multocida is an aerobic gram-negative coccobacillus. The organism has been recovered from the respiratory tracts of many domestic and wild mammals and birds, e.g., in 50 to 70 percent of cats and 12 to 66 percent of dogs. Most human infections are caused by animal bites, but infections have also been reported in pet owners, animal handlers, or other persons with frequent animal contact. In 5 to 15 percent of *Pasteurella* infections, there is no history of animal contact.

Clinical Manifestations, Diagnosis, and Treatment

Respiratory infections with *P. multocida* most often occur in patients with preexisting chronic obstructive pulmonary disease. The usual presentation is as a worsening of respiratory function. Alternatively, the disease may be manifest as an acute bacterial pneumonia, indistinguishable from pneumococcal pneumonia. Radiographically, the pneumonia characteristically spares the upper lobes. Diagnosis is made by culturing the organism from sputum or blood on conventional media.

Penicillin is considered the drug of choice for *Pasteurella* infections; third-generation cephalosporins, tetracyclines, or chloramphenicol may be used in the penicillin-allergic patient.

TULAREMIA

Tularemia is a disease characterized by high fevers and severe constitutional symptoms that is caused by *Francisella tularensis,* a gram-negative coccobacillus.

Epidemiology

F. tularensis is distributed throughout the Northern hemisphere in wild mammals, domestic animals, and arthropods. The most important vectors of the disease in the United States are rabbits, hares, and ticks. The seasonality of the disease depends on the geographic location. Tick-related disease predominates in the spring and summer months, whereas disease related to animal trapping are more likely to occur in the colder months.

Clinical Manifestations

The two most common forms of tularemia that have pleuropulmonary manifestations are the ulceroglandular and typhoidal syndromes. The ulceroglandular form, which makes up 75 to 85 percent of cases, has an ulcerated skin lesion and painful regional lymphadenopathy as its cardinal features. The typhoidal form (5 to 15 percent of cases) presents with fever, weight loss, and prostration without lymphadenopathy.

Overall, pneumonia is seen in about 50 percent of cases of typhoidal tularemia and 10 to 15 percent of ulceroglandular cases. The clinical presentation is one of a nonproductive cough, few physical findings in the lung, and patchy infiltrates on chest radiograph. In some patients, abnormalities can be detected on chest radiograph that are not detected clinically.

The organism usually arrives in the lung following a bacteremia and entrapment in the reticuloendothelial cells. Pathologically, there may be multiple necrotizing granulomas with alveolar destruction. Pneumonia may also result following inhalation of the organism, presenting with dry cough, fever, headache, and malaise.

Diagnosis and Treatment

The diagnosis of tularemia should be considered in any patient with pneumonia associated with painful lymphadenopathy, or with animal exposure in a region endemic for *F. tularensis.* The organism is rarely seen in Gram stains of sputum, pleural fluid, or suppurating lymph nodes. Most laboratories are reluctant to attempt to culture the organism because of the danger of creating infectious aerosols in the laboratory. The diagnosis is usually made by serologic methods. Fifty to 70 percent of patients will have positive agglutination titers within 2 weeks of illness. A 4-fold rise in titer or a single titer of > 1:160 is evidence of infection.

Streptomycin is the drug of choice for the treatment of tularemia, in a daily intramuscular dose of 15 to 20 mg/kg for 7 to 14 days. Clinical relapses are more common with tetracyclines or chloramphenicol. The overall mortality has decreased from 10 percent to 1 to 3 percent with adequate antimicrobial therapy.

The risk of tularemia can be minimized by using gloves when skinning or eviscerating animals and avoiding tick-infested areas if possible.

MELIODOSIS (PNEUMONIA CAUSED BY *PSEUDOMONAS PSEUDOMALLEI*)

Meliodosis is caused by *P. pseudomallei,* a small gram-negative rod that is a natural saprophyte endemic in Southeast Asia.

Epidemiology

P. pseudomallei can be isolated from soil, stagnant water, rice paddies, and produce in endemic areas. Human beings generally acquire disease via soil contamination of skin abrasions. Human-to-human transmission rarely occurs. Clinically recognized cases remain rare in this country, although serologic tests show evidence of subclinical infection in roughly 225,000 United States citizens who served in Vietnam. These individuals form a reservoir of latent disease that has the potential for reactivation years later. In troops returning to the United States, the prevalence of positive titers was related to the presence and extent of wounds.

Clinical Manifestations

The incubation period following exposure is as short as 2 to 3 days. The acute manifestations of meliodosis include cutaneous suppurative lesions, pneumonia, or septicemia. The acute pneumonia is characterized by fever, usually a nonproductive cough, tachypnea, and chest pain. There is usually upper lobe involvement, and cavitation is frequent. Patients who have the septicemic form complicating pneumonia have a very high mortality rate, often unaffected by therapy. The acute form of the disease is rarely seen in this country.

After leaving an area that is endemic for meliodosis, patients may develop subacute or chronic presentations of pulmonary disease, years after the initial exposure. This stage of disease can resemble tuberculosis both clinically and radiographically; significant weight loss, fever, chills, cough, and upper lobe cavitary infiltrates are characteristic. Skin manifestations are unusual during this stage. Other organs, including the brain, liver, joints, heart, and bones, may also be involved.

Diagnosis and Treatment

Meliodosis should be considered in the differential diagnosis of a febrile patient who has been in an area endemic for *P. pseudomallei,* particularly if the presentation includes respiratory failure, pustular skin lesions, or a radiographic appearance suggestive of tuberculosis without laboratory confirmation of tuberculosis. Sputum or other exudative material often contains poorly staining, gram-negative bacilli, with bipolar staining characteristics. The organism grows readily on most standard bacteriologic media. In the chronic forms of the disease, tissue biopsy may be necessary to make the diagnosis. Serologic methods also exist for making the diagnosis, although up to one third of culture-positive patients may have negative serologies at the time of diagnosis.

In patients with chronic disease who are not toxic, tetracycline, chloramphenicol, or trimethoprim-sulfamethoxazole have been used for 2 to 5 months. In patients who are more acutely ill, two drugs have been combined for the first month, followed by a prolonged course of trimethoprim-sulfamethoxazole. Surgical drainage of cavitary lesions is sometimes required. Imipenem can be used for patients with isolates resistant to trimethoprim-sulfamethoxazole. Patients with the more chronic forms of disease have a very good response rate with prolonged courses of antibiotics.

PULMONARY INFECTION WITH *STRONGYLOIDES STERCORALIS*

S. stercoralis infects human beings usually through skin contact with soil contaminated with filariform larvae. However, individuals may also be infected by the "autoinfection" cycle, whereby the larvae can transform into infective organisms during their passage with feces and reinfect either through the perianal region or the large intestine. The larvae then pass hematogenously to the lungs, into the alveolar spaces, up to the glottis, and then are swallowed into the small intestine. In temperate climates, the highest incidence of *S. stercoralis* infection is in institutions.

Clinical Manifestations

In immunocompetent patients, pulmonary disease due to *S. stercoralis* is unusual. However, in patients with abnormalities of cell-mediate immunity, e.g., related to lymphomas or leukemias, treatment with corticosteroids, or the acquired immunodeficiency syndrome, the hyperinfection syndrome may develop. In this setting, the transformation to infective larvae occurs within the host; the organisms subsequently invade the intestinal wall and widely disseminate to multiple organs including the lungs. This invasion is manifested by asthma, pulmonary infiltrates, and often by secondary infection with enteric gram-negative rods. The eosinophilia that is present in most immunocompetent patients with *Strongyloides* infection can be absent in the immunocompromised host.

Diagnosis and Treatment

In the hyperinfection syndrome, the mortality approaches 70 to 80 percent, despite treatment. Early diagnosis, by identification of larvae in stools, duodenal aspirates, or bronchial washings can be lifesaving if treatment with thiabendazole, 25 mg/kg twice daily, is initiated and continued for 2 to 3 weeks. Of utmost importance, patients who have a past history of exposure or potential exposure to *S. stercoralis* should be examined and treated before undergoing any immunosuppressive therapy.

BIBLIOGRAPHY

For a more detailed discussion, see Weinberg AN: Unusual bacterial pneumonias, in Fishman AP (ed), *Pulmonary Diseases and Disorders,* 2d ed. New York, McGraw-Hill, 1988, pp 1517–1534.

Agostini C, Trentin L, Zambello R, Semenzato G: HIV-1 and the lung. Am Rev Respir Dis 147:1038–1049, 1993.

Coulter C, Walker DG, Gunsberg M, Brown IG, Bligh JF, Prociv P: Successful treatment of disseminated strongyloidiasis. Med J Aust 157:331–332, 1992.

Mahmoud AAF: Helminthic diseases of the lungs, in Fishman AP (ed), *Pulmonary Diseases and Disorders,* 2d ed. New York, McGraw-Hill, 1988, pp 1719–1733.

Morris JT, McAllister CK: Bacteremia due to *Pasteurella multocida.* South Med J 85:442–443, 1992.

Weinberg AN: Respiratory infections transmitted from animals. Infect Dis Clin North Am 5:649–661, 1991.

Michael Beers

DEFINITION

The term *acute respiratory failure* (ARF) is used clinically to indicate a disease or disorder of the respiratory apparatus, fairly recent in onset, which has resulted in a level or pattern of external gas exchange that is inadequate for the metabolic needs of the body. This deficiency is reflected in arterial hypoxemia, hypercapnia, and (respiratory) acidosis. If the initiating mechanism is not arrested or reversed, the abnormalities in the blood gases are apt to progress to intolerable levels.

There is no precise level of arterial P_{O_2} or P_{CO_2} that defines ARF. However, an arterial $P_{O_2} < 50$ to 60 mmHg can be life threatening because further impairment of gas exchange can cause a drop in arterial P_{O_2} to levels that would compromise oxygen delivery to vital organs. A somewhat different threat is posed by an abrupt increase in arterial P_{CO_2} to about 50 mmHg or greater (and the accompanying acidosis); this acute hypercapnia and respiratory acidosis runs the risk of mental disturbances and depressed sensorium that may culminate in coma. To some extent, the effects of acute hypercapnia and of acute hypoxemia overlap. For example, both may severely compromise mental performance.

ETIOLOGY

With respect to etiology, the respiratory apparatus can be viewed as consisting of two components: (1) a *pump*, consisting of the entire ventilatory apparatus except for the pulmonary parenchyma, i.e., the respiratory centers in the brain and brain stem, the chest wall and respiratory muscles, and the conducting airways; and (2) a *gas exchanger*, the pulmonary parenchyma. This categorization enables distinction between two types of respiratory failure: (1) *pump failure,* characterized by CO_2 retention (hypercapnic respiratory failure); (2) *lung failure,* characterized by arterial hypoxemia (hypoxemic respiratory failure). The major causes of ARF are sorted into those two categories in Table 48-1.

PATHOPHYSIOLOGY

Underlying each clinical disorder listed in Table 48-1 is one or more of four pathogenetic mechanisms: alveolar hypoventilation, ventilation-perfusion ($\dot{V}/\dot{Q}$) mismatch, shunt, and diffusion abnormality (Table 48-2).

TABLE 48-1 Respiratory Disorders Associated with Acute Respiratory Failure

Lung failure (hypoxemic respiratory failure)
  Adult respiratory distress syndrome
  Respiratory distress syndrome of the newborn
  Cardiogenic (hemodynamic) pulmonary edema
  End-stage fibrotic lung disease
  Massive pulmonary thromboembolism
  Pneumonia

Pump failure (hypercapnic respiratory failure)
  Neuromuscular disease
    Guillain-Barré syndrome
    Myasthenia gravis
    Amyotrophic lateral sclerosis
    Cervical quadriplegia
    Botulism
    Poliomyelitis
    Bilateral diaphragmatic paralysis (including postcardioplegia)
    Hereditary myopathies
    Multiple sclerosis
    Collagen vascular disease (polymyositis)
  Central nervous disorders
    Drug overdose
    Head trauma
    Hypothyroidism
    Brain-stem infarction/neoplasm
  Disorders of the chest bellows
    Kyphoscoliosis
    Flail chest
    Tension pneumothorax
    Restrictive pleuritis
  Airway obstruction
    Asthma
    Chronic bronchitis and emphysema
    Anaphylaxis
    Cystic fibrosis
  Upper airway obstruction
    Epiglottitis
    Foreign body

PUMP FAILURE: HYPERCAPNIC RESPIRATORY FAILURE

Hypercapnia due to respiratory failure can arise in one of two ways: 1) alveolar hypoventilation secondary to a subnormal minute ventilation; and 2) $(\dot{V}/\dot{Q})$ mismatch.

TABLE 48-2 Pathogenetic Mechanisms in Acute Respiratory Failure

Mechanism	Type of failure	Feature
Global alveolar hypoventilation	Pump	Hypercapnia
Ventilation-perfusion mismatch	Pump and/or lung	Hypercapnia and/or hypoxemia
Shunt	Lung	Hypoxemia
Diffusion abnormality	Lung	Hypoxemia

In hypercapnia that originates in a subnormal minute ventilation, the alveolar and arterial P_{CO_2} is paralleled by a decrease in alveolar and arterial P_{O_2} in accord with the alveolar air equation:

$$P_{A_{O_2}} = P_{I_{O_2}} - P_{a_{CO_2}}/ R$$

where, $P_{A_{O_2}}$ = alveolar P_{O_2}, mmHg; $P_{I_{O_2}}$ = inspiratory P_{O_2}, mmHg; $P_{a_{CO_2}}$ = arterial P_{CO_2}, mmHg; and R = respiratory exchange ratio.

The major diagnostic feature of hypercapnic respiratory failure secondary to a subnormal minute and alveolar hypoventilation (global alveolar hypoventilation) is that *the normal alveolar-arterial difference in* P_{O_2} (the A-a O_2 gradient) is preserved.

There are many causes of alveolar hypoventilation due to subnormal minute ventilation ($\dot{V}_E$): central nervous system (CNS) depression, e.g., drugs, head trauma, or cerebrovascular accident; neuromuscular disorders, e.g., myasthenia gravis or Guillain-Barré syndrome; disorders of the chest bellows, e.g., traumatic flail chest; fatigue of the respiratory muscles, e.g., inordinate work of breathing during an acute exacerbation of chronic obstructive airways disease.

This preservation of the A-a O_2 gradient distinguishes the hypercapnia of global underventilation from that of $\dot{V}/\dot{Q}$ mismatch. $\dot{V}/\dot{Q}$ mismatch can cause hypercapnia by increasing the area that is ventilated but not perfused, i.e., by increasing the physiologic dead space. Such striking $\dot{V}/\dot{Q}$ abnormalities are apt to occur during an exacerbation of chronic obstructive airways disease (asthma, emphysema, and chronic bronchitis). The increase in dead space ventilation (and the resulting state of net [relative] alveolar hypoventilation) often occurs in the face of an increase in total minute ventilation ($\dot{V}_E$). Hypoxemia accompanies the hypercapnia. A cardinal feature, in contrast to the global alveolar hypoventilation that results from pump failure, is that the alveolar-arterial ΔP_{O_2} (the A-a O_2 gradient) widens due to $\dot{V}/\dot{Q}$ inequality.

LUNG FAILURE: HYPOXEMIC RESPIRATORY FAILURE

Hypoxemic respiratory failure is characterized by arterial hypoxemia and a markedly widened A-a O_2 gradient, usually associated with a normal or low arterial Pco_2. Three major mechanisms, singly or in concert, can contribute to hypoxemic respiratory failure: (1) *ventilation-perfusion ($\dot{V}/\dot{Q}$) mismatch;* (2) perfusion of nonventilated alveoli, i.e., the equivalent of a venoarterial shunt; and (3) diffusion limitation.

Ventilation-perfusion ($\dot{V}/\dot{Q}$) mismatch In addition to the increase in dead space ventilation that can result from $\dot{V}/\dot{Q}$, abnormalities during an exacerbation of chronic obstructive airways disease (see above), alveoli that are underventilated with respect to alveolar blood flow also occur in areas of *partial* atelectasis; the tendency to *partial* atelectasis is exaggerated by pneumothorax or pulmonary embolus. Arterial hypoxemia due to hypoventilated alveoli can usually be corrected with small increases in inspired oxygen.

Shunt (right to left) This designation refers to blood flow through nonventilated parts of the lung. Shunting (blood flow through nonventilated alveoli) can occur in pneumonia, congestive heart failure, and in the adult respiratory distress syndrome (ARDS). Clinically, shunt is distinguished from $\dot{V}/\dot{Q}$ mismatch by the failure of breathing of O_2-enriched air to relieve appreciably the arterial hypoxemia. The shunt can be quantified by applying a venous-admixture formula to blood-gas values obtained during 100% O_2 breathing.

Diffusion limitation is often a contributing, but rarely the predominant, factor in ARF.

CLINICAL MANIFESTATIONS

The signs and symptoms of ARF are usually not subtle but can often be misinterpreted.

Nonspecific Manifestations

The patient with impending ARF may simply look fatigued. Alternatively, the clinical picture can simulate primary disorders of organ systems other than the respiratory system. For example, arterial hypoxemia can manifest itself by abnormal mentation. Alternatively, it may elicit tachycardia and hypotension. Tachypnea is sometimes the striking feature. Conversely, reliance on cyanosis as a manifestation of ARF can be misleading because it only occurs when arterial hypoxemia is severe ($Po_2 < 40$ mmHg in a patient in whom the hemoglobin concentration is near normal).

Hypercapnia can also lead to misleading clinical manifestations in several different ways: (1) CNS disturbances, ranging from headache to narcosis, psychosis, lethargy, or even coma; (2) neuromuscular dysfunction manifested by muscle weakness, hyporeflexia, asterixis, tremor, or seizures; and (3) cardiovascular disturbances, e.g., tachycardia, hypertension and diaphoresis. Respiratory acidosis can compound the situation by causing cardiac dysrhythmias, hemodynamic instability, or altered mental function.

Specific Manifestations

In contrast to the nonspecific manifestations, certain clinical signs and symptoms direct attention to the respiratory system. For example, the patient with severe respiratory failure may be in obvious respiratory distress with poor air movement, use of the accessory muscles of breathing, paradoxical motion of the diaphragm, or an exaggerated breathing pattern (Kussmaul respirations). Also, the patient may manifest wheezing (either upper or lower airway), rales, lobar consolidation, cardiac gallops or murmurs (right or left sided), distended neck veins, or peripheral edema. Although these signs and symptoms may be telltale, the hallmark of ARF is the composition of the arterial blood, i.e., arterial hypoxemia or hypercapnia or both (Table 48-2).

Diagnostic Tests

Certain diagnostic studies can be helpful in defining the etiology of the ARF or in assisting with management.

General diagnostic measures Chest radiography is invaluable in demonstrating the nature and course of the disease and sometimes the etiology. Sputum examination, by Gram stain and culture, is indispensible for uncovering the etiology of a respiratory infection. The electrocardiogram can provide evidence of myocardial ischemia, arrhythmias, or pericardial disease as contributing factors. A drug/toxin screen is sometimes helpful in disclosing the etiology of unexplained acute hypercarbic respiratory failure.

Pulmonary function testing Certain bedside tests can be useful in quantifying the severity of respiratory dysfunction and in following the course of the illness. The choice of tests depends, in large part, on the underlying disease process. For example, in obstructive airways disease, flow rates (either peak expiratory flow or FEV_1), can be helpful. In neuromuscular disease, e.g., myasthenia gravis, forced vital capacity (FVC), maximum inspiratory pressure (MIP), and maximum expiratory pressure (MEP) can help to track the course of the illness.

MANAGEMENT

The management of ARF is both supportive and specific.

Supportive Interventions

In addition to supportive measures, certain measures are directed at improving gas exchange: (1) Establish and ensure an adequate airway. (2) Correct respiratory acidosis. Hypercapnia may be corrected by either increasing CO_2 output or decreasing CO_2 production. An increase in CO_2 output can be accomplished by increasing alveolar ventilation, e.g., by improving respiratory muscle function or mechanical ventilation; a decrease in CO_2 production can be accomplished by suppressing fever, treating infection and by decreasing carbohydrate intake. (3) Improve oxygenation. Oxygen therapy is directed at establishing tolerable levels of arterial oxygenation (arterial $Po_2 > 50$ to 60 mmHg or arterial saturations $> 90\%$) while avoiding O_2 toxicity. The administration of supplemental oxygen is discussed below. (4) Mechanical ventilation. Intubation via the oral or nasal route and mechanical ventilation are generally instituted when more conservative modalities prove ineffective and signs appear of respiratory muscle fatigue, i.e., unexplained increase in respiratory frequency, discoordinated breathing pattern, paradoxical movements of abdomen during breathing. (5) Treat the underlying disease process.

Specific Therapies

Successful management of ARF depends heavily on attention to the underlying pulmonary disorder and the pathogenetic mechanisms. Among the common underlying disorders are chronic obstructive pulmonary disease (COPD), cardiogenic pulmonary edema, ARDS, and neuromuscular diseases.

Chronic obstructive pulmonary disease (chronic obstructive airways disease, chronic bronchitis, and emphysema) The cardinal steps in the management of ARF in patients with these diseases are (1) arrest and reversal of the initiating mechanisms, e.g., infection or bronchospasm; (2) supportive measures, e.g., careful hydration, aminophylline administered intravenously, bronchodilators administered by inhalation, antibiotics, and corticosteroids; and (3) correction of hypoxemia by circumspect oxygen therapy.

Excessively enriched oxygen breathing mixtures can cause serious complications by abolishing the hypoxic stimulus to breathing, thereby worsening the hypercapnia and leading to respiratory arrest. By "controlled O_2 therapy," e.g., delivering 24% to 35% oxygen via a Venturi mask *(not via nasal canulae)*, arterial hypoxemia can generally be at least partially relieved. The goal is an arterial $Po_2 >$

50 while avoiding CO_2 retention; (4) correction of hypercapnia and acidosis.

The measures noted above often suffice to tide the patient over the early phase and to arrest the evolution of ARF. But, if the above measures fail, the patient must be intubated and mechanically ventilated to substitute for the fatigued and failing respiratory pump.

Cardiogenic pulmonary edema The cause of this syndrome is acute left ventricular failure. Management requires the delivery of supplemental oxygen while alleviating the underlying cardiac disorder. As a rule, intubation and assisted ventilation can be avoided by administering oxygen-rich inspired air and by implementing an effective cardiotonic regimen, e.g., diuretics, morphine, nitrates, and occasionally by rotating tourniquets. However, if arterial hypoxemia intensifies and CO_2 retention becomes evident, intubation and mechanical ventilation becomes necessary.

Adult respiratory distress syndrome ARDS is a syndrome of *acute* respiratory failure in which pulmonary edema caused by leaky pulmonary microvessels, is a major feature. The pulmonary pathology is a mixture of edema, atelectasis, and inflammation. The syndrome is manifested by bilateral pulmonary infiltrates on the chest radiograph, stiff lungs (a marked reduction in pulmonary compliance), and severe arterial hypoxemia that is refractory to the administration of oxygen-enriched inspired air (arterial Po_2 < 50 to 60 mmHg despite a concentration of O_2 in inspired air > 60%). Neither left heart failure nor volume overload is responsible for initiating the pulmonary edema.

Management is supportive while attempting to deal with the mechanism(s) that injured the pulmonary microvessels. High levels of supportive care in an intensive-care unit are required, including intubation, mechanical ventilation, and nutritional support. Several weeks to months may be required for the lungs to recover.

Neuromuscular respiratory failure In patients with ARF complicating neuromuscular disease, two clinical problems usually have to be addressed: (1) the neurologic diagnosis; and (2) the decision of when to intubate the patient with neurologic disease who is en route to ARF. With respect to the proper time for intubation and mechanical ventilation, bedside pulmonary function tests are extremely useful. Intubation is recommended when the forced vital capacity falls below two times the predicted tidal volume or the mean inspiratory pressure is < 20 cmH$_2$O.

The two most common neuromuscular disorders complicated by ARF are acute inflammatory polyneuropathy (the Guillain-Barré syndrome) and myasthenia gravis. In the Guillain-Barré syndrome, plasmapheresis begun early in the course of the disease decreases the duration of the need for mechanical ventilation; corticosteroids are of questionable benefit. The prognosis for this disease is excellent (85 percent functional recovery). In myasthenia gravis, corticosteroids (high dose) are the mainstay of therapy. In addition, it is important to avoid use of certain drugs known to exacerbate the crisis, e.g., the aminoglycosides, tetracycline, quinidine, procainamide, lidocaine, and Dilantin. Anticholinesterases (pyridostigmine) are ineffective in the acute stage but should be instituted during recovery.

NATURAL HISTORY AND PROGNOSIS

The natural history of ARF depends heavily on the underlying etiology and on minimizing complications during management. The in-hospital mortality from a single episode of ARF that requires mechanical ventilation can range from 10 to 40 percent (for COPD), to 50 percent (for ARDS), and up to 90 percent (for leukemia).

BIBLIOGRAPHY

For a more detailed discussion, see Hudson LD: Acute respiratory failure-overview, in Fishman AP (ed), *Pulmonary Diseases and Disorders,* 2d edition, New York, McGraw-Hill, 1988, pp 2189–2198.

Grippi MA, Fishman AP: Respiratory failure in structural and neuromuscular disorders involving the chest bellows, in Fishman AP (ed), *Pulmonary Diseases and Disorders,* 2d ed. New York, McGraw-Hill, 1988, pp 2299–2314.

Jeffrey AA, Warren PM, Flenley DC: Acute hypercapnic respiratory failure in patients with chronic obstructive lung disease: Risk factors and use of guidelines for management. Thorax 47:34–40, 1992.

Marini JJ: Recent advances in mechanical ventilation, in Fishman AP (ed), *Update: Pulmonary Diseases and Disorders,* New York, McGraw-Hill, 1992, pp 401–418.

Miro AM, Shivaram U, Hertig I: Continuous positive airway pressure in COPD patients in acute hypercapnic respiratory failure. Chest 103:266–268, 1993.

Ranieri VM, Giuliani R, Cinnella G, Pesce C, Brienza N, Ippolito EL, Pomo V, Fiore T, Gottfried SB, Brienza A: Physiologic effects of positive end-expiratory pressure in patients with chronic obstructive pulmonary disease during acute ventilatory failure and controlled mechanical ventilation. Am Rev Respir Dis 147:5–13, 1993.

| Acute Respiratory Distress Syndrome
(ARDS)

John Hansen-Flaschen

DEFINITION

The *acute respiratory distress syndrome* (ARDS) is defined as an
acute lung injury that results in widespread bilateral pulmonary
infiltrates, severe refractory hypoxemia, and a marked reduction in
lung compliance. Typical cases are recognized by experienced
clinicians with little difficulty. However, several related conditions
can be confused with this form of respiratory failure. For that
reason, certain aspects of the definition require special attention.

1. The term ARDS is reserved for clinical conditions in which the
   onset of respiratory failure results primarily from *acute injury to
   the lungs themselves.* Because left heart failure and intravascular
   fluid overload can cause a similar clinical pattern in the absence
   of any acute lung injury, right heart catheterization is often
   required to demonstrate that the pulmonary arterial wedge
   pressure is not elevated.
2. Damage to the lungs must be *acute* at onset. ARDS typically
   progresses to respiratory failure within 6 to 48 h after the initial
   injury to the lungs. Bleomycin toxicity and disseminated tuberculosis are examples of disorders that do not fit the definition of
   ARDS because they typically progress to respiratory failure over
   weeks rather than hours.
3. Pulmonary infiltrates need not be diffuse; however, they must be
   extensive and bilateral. Excluded by this criterion are focal
   conditions that can cause respiratory failure such as lobar
   pneumonia or unilateral lung contusion.
4. Disturbances in gas exchange must be *severe.* Criteria for severity
   vary somewhat; however, the term ARDS is generally reserved
   for episodes of acute lung injury that necessitate mechanical
   ventilation and administration of oxygen at a concentration >
   50%.

When respiratory failure associated with acute diffuse lung injury
was first described in the late 1960s, it was called *adult* respiratory
distress syndrome in contradistinction to the respiratory distress
syndrome of premature newborns. Since then, it has become clear
that ARDS occurs in children of all ages, including mature newborns. For that reason, *acute* respiratory distress syndrome is now
the preferred term for this condition.

Although ARDS is frequently accompanied by acute injury to

other organs, it should not be viewed exclusively as the pulmonary manifestation of the multiple organ failure syndrome (MOFS). ARDS occurs without concomitant failure of other organs in such diverse conditions as aspiration of gastric contents, *Pneumocystis carinii* pneumonia, and massive air embolism.

CAUSES AND ASSOCIATED DISORDERS

To date, > 50 causes of ARDS have been identified (Table 49-1). Many of the known causes are uncommon but readily apparent from the history. Others may be exceedingly difficult to prove, e.g., drug reactions and occult aspiration.

Epidemiologic studies have shown that most episodes of ARDS encountered in United States hospitals are associated with a few common causes or predisposing conditions, singly or in combination. *Sepsis syndrome* appears to be the single most important cause of ARDS in hospitalized patients. In fact, sepsis is so commonly implicated in ARDS, that this cause should be considered first in any patient who develops otherwise unexplained ARDS in association with a new fever, hypotension, or a clinical predisposition to serious infection. *Infectious pneumonia* may be the most common cause of ARDS in patients who develop ARDS outside of the hospital. Nosocomial pneumonias frequently cause ARDS as well. *Aspiration of gastric contents* is another common cause of ARDS. Approximately one third of hospitalized patients who experience a clinically recognized episode of gastric aspiration subsequently develop the syndrome.

Severe *trauma* and *surface burns* are frequently associated with the development of ARDS. Lung contusion is an important cause of ARDS that develops within 24 h after blunt injury to the chest. *Fat embolism* sometimes causes ARDS in patients with long bone fractures. This complication characteristically appears 12 to 48 h after the injury. It may be less common in the United States now than it was in the past because trauma victims are routinely and effectively immobilized before transport to the hospital. Sepsis syndrome is probably the most common cause of ARDS that develops several days or more after severe trauma or burn.

ARDS can be caused by *overdose of several common drugs,* including aspirin, opiates, phenothiazines, and tricyclic antidepressants. Idiosyncratic reactions to other drugs such as protamine and nitrofurantoin occasionally precipitate ARDS after therapeutic doses. *Radiologic contrast media* can also provoke ARDS in susceptible individuals. *Leukoagglutinin reactions* sometimes cause severe acute lung injury during or immediately after transfusion of a blood product. Most of these reactions are thought to result from the presence in the transfused blood product of antibodies directed against an antigen on the recipient's white blood cells.

TABLE 49-1 Causes of the Acute Respiratory Distress Syndrome

Cause	Frequency*	Cause	Frequency*
Infections		**Drugs and ingested toxins**	
Bacterial sepsis	F	Phenytoin	R
Gonococcemia	R	Protamine	R
Legionnaires' disease	I	Salicylates	I
Mycoplasma pneumonia	I	Toxic oil	I
Pneumococcal pneumonia	I	**Diagnostic and therapeutic**	
Adenovirus pneumonia	I	**agents**	
Babesiosis	R	Granulocyte transfusion	I
Blastomycosis	R	Leukoagglutinin transfusion	I
Coccidioidomycosis	I	reaction	
Cytomegalovirus pneumonia	I	Lymphangiography contrast	R
Falciparum malaria	I	medium	
Influenza pneumonia	I	Radiologic contrast media	R
Pneumocystis pneumonia	F	Thoracic radiotherapy	R
Rocky Mountain spotted fever	R	**Embolic disorders**	I
Tuberculosis	I	Amniotic fluid embolism	
Inhalation injuries		Fat embolism	F
Ammonia	I	Venous air embolism	I
Aspiration of gastric contents	F	**Inflammatory and neoplastic**	
Chlorine gas	I	**disorders**	
Near-drowning	F	Diffuse pulmonary	I
Nitrogen dioxide	I	hemorrhage	
Oxygen toxicity	I	Granulocytic leukemia	I
Phosgene	I	Pancreatitis	I
Smoke inhalation	I	Thrombotic	I
Sulfur dioxide	I	thrombocytopenic purpura	
Drugs and ingested toxins		**Physical injuries**	
Cytosine arabinoside	I	Bilateral lung contusion	F
Denatured rapeseed oil	I	Burns (extensive)	F
Ethchlorvynol	I	Heart lung transplantation	F
Ethylene glycol	I	Heat stroke	R
Hydrochlorothiazide	R	High altitude pulmonary	I
Lidocaine	R	edema	
Narcotics	I	Neurogenic pulmonary	I
Nitrofurantoin	I	edema	
Paraldehyde	R	Radiation	R
Paraquat	F	Reperfusion pulmonary	F
		Suicidal hanging	F
		Trauma	F

*Estimated frequency among individuals at risk: F = frequent; I = infrequent; R = rare.

SOURCE: Adapted from Hansen-Flaschen J, Fishman AP: Adult respiratory distress syndrome: Clinical features and pathogenesis, in Fishman AP (ed), *Pulmonary Diseases and Disorders,* 2d ed. New York, McGraw-Hill, 1988, 2206.

ARDS frequently develops in a setting of catastrophic acute illness or injury such that a single specific cause for the lung injury cannot be identified with certainty. Indeed, several precipitating factors may operate simultaneously. In such instances, presumptive treatment for sepsis is often justified.

DIFFERENTIAL DIAGNOSIS

In addition to ARDS, at least three other conditions cause acute, widespread pulmonary infiltrates and severe hypoxemia. They are hemodynamic pulmonary edema, diffuse alveolar hemorrhage, and metastatic cancer. These conditions resemble ARDS clinically, at least at onset, but none is accompanied by the alveolar inflammatory changes that characterize ARDS.

Hemodynamic pulmonary edema is distinguished from ARDS by an elevated pulmonary arterial wedge pressure (> 18 mmHg) and by rapid, complete clearing of pulmonary infiltrates after the wedge pressure has returned to normal. Hemodynamic edema accompanies ARDS in as many as 10 to 20 percent of cases, but in those instances, pulmonary infiltrates and hypoxemia persist for longer than 48 h after pulmonary capillary pressure is normalized.

Diffuse alveolar hemorrhage should be considered whenever sudden onset of widespread pulmonary infiltrates is accompanied by a dramatic fall in the hematocrit. Hemoptysis may be minimal or absent initially; however, airway fluid obtained after intubation is invariably bloody. On bronchoscopic examination, frothy red fluid is seen throughout the airways. Microscopic examination of fluid obtained by bronchoalveolar lavage discloses many hemosiderin-laden macrophages.

Metastatic cancer sometimes disseminates through the lungs with such rapidity that the clinical picture closely resembles ARDS. The distinction is important because, in contrast to ARDS, this condition is almost invariably fatal. The diagnosis can sometimes be made by cytologic examination of blood withdrawn from the pulmonary circulation through a Swan-Ganz catheter while the balloon is inflated. Bronchoscopy is the alternative diagnostic approach. If bronchoalveolar lavage does not yield the diagnosis of malignancy, transbronchial biopsy can be done even in mechanically ventilated patients, but at increased risk of complications. Occasionally, open lung biopsy is required to establish the diagnosis.

PATHOPHYSIOLOGY

ARDS is a form of acute respiratory failure characterized by several distinctive physiological disturbances. Once the lung injury has advanced to the stage requiring mechanical ventilation, all of these abnormalities are present, in varying degrees of severity, regardless of the precipitating cause. The following physiological disturbances in ARDS are readily identifiable at the bedside.

Hypoxemia Shunting of blood from right to left through atelectatic or fluid-filled alveoli causes a marked widening of the alveolar-to-arterial difference in P_{O_2}. The resultant hypoxemia is resistant to high concentrations of inspired oxygen but is often responsive to positive end-expiratory pressure (PEEP). Among survivors, hypoxemia is typically most severe during the first several days after the onset of ARDS. Some patients ultimately die of hypoxemia despite optimal therapy.

Increased physiologic dead space The physiologic dead space is typically increased in ARDS, frequently exceeding 60 percent of each breath. Consequently, a very large minute ventilation may be required to maintain tolerable levels of arterial P_{CO_2}. In some patients, improvement of the dead space abnormality lags behind the improvement in hypoxemia so that a persistent requirement for a large minute ventilation becomes the primary obstacle to weaning from mechanical ventilation.

Decreased pulmonary compliance The compliance of the congested, atelectatic lungs is invariably reduced in ARDS. The increased stiffness of the lungs is associated with corresponding reductions in lung volumes because alveolar airspaces are filled by exudate or obliterated by inflammatory changes. Because pulmonary compliance is reduced, high driving pressures are required to inflate the lungs during mechanical ventilation.

Increased airway resistance Airway resistance is difficult to measure in patients undergoing mechanical ventilation. Nevertheless, airway resistance appears to be increased in most patients with ARDS. In some instances, reversible bronchospasm may contribute to increased airway resistance.

Pulmonary hypertension As a rule, pulmonary hypertension is mild to moderate in ARDS even when the ARDS is severe. Often a difference of 5 to 10 mmHg or more can be demonstrated by right heart catheterization between the pulmonary artery diastolic pressure and the pulmonary arterial wedge pressure.

THE CLINICOPATHOLOGIC STAGES OF ARDS

Regardless of the initiating factors, ARDS tends to evolve, over days or weeks, along a common pathway marked by characteristic clinical, radiographic, and pathologic changes. Not all patients travel the entire pathway—many deviate along the way to recover or die. Nevertheless, the main route is well recognized and stereotypical.

In patients who develop the full-blown syndrome, ARDS typically progresses through three distinct but overlapping phases: an exudative phase, a proliferative and fibrotic phase, and, in survivors, a phase of repair and recovery.

Exudative Phase

ARDS begins with a physical or chemically mediated injury to the alveolar-capillary membranes of the lungs. This injury gives rise to the increased permeability pulmonary edema and acute inflammatory changes that characterize the exudative phase of the syndrome.

Considering the devastating consequences of the injury, the initial anatomic damage to the lungs is often surprisingly subtle. Indeed, the earliest structural abnormalities can be seen only with the aid of an electron microscope. At the outset, when the alveolar-capillary membranes still appear intact by light microscopy, ultrastructural studies show cytologic evidence of widespread injury to endothelial and epithelial cells. Damage to the endothelial and epithelial surfaces of the alveolar walls promotes leakage of protein-rich edema fluid into the interstitial spaces of the lungs. As the injury progresses, many of the alveoli fill with edema fluid, while others are collapsed by external compression or by alterations in surface tension. At this stage, ARDS is distinguished under the light microscope from hemodynamic pulmonary edema chiefly by the presence of hyaline membranes lining some of the alveolar surfaces.

Within hours after the initial insult, resident macrophages release a host of cytokines which act directly on pneumocytes to initiate or amplify the inflammatory response to acute lung injury. In response, circulating leukocytes adhere to the capillary walls and migrate into the lung. By 24 to 48 h, neutrophils are seen throughout the interstitial and alveolar spaces. Neutrophils are thought to play a major role in early progression of acute lung injury by releasing reactive metabolites of oxygen and several potent proteases that damage the lung. The coagulation system is also activated during the exudative phase of ARDS. Microthrombi form throughout the pulmonary microcirculation, interfering with gas exchange and contributing to the thrombocytopenia that is often observed during this phase.

The radiographic changes that occur during the exudative phase of ARDS are similar to those seen in hemodynamic pulmonary edema. Widespread alveolar infiltrates spread rapidly throughout both lungs. In severe cases, the pattern is sometimes referred to as a "bilateral white out" of the lungs.

Some patients recover quickly and completely after the exudative phase of ARDS. Certain forms of acute lung injury typically cause ARDS with rapid recovery, such as high-altitude pulmonary edema, fat embolism, and many acute drug reactions. In these conditions, the lungs may never develop the progressive inflammatory and proliferative changes that characterize the second phase of ARDS. Indeed, there is some question whether acute lung injury associated with rapid recovery should be included within the rubric of ARDS at all, because the prognosis is so much better than that associated with the full-blown syndrome.

Proliferation and Fibrosis

In patients who progress to the second phase of ARDS, proliferative changes are readily apparent in pathologic specimens obtained as early as 3 to 4 days after initial injury. Epithelial type II cells multiply to fill in the gaps along the alveolar epithelial surface left behind by the sloughing of necrotic type I epithelial cells. Within the adjacent interstitium, fibroblasts proliferate and begin to modify the extracellular connective tissue. Other fibroblasts migrate into the alveolar spaces and proliferate there, forming granulation tissue.

If appropriately regulated, the early proliferative changes in ARDS repair the damaged lungs and restore the structural integrity of the alveolar capillary membranes. In contrast, if the initial proliferative response continues without restorative modulation, progressive obliteration of the alveolar architecture ensues. Granulation tissue fills the alveolar spaces, preventing restoration of effective gas exchange and setting the stage for fibrotic remodeling of the alveolar capillary membranes.

Pulmonary fibrosis appears as early as 8 to 10 days after the onset of respiratory failure and progresses to a variable extent over the ensuing days or weeks. In advanced cases, the alveolar capillary membranes and the surfaces of alveolar ducts are progressively replaced by dense, irregular bands of fibrous tissue. Beyond 3 or 4 weeks, the most severely damaged areas of the lungs may resemble a sponge: innumerable cystic airspaces and dilated bronchioles are separated by thick walls of hypocellular connective tissue.

The radiographic appearance of the lungs changes dramatically during the proliferative and fibrotic phase of ARDS. Confluent alveolar infiltrates become less dense and homogeneous as edema fluid is resorbed and distal airspaces are reopened. Reticular infiltrates emerge in some areas, whereas ground-glass opacities predominate in others. Pulmonary barotrauma develops frequently during this phase, giving rise to pneumomediastinum and pneumothoraces. Multiple loculated pneumothoraces sometimes form during the advanced phase of proliferation and fibrosis.

Repair and Recovery

The lung function of many patients who enter the second phase of ARDS never seems to improve beyond a certain plateau. Either these patients are too sick for their lungs to heal, or the gas exchanging components of their lungs are so extensively destroyed that the healing process cannot restore an adequate blood-gas interface. These patients require mechanical ventilation and high concentrations of inspired oxygen until they die. Other patients do ultimately recover despite extensive fibrosis. The mechanical properties and gas exchanging function of their lungs returns toward normal during a third phase of ARDS that sometimes continues as long as 6 to 12 months after mechanical ventilation is discontinued.

Remarkably little is known about the reparative phase of advanced ARDS because few pathologic specimens are obtained during this time. Serial chest radiographs show progressive clearing of dense reticular infiltrates, suggesting that fibrous tissue is resorbed or rearranged. Months after the onset of ARDS, radiographic residua may be limited to a few linear densities or a shaggy appearance of the heart borders and diaphragm. The radiographic appearance of the lungs may even return to normal. Up to 75 percent of patients are left with a mild or moderate impairment in lung function, and occasional individuals are permanently disabled by severe chronic lung disease.

MANAGEMENT

To date, no pharmacologic agent has proven effective in lessening the severity or hastening the recovery of acute lung injury. Management of ARDS is directed at preventing or treating the underlying cause and at maintaining the general health of the patient with the hope that the injured lungs will heal. Successful treatment of ARDS requires frequent assessment and modification of cardiopulmonary function and meticulous attention to the many complications of intensive care.

Mechanical Ventilation

After intubation, volume-cycled mechanical ventilation is begun using the assist control mode with a tidal volume of 7 to 10 cc/kg and a respiratory rate of 10 to 25 breaths per minute. Then arterial blood gases and the breathing pattern of the patient are monitored closely to guide further adjustments of the ventilator.

Many acutely dyspneic patients with ARDS continue to make active respiratory efforts after initiation of mechanical ventilation even as arterial blood gases are restored toward normal. Active inspiratory effort and premature expiration cause the peak airway pressure to vary from breath to breath and may result in frequent, erratic sounding of the peak pressure alarm. Alveolar hypoventilation ensues because the patient receives less than the prescribed tidal volume each time the peak pressure alarm setting is exceeded. Also, excessive activity of the respiratory muscles can substantially increase production of CO_2 in critically ill patients. For these reasons, heavy sedation and paralysis are often necessary to suppress the respiratory efforts of the patient during the first several hours or days after mechanical ventilation is begun.

Rapid, complete paralysis can be achieved by giving pancuronium bromide intravenously at an initial dose of 0.1 mg/kg. Thereafter, incremental doses of 0.01 to 0.04 mg/kg are used as needed (typically every 1 to 2 h) to maintain paralysis. Continuous intravenous infusion of vecuronium or atracurium can also be used for this purpose. Generous doses of a benzodiazepine or an opiate should be given along with the paralyzing agent to induce amnesia. Intermittent injection of lorazepam and continuous infusion of morphine or fentanyl are cost-effective methods for sedating patients who are paralyzed. The need for continued paralysis should be reassessed daily or more often to minimize the many hazards associated with this therapy.

Current theories regarding the progression of lung injury during the proliferative and fibrotic stage of ARDS assign a key role to the high airway pressures typically required to ventilate the lungs during this time. High airway pressures are also thought to promote barotrauma. For these reasons, many authorities now recommend that peak airway pressures be kept as low as possible—ideally < 40 cmH_2O—during mechanical ventilation for ARDS.

Several strategies can be combined if necessary to accomplish this goal. Sedation and judicious use of paralyzing agents may be effective in lowering peak airway pressure if the patient is restless or agitated. Airway pressure can also be reduced by minimizing tidal volume and inspiratory flow rate. The tidal volume can be set as low as 7 to 8 cc/kg and the inspiratory flow rate can be reduced until the inspiratory-expiratory ratio increases to 1:1 or more. If necessary, inspiratory flow rate can be reduced further by reducing the respiratory rate until hypercapnia ensues. A P_{CO_2} > 70 mmHg can be tolerated if bicarbonate is administered to keep the pH > 7.30. One of the newer modes of mechanical ventilation, such as pressure-controlled or high-frequency ventilation, can also be used to reduce airway pressure.

No firm rule dictates how soon after intubation patients with ARDS should undergo tracheostomy. Prolonged translaryngeal intubation and tracheostomy both cause considerable injury to the upper airway. However, recent studies have shown that nasotracheal tubes are also frequently associated with development of sinusitis. Removal of the nasotracheal tube is generally necessary to clear the sinus infection. For this reason, and to improve the comfort of the patient, many clinicians perform tracheostomy after 2 or 3 weeks in patients with ARDS who are not likely to be extubated soon thereafter.

Oxygenation

Because an appreciable portion of the cardiac output flows through nonventilated lung units in ARDS, hypoxemia is invariably severe and responds poorly to supplemental oxygen. The goal of oxygen therapy in this condition is to maintain adequate oxygen delivery while avoiding the oxygen toxicity associated with high concentrations of inspired O_2. Unfortunately, neither the lowest acceptable PaO_2 nor the lowest tolerable inspired O_2 concentration can be determined with precision for individual patients. However, increasing the PaO_2 above 60 mmHg provides minimal additional benefit in O_2 delivery. Moreover, patients do recover completely from ARDS despite prolonged inspiration of O_2 at concentrations as high as 60% to 65%.

Immediately after the patient with ARDS is intubated, 100% O_2 is administered to ensure a margin of safety while the mechanical ventilator is adjusted and the condition of the patient is stabilized. Within 24 h after intubation, the inspired O_2 concentration is brought down to a nontoxic level, using PEEP, if necessary. PEEP improves arterial oxygenation in most, but not all, patients with ARDS by reexpanding atelectatic or fluid-filled alveoli, thereby decreasing the intrapulmonary shunting of blood. However, PEEP can also decrease cardiac output by impeding venous return to the right ventricle, particularly when the blood volume is low. These two physiologic effects have opposing influences on systemic O_2 delivery. For that reason, the level of PEEP must be adjusted carefully.

PEEP is generally begun at 5 cmH_2O, and the PaO_2 is measured 15 to 30 min later. This level of PEEP rarely causes an important reduction in cardiac output. If a higher level is required, a Swan-Ganz catheter is inserted and the cardiac output is monitored along with the PaO_2 as PEEP is increased in increments of 2 to 3 cmH_2O. Usually 5 to 15 cmH_2O PEEP is sufficient to achieve acceptable oxygenation. Occasionally, up to 20 to 25 cmH_2O PEEP is required. At higher levels of PEEP, it is often necessary to support the cardiac output by administering fluids intravenously or by resorting to an inotropic drug such as dobutamine.

Fluid Management

In general, patients with ARDS should be kept as dry as possible without compromising cardiac output to minimize accumulation of excess fluid in the lungs. This approach may be more important in the first stage of ARDS when leaky alveolar-capillary membranes characterize the lung pathology. Later on, when proliferation and fibrosis dominate the pathologic changes, the benefit of minimizing pulmonary capillary pressure is less certain.

Patients who develop ARDS immediately after trauma or major surgery may need massive amounts of fluid to maintain an adequate cardiac output. In these settings, circulatory considerations outweigh the goal of minimizing lung edema. Until loss of intravascular fluid slows, crystalloid or colloid should be infused aggressively to keep the pulmonary arterial wedge pressure above 10 mmHg. Several days later, excess fluid can be removed by diuresis or dialysis with the goal of reducing lung water and improving oxygenation.

Management of Barotrauma

Approximately 15 percent of patients with ARDS develop barotrauma. Clinical manifestations include subpleural air cysts, pneumomediastinum, pneumothorax, and subcutaneous emphysema. Pneumothorax can endanger the life of the patient with ARDS because positive pressure mechanical ventilation tends to drive air into the pleural space until increased intrathoracic pressure causes circulatory collapse (tension pneumothorax). For that reason, a chest tube should be placed as soon as a pneumothorax is recognized, regardless of its size.

ARDS is often accompanied by pleural inflammatory changes that cause loculation in the pleural space. In this circumstance, a chest tube may not prevent accumulation of air in ipsilateral pockets that do not communicate with the chest tube. Loculated pneumothoraces tend to form on the anterior surface of the lung in supine patients and can cause the disturbances associated with a tension pneumothorax. Sometimes as many as three or four chest tubes may be needed on an affected side to decompress loculated collections of air in the pleural space. In those who survive, the air leaks that gave rise to multiple pneumothoraces ultimately heal so that the chest tubes can be removed.

Recovery and Rehabilitation

The respiratory function of most patients who recover from ARDS begins to improve in the first few days. As arterial oxygenation improves, the inspired concentration of O_2 is reduced to 50% and then the level of PEEP is decreased. Many patients are ready to begin weaning from mechanical ventilation when they are able to tolerate an inspired O_2 concentration of 40% to 45% with 0 to 5 cmH_2O PEEP. Others require continued ventilatory support because of a persistent increase in physiologic dead space, an impairment in respiratory muscle function, or severe hemodynamic instability.

Many patients who recover from ARDS require supplemental oxygen for weeks after mechanical ventilation is discontinued. Some patients benefit from postural drainage and chest physical therapy after extubation because they have a weak or ineffective cough. Refeeding by mouth should be undertaken with caution because prolonged translaryngeal intubation can cause, or exacerbate, swallowing dysfunction that predisposes to aspiration. Some physicians routinely examine the larynx and obtain a pharyngoesophagram before allowing oral intake to resume.

Many patients who ultimately recover from ARDS are physically and mentally devastated by their disease. Enforced bed rest, continuous use of paralyzing agents, multiple surgical procedures, and recurrent episodes of sepsis can cause profound muscle weakness. Pain, neurologic injury, disruption of normal sleep-wake patterns, and adverse drug reactions often combine to precipitate severe psychiatric disturbances such as delirium and suicidal depression. For these patients, a comprehensive rehabilitation program is essential. Rehabilitation should be initiated as weaning from mechanical ventilation gets underway, and these efforts should be intensified soon after extubation. A coordinated transition from intensive care through an inpatient rehabilitation service to supervised convalescence at home is best achieved by a multidisciplinary team of rehabilitation specialists who work in close collaboration with the critical care team.

PROGNOSIS

Approximately 50 percent of patients with ARDS die before they leave the hospital. However, fewer than 20 percent actually succumb to respiratory failure. Instead, most of the nonsurvivors die early as a result of an underlying illness, or later because of sepsis or MOFS. Indeed, for most patients, the nature and severity of coexisting disorders appears to be more important than the cause or severity of the acute lung injury in determining survival. For example, the mortality rate for previously healthy patients who develop ARDS after near-drowning is < 10 percent, whereas the mortality rate for those who develop ARDS in association with septic shock generally exceeds 50 percent. Mortality approaches 100 percent for individuals who develop ARDS as a complication of severe hepatic dysfunction.

BIBLIOGRAPHY

For a more detailed discussion, see Hansen-Flaschen J, Fishman AP: Adult respiratory distress syndrome: Clinical features and pathogenesis, in Fishman AP (ed), *Pulmonary Diseases and Disorders,* 2d ed. New York, McGraw-Hill, 1988, pp 2201–2213.

Pattishall EN, Long WA: Surfactant treatment of adult respiratory distress syndrome, in Fishman AP (ed), *Update: Pulmonary Diseases and Disorders.* New York, McGraw-Hill, 1992, pp 225–236.

Suchyta MR, Clemmer TP, Elliott CG, Orme JF Jr, Weaver LK: The adult respiratory distress syndrome. A report of survival and modifying factors. Chest 101:1074–1079, 1992.

Wiedemann HP, Matthay MA, Matthay RA (eds): Adult respiratory distress syndrome. Clin Chest Med 11:575–811, 1990.

Zapol, WM, Lemaire F: *Adult Respiratory Distress Syndrome.* New York, Marcel Dekker, 1991, pp 1–432.

Oxygen therapy is used to correct arterial hypoxemia and to improve oxygen delivery to the tissues. However, the administration of oxygen, as in the case of any other medication, has to be viewed with respect to therapeutic versus toxic levels. Excess oxygen can have undesirable side effects and can cause toxicity that can be life threatening.

PHYSIOLOGIC EFFECTS OF OXYGEN BREATHING

Even in normal individuals, hyperoxia causes depression of the ventilatory drive, leading to mild hypercapnia. Although of little clinical consequence in the normal subject, this effect is greatly exaggerated in the chronically hypercapnic patient in whom a low arterial Po_2 contributes significantly to the ventilatory drive. Acute elimination of the hypoxic stimulus by oxygen breathing in this type of patient can rapidly precipitate respiratory failure.

By eliminating hypoxic pulmonary vasoconstriction, oxygen breathing worsens ventilation-perfusion relationships throughout the lungs. This mismatching contributes to the oxygen-induced CO_2 retention in patients with chronic obstructive pulmonary disease.

Breathing of pure oxygen leads to nitrogen washout from the alveoli. In poorly ventilated areas of the lung, the drop in alveolar nitrogen results in absorption atelectasis and an increased shunt fraction.

Hemodynamically, relief of acute hypoxia slows the heart rate and decreases both the cardiac output and right ventricular stroke work.

PULMONARY TOXICITY: PATHOGENESIS

The predominant manifestation of oxygen toxicity is acute lung injury. This effect depends on the partial pressure of oxygen in inspired air and duration of the exposure. Hyperbaric oxygenation accelerates the onset of pulmonary injury and leads to systemic manifestations of oxygen toxicity (see below).

Pulmonary oxygen toxicity is caused by the formation of reactive oxygen species ("free radicals") and their biochemical interactions at the cellular level. Oxygen radicals are extremely reactive due to their high affinity for additional electrons. Oxygen radicals inactivate proteins by reacting with sulfhydryl groups, cross-linking peptides, or oxidizing amino acids. By interacting with nucleotides and complex carbohydrates, they contribute to disruption of cell function. They also react with lipids to form lipid peroxides which, in turn, propagate the peroxidation process in a chain reaction, disrupting cell and organelle membranes.

Under normal conditions, antioxidant defense mechanisms, operating at the subcellular level, cope with the basal production of oxygen-free radicals, thereby avoiding cell damage. One line of defense is enzymatic: superoxide dismutase removes superoxide anion, catalase removes H_2O_2, and glutathione peroxidase removes both H_2O_2 and lipid peroxides. The oxidation-reduction cycle of glutathione, a tripeptide with a free sulfhydryl group, is essential in preventing oxidation of protein sulfhydryl groups. A second line of defense is nonenzymatic: free radical scavengers include ascorbic acid (vitamin C), α-tocopherol (vitamin E), and β-carotene (vitamin A).

Hyperoxia increases the production of oxygen radicals in the lung. Oxygen toxicity results when the production of free radicals overwhelms the antioxidant protective mechanisms of the lung. In addition to the direct effects of oxygen radicals on cells, oxygen toxicity is associated with the influx of macrophage and neutrophils and resultant inflammatory changes, increased levels of circulating vasoactive substances, altered surfactant synthesis, and impaired mucociliary clearance promoting bacterial superinfection.

HISTOPATHOLOGY

The histologic changes associated with prolonged exposure to hyperoxia have been most clearly demonstrated in laboratory animals; limited human studies are available which support the experimental findings. The pulmonary injury caused by oxygen toxicity is characterized by diffuse alveolar damage. An exudative phase occurs early on, characterized by widespread injury to the alveolar capillary barrier with resultant accumulation of proteinaceous fluid and red cells in the alveolar airspaces and formation of hyaline membranes. This is followed by the accumulation of neutrophils and macrophages in the interstitium and airspaces, along with influx of platelets in the capillaries and deposition of fibrin thrombi.

The exudative phase of hyperoxic lung injury is succeeded by cellular proliferation and fibrosis: type II pneumocytes proliferate and line the alveoli, while macrophages, monocytes and fibroblasts proliferate in the interstitium. With continued exposure to hyperoxia, widespread fibrosis and complete disruption of normal parenchymal architecture ensues, ultimately leading to death. Removal of the hyperoxic insult at a sublethal phase permits reparation of lung injury, leading unpredictably to either full restoration of normal lung architecture or to varying degrees of fibrosis and emphysema.

CLINICAL MANIFESTATIONS OF PULMONARY TOXICITY

Limited human studies have demonstrated that administration of oxygen at a concentration of 50% or less is well tolerated for prolonged periods without significant toxicity. Breathing 100% O_2, on the other hand, is potentially quite toxic. Exposure to 100% O_2 for longer than 12 to 24 h results in an acute tracheobronchitis, manifest clinically by cough and retrosternal chest pain. Inflammatory changes are present in the tracheobronchial mucosa and mucociliary clearance is diminished. After 24 h of breathing 100% O_2, the vital capacity decreases significantly; after 48 h, static lung compliance and diffusing capacity decrease along with an increase in the alveolar-arterial oxygen gradient.

Exposure to 100% O_2 for more than 100 h leads to progressive lung injury that clinically and radiographically resembles the acute respiratory distress syndrome (ARDS). Patients may note worsening dyspnea, and physical examination may reveal low-grade fever, tachypnea, and inspiratory rales. The chest radiograph initially demonstrates interstitial infiltrates which rapidly progress to an alveolar-filling pattern. Unfortunately, the clinical manifestations of oxygen toxicity are rarely clear-cut. Patients most prone to develop oxygen toxicity are those with preexisting acute lung injury who require use of high concentrations of supplemental oxygen to correct arterial hypoxemia. In this setting, it may be virtually impossible to distinguish those features ascribable to oxygen toxicity from those due to the underlying disease process.

Unless the process of oxygen toxicity can be arrested, pulmonary function decreases progressively leading to death or permanent disability. Although decreasing the partial pressure of oxygen in the inspired air to that of ambient air can lead to gradual resolution of the pulmonary injury and full restoration of function, this is often not feasible in the critically ill patient whose lungs have been severely damaged.

SYSTEMIC TOXICITY

In neonates, the administration of 50% to 100% O_2 can cause a serious form of retinopathy (retrolental fibroplasia). This damage is attributed to hyperoxic vasoconstriction of the retinal vessels, endothelial cell damage, and cessation of vascularization to the periphery of the retina. Return to normoxic breathing mixtures is followed by disorganized vascular proliferation, subsequent hemorrhage, and fibrosis. The end result is retinal detachment and irreversible blindness.

In adults, progressive myopia has occurred in some patients receiving hyperbaric oxygen therapy. The cause is believed to be oxygen-induced changes in lens shape and metabolism. This condition is totally reversible after the course of hyperbaric oxygen therapy has been completed.

Manifestations of central nervous system toxicity are uncommon until high levels of hyperbaric oxygenation are reached, e.g., 100% O_2 at 3 atmospheres pressure. At these high levels, the manifestations include changes in mental status, visual field abnormalities, tinnitus, gustatory and olfactory sensations, nausea and vomiting, muscle twitching, and grand mal seizures.

DIAGNOSIS

Diagnosing oxygen toxicity is frequently a formidable challenge because the clinical, physiologic, histologic, and radiographic features may be indistinguishable from those of the underlying lung injury for which high levels of oxygen are being used. No tests are specific for oxygen poisoning. The diagnosis is generally based on a high index of suspicion in the patient who demonstrates progressive respiratory deterioration after prolonged exposure to high oxygen mixtures.

Routine diagnostic studies are nonspecific. The vital capacity and pulmonary compliance are decreased in association with a decrease in the diffusing capacity. The arterial-alveolar oxygen gradient is widened. Serial chest radiographs show progressive alveolar infiltrates. The pulmonary capillary wedge pressure, determined by use of a Swan-Ganz catheter, is low, consistent with noncardiogenic pulmonary edema. Concentrations of albumin and transferrin in bronchoalveolar lavage fluid are increased, suggesting increased capillary permeability.

Biochemical tests have recently been developed as possible indicators of early oxidative damage. For example, pentane and ethane, by-products of lipid peroxidation, can be detected in expired respiratory gases during oxygen poisoning. A decrease in the lung's ability to metabolize biogenic amines, polypeptides, and prostaglandins may also signal the onset of oxygen toxicity. However, these tests are still experimental and unavailable for clinical use.

TREATMENT

There is no specific medical therapy for oxygen toxicity. Efforts are directed at avoiding or minimizing oxygen exposures that may evoke toxicity. The following guidelines are suggested:

1. 100% O_2 can be used safely for up to 24 h in emergency situations, such as cardiopulmonary arrest and shock.
2. Thereafter, inspired oxygen concentrations should be maintained at no more than 50% to 60%. The lowest concentration required to achieve adequate oxygenation ($Pao_2 > 60$, or HbO_2 saturation > 90%) should be used.

3. If > 60% inspired oxygen is required, positive end-expiratory pressure (PEEP) should be applied during mechanical ventilation. This will reopen collapsed alveoli, decrease intrapulmonary shunting, and improve oxygenation, thus allowing further decrements in the inspired oxygen concentration.

4. To permit tolerance of marginal arterial oxygen tensions which may result from limiting the concentration of inspired oxygen, oxygen consumption by peripheral tissues should be minimized and oxygen delivery optimized. Oxygen consumption can be diminished by lowering fever with antipyretics, controlling agitation with sedatives, and instituting muscle paralysis. On occasion, induced hypothermia can also be used to decrease oxygen demands. Oxygen delivery to the tissues can be improved by increasing cardiac output by administering inotropic agents and by maintaining high normal hemoglobin levels with blood transfusions.

5. Maintenance of adequate nutrition is essential. Susceptibility to pulmonary oxygen toxicity is potentially exacerbated by dietary deficiencies. Protein malnutrition leads to inadequate glutathione synthesis. Deficiencies of vitamins and trace minerals disrupt antioxidant defense mechanisms.

6. Synergistic effects of oxygen-induced pulmonary toxicity have been reported with medications (disulfiram and nitrofurantoin) and chemotherapeutic agents (bleomycin, mitomycin, and cyclophosphamide). History of exposure to these agents should prompt attempts at minimizing exposure to high concentrations, e.g., during general anesthesia.

7. Corticosteroids have not been effective in alleviating oxygen toxicity, whereas they may increase the incidence and severity of infectious complications in patients with acute lung injury.

8. Although the administration of exogenous antioxidants, e.g., superoxide, catalase, vitamins A, E, C, N-acetylcysteine, deferoxamine, has improved oxygen tolerance in animal models, these agents are not available for clinical use.

BIBLIOGRAPHY

For a more detailed discussion, see Fisher AB: Pulmonary oxygen toxicity, in Fishman AP (ed), *Pulmonary Diseases and Disorders*, 2d ed. New York, McGraw-Hill, 1988, pp 2331–2338.

Griffith DE, Garcia JG, James HL, Callahan KS, Iriana S, Holiday D: Hyperoxic exposure in humans. Effects of 50 percent oxygen on alveolar macrophage leukotriene B4 synthesis. Chest 101:392–397, 1992.

Jacobson JM, Michael JR, Jafri MH, Gurtner GH: Antioxidants and antioxidant enzymes protect against pulmonary oxygen toxicity in the rabbit. J Appl Physiol 68:1252–1259, 1990.

Klein J: Normobaric pulmonary oxygen toxicity. Anesth Analg 70:195–207, 1990.

McNamara JO, Fridovich I: Did radicals stroke Lou Gehrig? Nature 362:20–21, 1993.

Risberg B, Smith L, Ortenwall P: Oxygen radicals and lung injury. Acta Anaesthesiol Scand Suppl 95:106–116, 1991.

Stogner SW, Payne DK: Oxygen toxicity. Ann Pharmacother 26:1554–1562, 1992.

| Mechanical Ventilation

Horace M. DeLisser

The primary use of mechanical ventilation is to enable the elimination of metabolic CO_2 when spontaneous ventilation no longer suffices, e.g., hypercapnic respiratory failure. It can also be useful in treating hypoxic respiratory failure by enabling the administration of O_2-enriched inspired mixtures. In disorders of the respiratory apparatus in which the work of breathing is inordinately high, mechanical ventilation decreases the work and O_2 cost of breathing, thereby decreasing total metabolic need for O_2 and decreasing the CO_2 load to be eliminated by the lungs.

Physiologic measurements which typify the respiratory abnormalities in patients subjected to mechanical ventilation are summarized in Table 51-1. Not all of these measurements are indicated in a particular patient, and not all are equally useful in tracking the course of the patient. Certain of these measurements can be useful in one circumstance, whereas others are useful in other circumstances. Proper use of these measurements requires clinical judgment, and their trends are generally more significant than their absolute values.

TABLE 51-1 Some Physiological Derangements in Patients Subjected to Mechanical Ventilation

Parameter	Normal range	Mechanical ventilation indicated
Pulmonary Mechanics		
Vital capacity mL/kg	65–70	< 10–15 (or < 1.0 L)
FEV_1 mL/kg	50–60	< 10 (or < 0.5 L)
Inspiratory force, cmH_2O	80–100	< 20–30
Ventilation		
Respiratory rate, breaths/min	10–20	> 35
Tidal volume mL/kg	5–8	< 5
Minute ventilation L/min	5–8	> 10–15 (or > 50% of MVV)
Maximal voluntary ventilation (MVV), L/min	> 100	< 20
Pa_{CO_2}, mmHg	36–44	> 55 mmHg
pH	7.36–7.44	< 7.30
Oxygenation		
Sa_{O_2}, %	> 95	< 90 on maximal FI_{O_2}
Pa_{O_2}, mmHg	> 300	< 60 on maximal FI_{O_2}
$PA_{O_2} - Pa_{O_2}$, mmHg	25–65	> 350–450 on 100% FI_{O_2}

TYPES OF MECHANICAL VENTILATORS

Mechanical ventilators can be divided into two main types based on the method by which pressure is applied to achieve lung inflation: negative pressure and positive pressure.

Negative Pressure Ventilators

Negative pressure ventilators (tank ventilators or body suits) inflate the lungs by generating a subatmospheric pressure intermittently around the chest. Historically, they were the first to achieve widespread use in the treatment of patients with respiratory failure, particularly that due to poliomyelitis. Although these tank ventilators do obviate the need for endotracheal intubation, they have several limitations. The respiratory rate has to be set manually and readjusted manually; nursing care is difficult; the rigid enclosure around the patient's body may pose psychological problems; and an adequate minute ventilation can be difficult to achieve in the patient in whom airway resistance is very high or lung compliance is very low. Because of these problems, negative pressure ventilators are uncommonly used in the acute care setting. More often, they are used in patients with chronic respiratory failure secondary to neuromuscular disease.

Positive Pressure Ventilators

Positive pressure ventilators are now the mainstay of modern respiratory support. The lungs are inflated intermittently by applying positive pressure to the airways. These ventilators are divided into three groups according to the mechanism for terminating the flow of gas during inflation: pressure cycled, time cycled, and volume cycled.

Pressure cycled The earliest positive pressure machines were pressure cycled. In their simplest form, they allow gas to flow into the lungs until a preset pressure limit is reached; at that juncture, the flow of air into the lungs cuts off and the expiratory phase begins. However, because the imposed pressure is fixed, the inflow of gas ceases when the prefixed pressure is reached. Therefore, the volume delivered depends on changes in lung compliance and airway resistance. These ventilators are not well suited for hospitalized patients on continuous ventilator support in whom respiratory mechanics are changing. In addition, most pressure-cycled ventilators lack a mechanism by which the concentration of O_2 in inspired air can be controlled or a mechanism to enable the application of positive end-expiratory pressure. Therefore, their use has been reserved for *intermittent* positive pressure breathing (IPPB) therapy and for ventilation of stable comatose patients with relatively normal lungs who are ventilator dependent. The one exception is in the neonatal intensive care unit where, for a number of reasons, pressure-cycled ventilators are the preferred method of positive pressure ventilation.

Time cycled In a time-cycled ventilator, the inspiratory flow of gas is delivered for a preset inspiratory time. The tidal volume is set by adjusting the flow rate and inspiratory time. Although these machines can be used to manage seriously ill patients, the volume of gas delivered varies with changing respiratory mechanics.

Volume cycled Virtually all ventilators currently used for continuous respiratory support in adults are volume-cycled machines. They deliver a predetermined volume unless a specified (pop-off) pressure is exceeded. Because the volume delivered is fixed, the inspiratory pressure generated varies with the compliance and resistance characteristics of the patient and the ventilator circuit. The popularity of these machines resides in their capacity to deliver a fixed tidal volume despite fluctuating lung mechanics. Their effectiveness depends on the integrity of the closed circuit between machine and the airways; an air leak decreases the volume delivered to the lungs.

MODES OF POSITIVE PRESSURE VENTILATION

Distinction between different modes of ventilators is based on the timing and triggering of the breath delivered by the machine. The following modes are currently in use: controlled mechanical ventilation, assist-control ventilation, intermittent mandatory ventilation, and pressure support ventilation.

Controlled mechanical ventilation (CMV) During CMV, a preset volume of pressure is delivered at a predetermined rate regardless of the patient's effort. This method is extremely uncomfortable for the awake patient. Therefore, it is used almost exclusively in patients who are apneic as a result of brain damage, drug overdose, sedation, or muscle paralysis.

Assist-control ventilation (ACV) In this method, an inspiratory effort triggers the ventilator at a frequency set by the patient's spontaneous breathing rate. If the patient's spontaneous rate falls below a preset (back-up) rate, the machine will cycle automatically at the back-up rate, thereby ensuring a minimum minute ventilation. This method allows the patient to interact with the ventilator; from the viewpoint of the patient, it is more comfortable than CMV. ACV is the usual method for initiating mechanical ventilation.

Intermittent mandatory ventilation (IMV) This method combines spontaneous and mechanical ventilation. The patient's spontaneous breaths are supplemented by machine-delivered breaths. If the breaths from the ventilator are timed to coincide with spontaneous effort, the method is termed *synchronized IMV* (SIMV). This method allows the ventilator to assist the patient's spontaneous efforts without the risk of overventilation. Proponents of IMV envisage a decrease in adverse cardiovascular responses from positive end-expiratory pressure (PEEP), less barotrauma because of the use of lower mean airway pressures, a reduced need for patient sedation, a reduction in respiratory muscle fatigue, and more rapid weaning from mechanical ventilation. These putative benefits still await confirmation. At high rates of machine cycles, SIMV can be used for full support of the ventilation. More often, it is used at low rates for the partial support of the ventilation in the course of weaning.

Pressure support ventilation (PSV) This is a new method which has quickly gained widespread acceptance. With PSV, each spontaneous breath is augmented by a clinician-specified amount of positive pressure during inspiration. This inspiratory pressure support is maintained as long as the patient maintains a minimal inspiratory effort. Although the clinician sets the level of pressure support, the patient sets the respiratory rate, the flow rate, and inspiratory time. It has been suggested that PSV may improve respiratory muscle function and patient-ventilator synchrony. Although PSV requires the patient to initiate ventilation, it cannot adjust to variations in lung mechanics. Consequently, PSV is not suitable for patients with an unreliable ventilatory drive or variable airway resistance or pulmonary compliance. It is used most often as a weaning mode.

VENTILATOR SETTINGS

To optimize the delivery and exchange of gas, a number of parameters are adjusted during the operation of the ventilator by the clinician.

Fraction of oxygen in inspired air (FIO_2) At the onset of O_2 therapy, the FIO_2 is set at a high concentration (often at 1.0) to ensure adequate oxygenation. Subsequently, the FIO_2 is adjusted according to the results of arterial blood-gas analysis: the FIO_2 is chosen to maintain the arterial PO_2 > 60 mmHg or the O_2 saturation > 90%. This level of FIO_2 avoids certain adverse effects: tracheobronchitis, decreased mucociliary clearance, decreased macrophage function, and parenchymal tissue injury and fibrosis.

Tidal volume and "sighing" A tidal volume of 10 to 12 ml/kg of body weight is desirable. In the conscious spontaneous breathing individual, sighs or yawns prevent the development of atelectasis. Ventilators carry a sigh mode to hyperinflate the lungs periodically, i.e., to mimic a sigh. The patient should be sighed every few minutes at two to three times the tidal volume.

Respiratory rate The respiratory rate that is selected depends on the desired minute ventilation and the type of ventilator. In the patient who is breathing spontaneously and maintaining an adequate pH while on ACV, the back-up rate is set at 2 to 4 breaths per minute below the spontaneous rate; this back-up rate will offer protection in case the patient fails to trigger the ventilator. However, if the spontaneous ventilation is inadequate, the rate (and tidal volume) are set at a frequency that will produce a minute ventilation sufficient to maintain an acceptable pH. For the IMV mode, the ventilator is set at a rate close to that being used by the patient; subsequently, the rate can be decreased according to the clinical and laboratory status.

Inspiratory flow rate (IFR) Generally, an IFR of 40 to 60 L/min is ideal. A faster flow rate decreases inspiratory time and interferes less with venous return, but may cause less uniform distribution of tidal ventilation. In patients with airway obstruction, higher flow rates, by shortening inspiration and thus allowing more time for exhalation, can significantly reduce air trapping.

Inspiration-expiration ratio (I:E ratio) On some pressure-limited and time-cycled ventilators, the ratio of inspiratory to expiratory time can be adjusted. However, for volume-cycled ventilators, the I:E ratio is determined indirectly by setting the tidal volume, ventilator frequency, and IFR. In general, short I:E ratios are used to allow more time for exhalation and thus minimize air trapping and lower mean intrathoracic pressure.

Alarm (pop-off) pressure For volume-cycled ventilators, the peak airway pressure depends not only on the tidal volume, but also on the inspiratory flow rate, the airway resistance, and the compliance of the thorax. Typically, the pop-off pressure is set at 10 to 20 cmH$_2$O above the peak pressure observed during normal cycling. An isolated pop-off cycle is usually due to patient coughing or splinting and is of little concern. However, if the ventilator alarms sound repeatedly, the patient should be removed from the machine and manually ventilated while being evaluated for a complication: plugging of the endotracheal tube and trachea (by passing a suctioning catheter), increased airway resistance, or a pneumothorax.

Positive end-expiratory pressure   PEEP refers to the maintenance of positive (above atmospheric) pressure at the end of expiration. By opening collapsed airways and recruiting alveoli that would otherwise be atelectatic or fluid filled, the functional residual capacity and gas exchanging surface increase, thereby improving ventilation-perfusion relationships and arterial oxygenation. Although PEEP may redistribute pulmonary edema, it does not drive the excess fluid out of the lung. PEEP is used in patients with diffuse acute pulmonary disease who develop severe hypoxemia despite high, and potentially toxic, concentrations of inspired oxygen, e.g., the adult respiratory distress syndrome (ARDS), massive congestive heart failure, or diffuse pneumonia. It has not been shown to prevent ARDS or postoperative atelectasis. The major complications of PEEP generally occur at high inspiratory pressures and include decreases in cardiac output due to impaired venous return and barotrauma. Therefore, caution should be exercised in applying PEEP to patients with hypovolemia, low cardiac output, hypotension, and evidence of barotrauma or emphysematous lung disease.

NONCONVENTIONAL FORMS OF VENTILATION

Recently, a number of new modes of ventilation have been introduced into clinical practice. Among these are high-frequency ventilation (HFV) and inverse ratio ventilation.

High-Frequency Ventilation

HFV is a type of mechanical ventilation in which tidal volumes equal to, or less than, the dead space are breathed at frequencies between 60 and 3600 breaths per minute. Three types of HFV have been evaluated clinically: high-frequency positive pressure ventilation (HFPPV), high-frequency oscillation (HFO), and high-frequency jet ventilation (HFJV).

HFPPV can be applied using conventional positive pressure ventilators which administer tidal volumes of 200 to 300 ml, at rates ranging from 60 to 100 breaths per minute. In HFO, a very small volume (1 to 3 ml/kg) is moved in and out of the lung at high frequencies (500 to 3000 cycles per minute) by a piston pump. Finally, in HFJV, pulses (jets) of gas are delivered via a narrow catheter positioned in the endotracheal tube or trachea. HFV has been used for ventilator support of patients with hypoxemia due to lung injury or barotrauma. Despite theoretical advantages to HFV, it has not proved to be superior to conventional ventilation using PEEP with respect to physiologic parameters (accumulation of lung water, cardiovascular function, gas exchange), morbidity, and mortality.

Inverse Ratio Ventilation (IRV)

This is a ventilatory technique in which the I:E ratio is adjusted to be > 1. This contrasts with conventional mechanical ventilation in which the I:E ratio is < 1. During volume-cycled ventilation, IRV can be achieved by introducing an inspiratory pause to slow the rate of inspiratory gas flow; during pressure-cycled ventilation, the inspiratory time can be increased. It has been proposed that IRV improves oxygenation by, in effect, creating "auto-PEEP" and thus recruiting collapsed alveoli. Also, some reports indicate that IRV may improve oxygenation in patients with acute lung injury who have failed to respond to conventional I:E ratios or PEEP. However, the higher mean intrathoracic pressure during IRV may interfere with venous return and increase the risk of barotrauma. Also, IRV is often uncomfortable, therefore requiring sedation and paralysis.

DISCONTINUATION OF MECHANICAL VENTILATION (WEANING)

Removal of the patient from mechanical ventilation (weaning) should begin only when the patient's clinical state is stable and the indication(s) for mechanical ventilation have been resolved or brought under control. Certain key factors must be considered. The patient should be hemodynamically stable and not require the intravenous administration of vasopressors or inotropic medications. The patient should be able to trigger the ventilator if the machine is in an ACV mode or breathe spontaneously if the ventilator is in an IMV mode. Ideally, the patient should be awake and alert to cooperate maximally with weaning efforts. Fluid status, electrolytes, and pH should be in balance, and gas exchange should be adequate, i.e., PO_2 > 60 mmHg on an $FIO_2 \leq 0.5$.

In addition to the above, a number of measured and calculated indices are useful in predicting the outcome of attempts to discontinue mechanical ventilation. Indices generally predictive of success include: (1) resting minute ventilation $\leq$ 10 L/min; (2) a maximal voluntary ventilation $\geq 2\times$ minute ventilation; (3) vital capacity > 1 L; (4) a negative inspiratory pressure ≤ -30 cmH$_2$O; and (5) a spontaneous respiratory rate < 30 breaths per minute. Although these criteria are helpful, up to 30 percent of patients who fail to meet these criteria will still be able to be weaned from mechanical ventilation. Because these criteria were developed for patients requiring short-term ventilator support, they fall short of predicting success in patients on prolonged ventilator support.

Newer predictors of failure to wean continue to be proposed. Most recently, Yang and Tobin have proposed two new predictive indexes. The first is the ratio of respiratory frequency (f) to tidal volume (V_T), which provides a measure of the extent of rapid shallow breathing. The second index, termed CROP, integrates thoracic Compliance, respiratory Rate, arterial Oxygenation, and maximal inspiratory Pressure. Prospectively these were shown to be superior to traditional predictors of weaning outcome. Although promising, the general applicability of these criteria remains to be proven.

As noted above, an appreciable number of patients in whom weaning parameters predict failure to wean can be weaned. However, patients of this type need to be observed with extraordinary caution during the weaning process.

For the patients on short-term ventilatory support, particularly those with good weaning parameters, it is common practice to have the patient undergo a trial of spontaneous breathing through a T-piece circuit. During this T-piece trial, the patient's level of comfort, blood pressure, pulse, respiratory rate, electrocardiographic rhythm, oxygen saturation, and arterial blood-gas levels are monitored for signs of deterioration, particularly in the first 30 minutes. Signs of failure include an increase or decrease in diastolic blood pressure of 20 mmHg; an increase or decrease in heart rate of 30 beats per minute; an increase in respiratory rate of 10 breaths per minute; a decrease in O_2 saturation; the occurrence of arrhythmias; and the development of intolerable dyspnea or changes in mental status. If the patient can breathe spontaneously for 1 to 2 h, mechanical ventilation can be discontinued because the patient will probably not deteriorate acutely.

For individuals who fail a T-piece trial, or in whom the weaning parameters are poor, or who have required prolonged mechanical ventilation, the weaning process is more gradual. Currently there are three techniques of weaning that are in widespread use: T-piece weaning, IMV weaning, and pressure support weaning.

During *T-piece weaning,* the patient is placed intermittently on a T-piece circuit and allowed to breathe spontaneously; the duration of T-piece breathing is increased progressively based on patient response. T-piece weaning induces periods of stress separated by recovery periods of complete rest (ranging from 1 to 3 h). Although this strategy is conventional for weaning, the abrupt transition between ventilator support and spontaneous breathing may not be well-tolerated in some patients, e.g., those who are anxiety prone.

For *IMV weaning,* the ventilator is set in the IMV mode and the rate is progressively decreased, e.g., by 2 to 4 breaths per minute in accord with the patient's tolerance. In this way, the abrupt changes that occur with T-piece weaning are avoided, and the patient is allowed to gradually assume the burden of ventilation. However, depending on the ventilator, considerable work may be required during spontaneous breathing to initiate flow through the IMV circuit. Low levels of positive pressure support may help to eliminate the inspiratory work imposed by ventilator demand valves during IMV weaning.

Pressure support weaning represents the newest weaning technique. In this approach, a level of pressure is set that produces a targeted tidal volume. The pressure is then decreased gradually while ensuring that the tidal volume remains adequate. Patients tolerating pressure support of 5 cmH$_2$O are ready for extubation. This weaning mode is unsuitable for patients with variable respiratory drive or with fluctuating respiratory mechanics.

Although there has been much debate over the advantages and disadvantages of the different weaning techniques, currently no controlled randomized data indicate that any one strategy is superior to the others. Consequently, decisions regarding the technique used must reflect physician experience and the specific needs of the individual patient.

A number of factors may contribute to the inability to wean a patient. These include acid-base abnormalities, electrolyte depletion (calcium, potassium, magnesium, phosphate), inadequate or improper nutrition, hormonal imbalance (thyroid or steroid), deconditioning, excessive patient fear and anxiety, inadequate rest, and poor patient positioning. In the patient who is weaning poorly, these factors should be considered and corrected.

BIBLIOGRAPHY

For a more detailed discussion, see Lanken PN: Mechanical ventilation, in Fishman AP (ed), *Pulmonary Diseases and Disorders,* 2d ed. New York, McGraw-Hill, 1988, pp 2373–2386.

Hinson JR, Marini JJ: Principles of mechanical ventilator use in respiratory failure. Annu Rev Med 43:341–361, 1992.

MacIntyre NR: New forms of mechanical ventilation in the adult. Clin Chest Med 9:47–54, 1988.

Marini JJ: Recent advances in mechanical ventilation, in Fishman AP (ed), *Update: Pulmonary Diseases and Disorders.* New York, McGraw-Hill, 1992, pp 401–418.

Tobin MJ, Carlson RW, Gehab MA: Mechanical ventilation. Crit Care Clin 6:489–811, 1990.

Yang KL, Tobin MR: A prospective study of indexes predicting the outcome of trials of weaning from mechanical ventilation. N Engl J Med 324:1445–1450, 1991.

Richard Schwab

ENDOTRACHEAL TUBE COMPLICATIONS

Complications Relating to Tracheal Intubation

Mechanical ventilation can be associated with complications at each stage of the process: during intubation, while the endotracheal tube is in place, during extubation, and after extubation.

Complications During Intubation

Most complications that occur during intubation are attributable to inexperience in intubation. For example, intubation is apt to be unduly prolonged (> 2 to 3 minutes), or the right main-stem bronchus may be inadvertently intubated, leading to pneumothorax, alveolar hyperventilation, and atelectasis. Also, cardiac arrhythmias and pulmonary aspiration are common during intubation. Nasal bleeding and tooth avulsions may complicate nasal and oral intubation, respectively. A comparison of the pros and cons of orotracheal and nasotracheal intubation is presented in Table 52-1.

Complications with the Endotracheal Tube in Place

Injury to the larynx or trachea can develop while the endotracheal tube is in place. Both the tube and the cuff can damage the mucosa. Injury to the larynx usually manifests itself as laryngeal ulceration, edema or inflammation; tracheal injury occurs primarily at the cuff site but can also occur at the tip of the tube. Injury at the cuff site is secondary to ischemia of the tracheal mucosa which causes mucosal ulceration and necrosis; in turn, the local ulceration and necrosis may lead to tracheal stenosis. Occasionally a fistula develops between the trachea and esophagus resulting in gastric distention which can be dramatic.

Mechanical problems, including obstruction of the tube and disconnection from the ventilator, occurs in about 6 percent of intubated patients. Cuff leaks develop in about 20 percent of intubated patients. In the intensive-care unit, self-extubation occurs in about 13 percent of intubated patients.

The risk of pulmonary aspiration is always present while the endotracheal tube is in place, even though the cuff is adequately inflated. A simple and effective way of reducing the risk of aspiration is to maintain the patient in a semierect position, particularly during periods of enteral feeding.

TABLE 52-1 Comparison of Orotracheal and Nasotracheal Intubation

Orotracheal Intubation
  Advantages
    Direct laryngeal visualization
    Allows intubation with short large-bore tubes
    Easily suctioned
  Disadvantages
    Not easily fixed—mouth care difficult
    More difficult in awake patients
Nasotracheal Intubation
  Advantages
    Permits intubation without laryngeal visualization
    Tube is relatively fixed
    Good mouth care
    May be performed in awake patients with minimal sedation if adequate
      topical anesthesia is used
  Disadvantages
    Long small-bore tube may be necessary
    Success rate lower than with oral intubation
    Suctioning may be more difficult because of small bore or kinking
    May precipitate nosebleeds, erosion of alae nasi and nasal cartilages,
      and sinus infection

SOURCE: Geer RT: Intubation and management of the airways, in Fishman AP(ed), Pulmonary Diseases and Disorders, 2d ed. New York, McGraw-Hill, 1988, pp 2342.

Edema caused by an indwelling nasotracheal tube can lead to an acute purulent sinusitis by obstructing the ostia of the nasal sinuses, thereby impairing drainage. An unexplained fever is often the only sign of this complication. The diagnosis of an acute purulent sinus is most readily made by a computed tomography (CT) scan of the paranasal sinuses; conventional radiographs of the sinuses are often inadequate in critically ill patients because they cannot be positioned adequately. The presence of acute sinusitis calls for removal of the nasotracheal tube and either replacement by an orotracheal tube or a tracheostomy. A course of antibiotics should be initiated.

Complications During Extubation

Complications during extubation are infrequent. Stridor occurs in about 1 percent of patients after they are extubated; usually the stridor is secondary to laryngeal edema. If the laryngeal edema does not severely compromise the lumen of the upper airway, it can be treated conservatively with nebulized racemic epinephrine. However, if the stenosis is sufficiently severe to cause respiratory distress, reintubation has to be undertaken. Corticosteroids should then be continued for 24 to 48 h. When extubation is once again to be attempted, an experienced anesthesiologist and otolaryngologist should be at hand. In severe laryngeal stenosis, tracheostomy may be necessary to remove the endotracheal tube and to permit sufficient time for the edema and upper airway obstruction to subside.

Laryngeal spasm is responsible less often than laryngeal edema for postextubation stridor. In contrast to laryngeal edema, laryngospasm is a transient event which is rapidly reversed with positive pressure bagging. On rare occasion, the use of a short-acting neuromuscular blocking agent, e.g., succinylcholine, may be required to relieve laryngospasm.

Complications After Extubation

Hoarseness is the most common complication after extubation, occurring in up to 80 percent of patients; usually it resolves within a few days. Tracheal stenosis, usually at the cuff site, develops in up to 20 percent of patients after endotracheal intubation. In most instances, the tracheal stenosis is mild and does not cause clinically significant morbidity. However, stenosis sufficient to elicit clinically significant obstruction of the upper airway does occasionally occur. The risk of causing tracheal injury that leads to stenosis can be minimized by maintaining cuff pressures at < 25 mmHg.

Aspiration is a common and often unappreciated complication of the postextubation period. At this juncture, patients are prone to aspiration for a variety of reasons: ulceration and the resultant incomplete apposition of the vocal cords, impaired gag reflex, and vocal cord paralysis. In most patients, the withholding of oral feedings for 12 to 24 h will permit return of normal swallowing function. However, feedings should not be restarted until a normal gag reflex can be demonstrated. The first feeding should be under direct observation to ensure that the patient does not appear to be aspirating. If doubt remains, evaluation by a speech pathologist and by barium esophagram should be undertaken.

COMPLICATIONS ASSOCIATED WITH TRACHEOSTOMY

Operative complications associated with tracheostomy include postoperative bleeding, pneumothorax, and subcutaneous or mediastinal emphysema. Life-threatening complications of an indwelling tracheostomy tube include tracheoesophageal fistula and tracheoinnominate artery fistula. Tracheal stenosis remains the most serious complication after the tracheal cannula is removed. Most often, the stenosis occurs at the stomal site but it may also occur at the site of the cuff. The incidence of tracheal stenosis following tracheostomy ranges from 17 to 75 percent, the wide variation in incidence reflecting the varying criteria used to define stenosis.

The ideal time for tracheostomy in the intubated patient remains debatable. At many institutions, endotracheal tubes are left in place up to 3 weeks before tracheostomy is considered. The decision must be individualized and should take into account if the patient will soon be weaned from the mechanical ventilator; conversely, if it is anticipated that mechanical ventilation is to be prolonged, the tracheostomy need not be delayed in the hope of early extubation. The advantages and disadvantages of translaryngeal intubation and tracheostomy are compared in Table 52-2.

COMPLICATIONS ATTRIBUTABLE TO VENTILATOR MALFUNCTION

Malfunction of the ventilator or the tubing circuit can lead to complications of mechanical ventilation. So can human error. Mechanical failure can affect the components of the ventilator (alarms, compressor, control switches, or indicators) or the components of the breathing circuit (leaks in the tubing, malfunction of the exhalation valve, and disconnection of the circuitry). Electrical failure from overloaded circuits or electromagnetic interference can cause the ventilator to become inoperative. Many episodes of ventilator malfunction are caused by the inadvertent turn-off of

TABLE 52-2
Comparison of Translaryngeal Intubation and Tracheostomy

Translaryngeal Intubation
 Advantages
  A simple rapid procedure
  Avoids surgery
  Avoids stomal injury
 Disadvantages
  Less comfortable
  Causes laryngeal injury and late subglottic stenosis
  Causes injury to mouth, nose, and pharynx
  More difficult to suction
Tracheotomy
 Advantages
  More secure
  Easier suctioning and care
  Allows easier oral intake
  Permits speech
 Disadvantages
  Significant operative morbidity
  Higher incidence of lung infection
  Delayed morbidity, tracheal stricture, and hemorrhage

SOURCE: Geer RT: Intubation and management of the airways, in Fishman AP(ed), Pulmonary Diseases and Disorders, 2d ed. New York, McGraw-Hill, 1988, pp 2343.

alarms or human error. In most instances, equipment failure causes an alarm to be triggered. For example, a leak in the circuit or in the exhalation valve triggers the alarm for low exhaled volumes, whereas the alarm for high inspiratory pressure is triggered if the exhalation valve becomes stuck in the closed position. If the sensitivity of the ventilator is dialed down excessively, the ventilator may autocycle, causing relative hyperventilation. In *all* instances, if the ventilator is malfunctioning and the cause of the malfunction is not immediately obvious, the patient should be disconnected from the ventilator and ventilation maintained via a mask and resuscitation bag until the problem is corrected.

BAROTRAUMA

Pulmonary barotrauma, caused by the application of excessive positive pressure to the airways, causes rupture of overdistended alveoli and can result in one or more of the following: pulmonary interstitial emphysema (PIE), pneumomediastinum, subcutaneous emphysema, pneumoperitoneum, pneumopericardium, pneumothorax, and subpleural air cysts.

The earliest sign of barotrauma is usually manifested as the accumulation of extra-alveolar air in the interstitium of the lung, i.e., PIE. The radiographic findings of PIE include large and small parenchymal air cysts, linear streaks of air directed toward the hilum, circumferential air pockets around the pulmonary vessels, and enlarging subpleural air cysts. PIE should be considered a harbinger of pneumothorax and efforts exerted to prevent further barotrauma. Similarly, the presence of mediastinal, pericardial, or subcutaneous emphysema (which, per se, usually cause no harm to the patient) should all be regarded as portents of a subsequent pneumothorax. A pneumothorax which develops while on positive pressure ventilation can rapidly become a life-threatening event as pressure within the thorax exceeds atmospheric, i.e., a tension pneumothorax impairs cardiac filling, decreases cardiac output, and leads to systemic hypotension.

Another complication of barotrauma can be systemic air embolism which is manifested as a stroke, cardiac dysfunction, and livedo reticularis of the lower extremities.

The incidence of ventilator-induced barotrauma is about 15 percent (range of 4 to 48 percent). The factors responsible for ventilator-induced barotrauma include high peak and mean inspiratory airway pressures, large tidal volumes, high levels of positive end-expiratory pressure (PEEP), and hyperinflation of the lungs. The risk of barotrauma is high in patients with necrotizing pneumonia, adult respiratory distress syndrome (ARDS), and preexisting alveolar overdistention, such as asthma and emphysema.

The role of peak inspiratory pressure has been extensively studied as a risk factor for ventilator-induced barotrauma. In one study, primarily of patients with ARDS, the importance of the level of peak pressure was dramatically shown: 43 percent when the peak inspiratory pressures were > 70 cmH$_2$O, 8 percent when peak inspiratory pressures ranged from 50 to 70 cmH$_2$O, and zero when peak pressures were < 50 cmH$_2$O. In patients with normally compliant lungs, e.g., asthmatics, the risk of barotrauma appears to correlate more with the degree of hyperinflation of the lungs (see Auto-PEEP below) than with peak inspiratory pressures.

Strategies that avoid inordinate peak inspiratory pressures decrease the risk of barotrauma. These include sedation and paralysis of the patient, changing the ventilator mode (switching from assist-control to intermittent mandatory ventilation), reducing inspiratory flow rates (although this runs the risk of promoting hyperinflation), and smaller tidal volumes. In asthmatics, auto-PEEP can be minimized by prolonging expiration, along with *increasing* the inspiratory flow rate, decreasing the tidal volume, and decreasing the respiratory rate. If these relatively simple measures fail to limit inspiratory pressures or auto-PEEP, controlled hypoventilation can be used accompanied by the administration of sodium bicarbonate to maintain a tolerable blood pH.

The treatment of choice for pneumothorax is a tube thoracostomy. Intervention usually has to be rapid to prevent circulatory collapse. It is not uncommon for patients with ARDS to develop multiple, loculated pneumothoraces that require placement of multiple chest tubes. The use of prophylactic chest tubes in a patient with pulmonary barotrauma, but without a pneumothorax, is not recommended.

AUTO-PEEP

Auto-PEEP or intrinsic PEEP refers to the automatic maintenance by the patient of PEEP in the alveoli because they are incompletely emptied by the time that expiration is over. At high risk for developing auto-PEEP are patients with obstructive airways disease who are being mechanically ventilated or patients with other types of lung disease who are ventilated at high frequencies and tidal volumes. By manually occluding the expiratory port at end-exhalation, pressure throughout the system equilibrates so that the manometer will register the level of positive pressure in the alveoli, i.e., the level of auto-PEEP.

The physiological consequences of auto-PEEP are the same as those caused by ventilator-delivered PEEP. In particular, venous return to the heart is impeded, leading to inadequate filling pressures and diminished cardiac output. Importantly, the level of auto-PEEP is also superimposed on the pulmonary capillary wedge pressure, thereby artificially elevating it. Auto-PEEP is a treatable cause of hypotension. As indicated above with respect to minimizing peak inspiratory pressures, in the face of circulatory compromise, auto-PEEP should be minimized by prolonging the expiratory time (along with decreasing the respiratory rate and tidal volume, and increasing the inspiratory flow rate). Expansion of the circulating blood volume by administering fluids intravenously is also helpful in treating PEEP-induced systemic hypotension. Continued medical therapy to relieve airflow obstruction (bronchodilators, corticosteroids) is also an essential component of management.

NOSOCOMIAL PNEUMONIA

Nosocomial pneumonia is a common complication of mechanical ventilation, i.e., an incidence of approximately 30 percent. The major pathogenetic mechanism for nosocomial pneumonia in patients undergoing mechanical ventilation is colonization of the oropharynx and gastrointestinal tract, followed by aspiration into the tracheobronchial tree. Impaired cough and impaired mucociliary clearance add to the risk of infection. The risk of nosocomial pneumonia also appears to be enhanced by use of antacids and H_2-blockers which alkalinize the stomach and promote bacterial growth. Another mechanism for colonization and the development of nosocomial pneumonia is direct inoculation of the tracheobronchial tree from environmental sources, such as the endotracheal tube, the ventilator circuit, respiratory therapy equipment, or the hands of medical personnel. Because the condensate in the ventilator tubing can rapidly become colonized with gram-negative rods, the ventilator tubing should be changed every 24 to 48 h as a measure for preventing ventilator-associated pneumonia.

Recognition of nosocomial pneumonia in the ventilated patient can be problematic, particularly in the patient with ARDS in whom the underlying disease has produced widespread abnormalities on the chest radiograph. Although sputum cultures are frequently positive in mechanically ventilated patients, they fail to distinguish between colonization and infection. One strategy to circumvent this difficulty in bronchoscopy is with the use of a protected catheter brush or bronchoalveolar lavage, in concert with quantitative culture techniques. In principle, this approach can provide uncontaminated samples from the lower respiratory tract for the diagnosis of nosocomial pneumonia in the ventilated patient. However, further clinical studies are required to define the sensitivity and specificity of this technique.

One additional measure for preventing nosocomial pneumonia in patients on ventilators has been the use of antibiotics, administered prophylactically by the oral route or aerosolization, in the attempt to minimize tracheobronchial colonization. Another has been the use of gastrointestinal decontamination regimens. However, there is as yet no consensus about the effectiveness of these approaches.

MISCELLANEOUS MEDICAL COMPLICATIONS OF MECHANICAL VENTILATION

Inadvertent alveolar hyperventilation and hypoventilation commonly occur during mechanical ventilation. Frequent monitoring of arterial blood gases with adjustment of the machine-delivered minute ventilation can avoid these problems. Airway pressures generated by an agitated patient whose respiratory efforts are asynchronous with the ventilator (commonly referred to as "bucking the ventilator") frequently exceed the pressure ceiling of the ventilator, causing the breath delivered by the machine to end prematurely, thereby decreasing minute ventilation and leading to worsening hypercapnia. In this circumstance, sedation often restores patient-ventilator synchrony, permitting delivery of the appropriate minute ventilation and correcting hypercapnia. If sedation does not suffice, paralysis may be required.

Atelectasis is a frequent complication of mechanical ventilation. Often it is associated with intubation of a main-stem bronchus or retained secretions. Fluid retention, hyponatremia, and a reduction in urine output occur in patients on mechanical ventilation; these effects are generally related to the release of antidiuretic hormone and of atrial natriuretic factor and to a reduction in cardiac output secondary to positive pressure ventilation. Massive gastric distention can sometimes develop and should be decompressed by a nasogastric tube. Delayed gastric emptying (which may predispose to aspiration), ileus, gastrointestinal bleeding, and pseudo-obstruction are common occurrences in mechanically ventilated patients and can compromise enteral feedings. Finally, positive pressure ventilation can increase intracranial pressure in patients with central nervous system injury.

BIBLIOGRAPHY

For a more detailed discussion, see Geer RT: Intubation and management of the airways, in Fishman AP (ed), *Pulmonary Diseases and Disorders,* 2d ed. New York, McGraw-Hill, 1988, pp 2339–2346.

McCulloch TM, Bishop MJ: Complications of translaryngeal intubation. Clin Chest Med 12:507–521, 1991.

Pierson DJ: Complications associated with mechanical ventilation. Crit Care Clin 6:711–724, 1990.

Rivera R, Tibballs J: Complications of endotracheal intubation and mechanical ventilation in infants and children. Crit Care Med 20:193–199, 1992.

Harold I. Palevsky

Hemodynamic monitoring is an essential feature of the intensive care unit where it is used for determining the stability of the circulation, to signal the onset of deterioration, and to assess the efficacy of therapeutic interventions. Current enthusiasm for, and the widespread use of, hemodynamic monitoring has to be tempered with two caveats: (1) the less experienced the operator, the more likely the occurrence of complications; and (2) interpretation is not simply a matter of translating numbers into words; traps exist in the equipment, the techniques, the calculations, and in the final analysis.

SYSTEMIC ARTERIAL CATHETERIZATION

Patients who are hemodynamically unstable or who need frequent sampling of arterial blood for gases (more than four samples per 24 h) are candidates for an indwelling arterial cannula. Arterial cannulation affords three advantages over repeated arterial puncture: (1) continuous monitoring of systemic arterial blood pressure and access to arterial blood for gas analysis; (2) greater reproducibility of the results of blood-gas analyses; and (3) fewer complications.

Although catheters can be placed into a radial, brachial, axillary, femoral, or dorsalis pedis artery, the radial artery is usually used because of its accessibility and its ample collateral circulation. To ensure that the radial artery is not the dominant source of blood to the hand and that the collateral circulation to the hand will suffice if the radial artery should inadvertently be interrupted as a complication of arterial cannulation, an Allen's test is performed before cannulation. In this test, both the radial and ulnar arteries of the hand are compressed until the hand blanches; the ulnar artery is then released and the time required for return of color is noted. If reperfusion occurs within 5 s, the collateral circulation is adequate and the risk of distal ischemia is small, even if the radial artery should occlude. A reperfusion time of > 7 s indicates marginal collateral supply and dictates that another catheter site should be chosen. Once the adequacy of collateral circulation has been established, a small-bore Teflon catheter is inserted percutaneously into the artery and connected to the transducer using noncompliant tubing; the "line" also includes stopcocks for blood sampling and a flushing device that maintains patency of the system by continuous flow of heparinized saline.

There are two major complications of systemic arterial cannulation: bacteremia and ischemia of the hand (Table 53-1). The risk of

TABLE 53-1
Major Complications of Systemic Artery Catheterization

Infection: local and systemic
Vascular compromise: flow reduction, arterial occlusion, distal ischemia, and necrosis
Hematoma
Compressive neuropathy
Aneurysm or pseudoaneurysm
Arteriovenous fistula
Antegrade embolization of air or thrombus
Hemorrhage

bacteremia increases the longer the cannula is left in place; it also increases if surgical exposure of the vessel was used to insert the cannula and if the local area becomes infected. Although overt ischemia secondary to either thrombosis or embolization is uncommon (occurring in < 0.6% of arterial cannulations), reduced arterial blood flow to the hand or occult arterial occlusion is found in up to one half of arteries within 1 week after removing the catheter. Among the factors predisposing to ischema are preexisting peripheral vascular disease, systemic hypotension, and a low cardiac output. Others are the use of a wide-bore catheter for cannulation, a small artery (as in women and children), damage to the artery during insertion of the catheter (as often follows repeated attempts to introduce the catheter), and leaving the catheter in place for days. When catheters are left in place for 3 days or less, the incidence of reduced flow to the hand is 11 percent and local infection is rare. More than 4 days of cannulation is associated with an increasing incidence of both arterial occlusion and local infection. Nonetheless, because the process of introducing the catheter is associated with complications, it is generally preferable to leave a well-functioning, closely monitored catheter in place than to replace it. In some instances, an arteriovenous fistula forms, particularly if an adjacent vein has been cannulated or manipulated.

Antegrade embolization of air or thrombus occasionally occurs during catheter flushing. Also, accidental disconnection of the tubing from the arterial catheter can result in life-threatening blood loss, i.e., up to 500 ml/min.

CENTRAL VENOUS CATHETERIZATION

Central venous catheterization (with the catheter tip just proximal to the right atrium) is useful in providing a direct measure of the filling pressure of the right ventricle (right atrial pressure) and an access route for intravenous infusion of vasoactive agents and parenteral nutrients. However, a catheter lodged proximal to the right atrium, i.e., that stops short of the pulmonary artery, has little role in monitoring patients with cardiac or respiratory failure because it fails to provide several different types of hemodynamic information: (1) right ventricular afterload; (2) left ventricular filling pressures; and (3) mixed venous blood either for determining the cardiac output by the Fick principle or for determining the systemic arteriovenous difference in O_2 content.

PULMONARY ARTERIAL CATHETERIZATION

The flow-directed, balloon-tipped pulmonary arterial catheter (Swan-Ganz catheter) has revolutionized the monitoring of critically ill patients.

The Catheter

The balloon flotation (Swan-Ganz) catheter most often used is a triple-lumen, 110-cm catheter that is marked externally at 10-cm intervals. The lumens open respectively at the distal tip, 30 cm proximally, and into the flotation balloon adjacent to the catheter tip; when properly lodged in the pulmonary artery, the distal lumen opens into the pulmonary artery and the proximal lumen into the right atrium. Pressures can be recorded and samples can be drawn from each lumen separately. The standard catheter is also designed for determination of cardiac output by the thermodilution technique. For this purpose, a wire extending from a thermistor lead, 1 to 5 cm from the tip, leads externally to a cardiac output computer.

An essential feature of this self-guiding catheter is the latex balloon, adjacent to the tip, between 1.0 and 1.5 ml in capacity; it engulfs the tip when inflated, providing a large surface that minimizes the likelihood of endocardial irritation and arrhythmia. The balloon is inflated when the catheter tip has passed beyond the introducer and into a large vein of the thorax or an iliac vein. The balloon is inflated in the right atrium using a volume dictated by the manufacturer. The inflated balloon floats the catheter into the main pulmonary artery and then into one of the pulmonary arterial branches. Occlusion of a pulmonary arterial branch by the inflated balloon enables the pulmonary arterial wedge pressure (postocclusive balloon pressure) to be recorded. Modifications of the Swan-Ganz catheter provide for electrodes, either to record the intracavitary electrocardiogram (ECG) or to pace the heart, and for an oximetric system, using fiberoptics, to determine O_2 saturation.

Indications

Catheterization of the pulmonary artery is often indispensable for management of patients with acute respiratory distress syndrome

(ARDS), pulmonary hypertension, or cardiac instability after myocardial infarction; in contrast, it is generally unwarranted in uncomplicated myocardial infarction. It is often useful as a guide to achieving an important hemodynamic balance in patients who require the intravenous administration of fluids to sustain cardiac output and oxygen delivery to the tissues. On the one hand, the rate and volume of fluid are adjusted to sustain left ventricular filling pressures; on the other hand, the fluid load must not increase pulmonary capillary pressures to levels that run the risk of pulmonary edema. Although pulmonary artery catheterization does entail complications and risk (Table 53-2), the risk-benefit ratio of doing the procedure in appropriate patients is generally much more favorable than that of management without benefit of the hemodynamic data that the catheter provides.

Insertion

The catheter can be introduced percutaneously through the internal jugular, external jugular, subclavian, femoral, or antecubital (basilic system) veins (Table 53-3); a cutdown may be required if the catheter is to be introduced into an antecubital vein. The particular site chosen for catheterization is usually dictated by the prior experience of the operator and the availability of suitable veins.

The pulmonary artery can be catheterized at the bedside using the ECG to monitor for arrhythmias and pressure recording from the distal tip to identify the consecutive cardiac chambers traversed by the catheter, i.e., right atrium to right ventricle to pulmonary

---

TABLE 53-2 Major Complications of Pulmonary Artery Catheterization

Complications of central venous cannulation, i.e., pneumothorax, arterial puncture, air embolus

Infection: local and/or systemic

Thrombophlebitis: at insertion site, in central veins, in pulmonary artery

Pulmonary embolus

Pulmonary infarction: secondary to catheter migration and persistent wedging and/or pulmonary embolus

Ventricular arrhythmias: transient or persistent

Atrial arrhythmias

Right bundle branch block

Endocarditis: marantic and septic

Perforation or rupture of the pulmonary artery

Trauma to tricuspid apparatus with resultant insufficiency

Air embolus

Catheter knotting

Balloon rupture

TABLE 53-3
Choice of Venous Access for Right Heart Catheterization

Site	Advantages	Disadvantages	Approximate distance to right atrium
Internal jugular vein	Large vein, easy to cannulate Constant anatomy Easy to float catheter (especially from right side) Best approach for patient on mechanical ventilator	Risk of pneumothorax (less than subclavian approach) Thoracic duct injury Carotid puncture	15–20 cm
Subclavian vein	Large vein, easy to cannulate Constant anatomy Easy to float catheter (especially from left side)	Risk of pneumothorax Hemothorax Thoracic duct injury Subclavian artery puncture	15–20 cm
Antecubital vein (basilic system)	Safest method if patient anticoagulated or if bleeding diathesis Patient need not be supine for vascular access	Difficulty entering intrathoracic vein Venospasm Phlebitis Limited reuse of vein Spontaneous wedging	40 cm from right side 50 cm from left side
Femoral vein	Large vein, easy to cannulate	May require fluoroscopy to float catheter Risk of infection Risk of thrombophlebitis	30 cm

artery (Fig. 53-1). The right ventricle should be traversed as quickly as possible because delay of the catheter tip in this chamber increases the prospect of triggering a serious arrhythmia. If the right atrium or ventricle is dilated, if the tricuspid valve is insufficient, or if pulmonary arterial hypertension is present, fluoroscopy may be needed to direct the catheter tip through the heart. A chest radiograph is obtained after the insertion to confirm the final position of the catheter.

After the inflated balloon has lodged in a distal pulmonary arterial branch, certain criteria are useful in establishing that the catheter is properly wedged: (1) the catheter system flushes freely; (2) a distinctive low amplitude waveform appears promptly when the balloon is inflated and reverts quickly to a pulmonary arterial

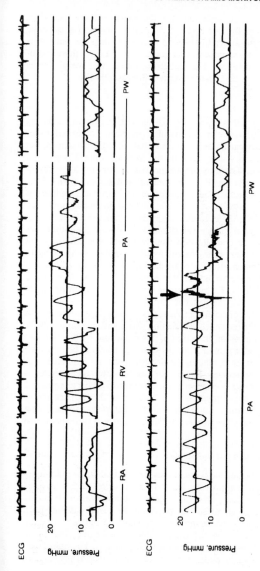

FIG. 53-1 Continuous ECG and pressure tracing during placement of a pulmonary artery catheter. *Top:* Pressures are recorded sequentially as the catheter is advanced from the right atrium (RA), right ventricle (RV), and pulmonary artery (PA) into wedge position (PW). *Bottom:* Inflation of the catheter balloon (arrow) is accompanied by a change in the contour and level of pressure. Horizontal lines at the end of the PA and PW tracings are mean pressures.
SOURCE: Palevsky HI, Fishman AP: Hemodynamic monitoring in acute respiratory failure. *Pulmonary Diseases and Disorders,* 1988, p 2351.

pressure tracing on deflation; (3) the mean balloon occlusion pressure is lower than or equal to the pulmonary arterial diastolic pressure; and (4) arterialized blood aspirated while the balloon is inflated has an O_2 saturation that is equal to or higher than that of systemic arterial blood. The catheter position, i.e., wedge versus pulmonary artery, can also be verified fluoroscopically.

Complications

Ventricular arrhythmias, usually self-limited, are common during insertion of the catheter. Ventricular premature contractions or ventricular tachycardia occur in up to half of catheterizations, but treatment for arrhythmias is required in fewer than 3 percent of catheterizations. The most important risk factors for arrhythmias are arterial hypoxemia ($Po_2 < 60$ mmHg) and acidosis (pH < 7.0).

Pulmonary infarction can follow either prolonged or spontaneous wedging of the catheter or a catheter-induced pulmonary embolus.

Inflation of the balloon after the catheter has moved out into a pulmonary arterial branch can damage or rupture the pulmonary arterial branch, a complication usually heralded by the onset of hemoptysis. Rupture of the catheter balloon makes it impossible to wedge the catheter. It also engenders the risk of air embolus if attempts are made to inflate the ruptured balloon. A ruptured balloon can be extremely dangerous if right-to-left shunting allows injected air to enter the systemic circulation.

Infections are common complications of indwelling catheters. As noted above, the incidence of infection varies with the time that the catheter is left in place. In addition, it is influenced by the extent to which the catheter is manipulated. Although bacterial colonization of the catheter is common, occurring in up to 35 percent of catheterizations, spiking fevers that resolve after the catheter is removed occur in 8 percent of catheterizations and bacteremia in 2 percent. Scrupulous attention to the sterility of the catheter and of the insertion site and prompt removal of catheters that are no longer clinically necessary help to decrease the incidence of catheter-related infection.

Measurements and Determinations

Table 53-4 indicates the types of measurements that the pulmonary arterial catheter can provide. Right atrial pressure can be measured by using the proximal port of the catheter; pulmonary arterial systolic, diastolic, and mean pressures, by using the distal catheter port. Cardiac output is determined by applying the indicator-dilution principle, generally by the thermodilution technique; less often, cardiac output is determined by the Fick principle. The pulmonary arterial occlusion or wedge pressure (discussed below) provides an

TABLE 53-4
Measurements Obtained with a Pulmonary Arterial Catheter

Pressures
Right atrial pressure
Right ventricular pressures
Pulmonary artery pressures (systolic, diastolic, mean)
Pulmonary artery occlusion or wedge pressure
Flow
Cardiac output
Blood Sampling
Mixed venous blood
Pulmonary capillary blood (wedge catheter)
Consecutive cardiac chambers for evidence of shunts, e.g., abrupt increase in oxygenation

estimate of left ventricular filling pressure. From these measurements, and the hemodynamic and blood-gas determinations obtained via systemic arterial catheterization, the basic physiologic parameters of cardiovascular function can be calculated (Table 53-5).

Pulmonary arterial wedge pressure In normal individuals, the balloon occlusion (wedge) pressure approximates left atrial pressure (Pla) and left ventricular end-diastolic pressure (LVEDP). The wedge pressure is most often used as an estimate of left ventricular preload. However, discrepancies between the wedge pressure recorded distal to an inflation balloon and mean Pla occur in several situations: (1) obstruction of the pulmonary veins by tumor, vasculitis, or mediastinal fibrosis; (2) in diseases in which abnormally high airway pressures are transmitted to the vascular bed, e.g., obstructive airway disease; and (3) during positive pressure ventilation, especially with the use of positive end-expiratory pressure (PEEP). In conditions that alter the relationship between Pla and LVEDP, e.g., mitral stenosis, the wedge pressure will also no longer reflect LVEDP.

It is worth emphasizing that even in the normal lung, the wedge pressure only provides a meaningful measure of Pla in that part of the lung operating under zone 3 conditions (Fig. 53-2), i.e., when the column of blood between the balloon and the pulmonary vein is continuous. As a rule, the flow-directed catheter floats into an area that satisfies the hemodynamic criteria for zone 3. However, therapeutic interventions can change the boundaries of zone 3, e.g., a diuresis that decreases the pulmonary venous pressure or positive pressure ventilation using PEEP that enlarges zones 1 and 2 at the expense of zone 3.

Certain characteristics of the wedge pressure tracing can arouse suspicion that the catheter is not lodged in zone 3: (1) pronounced variations in the wedge tracing accompanying changes in respiratory pattern; (2) the absence of cardiac events in the wedge tracing, e.g.,

TABLE 53-5
Calculations Based on Pulmonary Artery Catheter Measurements

Cardiac Index (L/min/m^2)

$CI = \dfrac{\dot{Q}_T}{BSA}$, where $\dot{Q}_T$ is cardiac output in L/min and BSA (body surface area) is in m^2.

Pulmonary Vascular Resistance (dyn • s / cm^5)

$PVR = \dfrac{\overline{P}pa - \overline{P}w}{\dot{Q}_T} \times 79.9$,

where $\overline{P}pa$ is mean pulmonary arterial pressure in mmHg; $\overline{P}w$ is mean pulmonary wedge pressure in mmHg; $\dot{Q}_T$ is cardiac output in L/min; 79.9 is a conversion factor for adjusting to the proper units (dyn • s / cm^5).

Systemic Vascular Resistance (dyn • s / cm^5)

$SVR = \dfrac{\overline{P}pa - \overline{P}ra}{\dot{Q}_T} \times 79.9$,

where $\overline{P}a$ is mean systemic arterial pressure in mmHg; $\overline{P}ra$ is mean right atrial pressure in mmHg; is cardiac output in L/min; 79.9 is a conversion factor for adjusting to the proper units (dyn • s / cm^5).

Stroke Volume Index (ml/beat/m^2)

$SVI = \dfrac{\dot{Q}_T/HR}{BSA}$, where $\dot{Q}_T$ is cardiac output in ml/min; HR is heart rate in beats per minute; and BSA is body surface area in m^2.

Right Ventricular Stroke Work Index (g • m/m^2)

$RVSWI = SVI \times (\overline{P}pa - \overline{P}w) \times 0.0136$,

where SVI is stroke volume index in ml/beats/m^2; $\overline{P}pa$ is mean pulmonary arterial pressure in mmHg; $\overline{P}w$ is mean pulmonary wedge pressure in mmHg; and 0.0136 is a conversion factor for adjusting to the proper units (g • m/m^2).

Left Ventricular Stroke Work Index (g • m/m^2)

$LVSWI = SVI \times (\overline{P}a - \overline{P}ra) \times 0.0136$,

where SVI is stroke volume index in ml/beat/m^2; $\overline{P}a$ is mean systemic arterial pressure in mmHg; $\overline{P}ra$ is mean right atrial pressure in mmHg; and 0.0136 is a conversion factor for adjusting to the proper units (g • m/m^2).

Arteriovenous Difference in O$_2$ Content (Vols %)

$(a - v) Do_2 = Cao_2 - Cvo_2$, where O_2 content = (Hgb $\times$ 1.34 $\times$ % saturation) + 0.0031 $\times$ Po_2 for both arterial (Cao_2) and mixed venous (Cvo_2) specimens.

Shunt Fraction (%)

$\dfrac{\dot{Q}_S}{\dot{Q}_T} = \dfrac{Cco_2 - Cao_2}{Cco_2 - C\overline{v}o_2}$, where Cc$o_2$ is pulmonary capillary O_2 content; Cao_2 is systemic arterial O_2 content; and C$\overline{v}o_2$ is mixed venous O_2 content.

Fick Equation for Cardiac Output (L/min)*

Systematic Blood Flow = $\dfrac{\dot{V}o_2}{Cao_2 - C\overline{v}o_2}$,

TABLE 53-5   (*Continued*)

where $\dot{V}_{O_2}$ is oxygen consumption in ml/min; Ca_{O_2} is systemic arterial O_2 content in ml/L; and $C\bar{v}_{O_2}$ is mixed venous O_2 content in ml/L.

$$\text{Pulmonary Blood Flow} = \frac{\dot{V}_{O_2}}{Cpv_{O_2} - Cpa_{O_2}},$$

where, $\dot{V}_{O_2}$ is oxygen consumption in ml/min; Cpv_{O_2} is pulmonary venous O_2 content in ml/L; and Cpa_{O_2} is pulmonary arterial O_2 content in ml/L.

*If a measured O_2 consumption is used in the calculation, this is a Fick determination of cardiac output. If O_2 consumption is estimated, then the calculation provides an "estimated" determination of cardiac output using the Fick principle.

The difference between pulmonary blood flow and systemic blood flow can be used to detect the presence of left-to-right intracardiac shunt.

---

a waves or *v* waves; (3) a higher wedge pressure than the pulmonary arterial diastolic pressure; and (4) an inordinate increase in wedge pressure as PEEP is applied, i.e., the wedge pressure increases by 50 percent of the imposed increment in PEEP.

PEEP has multiple effects on cardiac function and the wedge pressure. PEEP often depresses cardiac output, in part by interfering with venous return. Also, it is transmitted in variable degree to the wedge pressure measurement.

Finally, PEEP raises peri-pericardial pressure, thereby decreasing the left ventricular transmural pressure. The increase in the peri-pericardial pressure causes the left ventricle to act as though it were less compliant, even though its inherent mechanics have not changed. As a result, both end-diastolic pressure in the left ventricle (referred to atmospheric pressure) and wedge pressure increase, suggesting myocardial depression either due to PEEP or to the underlying disorder, e.g., ARDS. The increased peri-pericardial pressures and the limited distensibility of the ventricular wall can cause the recorded wedge pressure to be dependent on the heart rate : during *bradycardia,* wedge pressure along with left ventricular end-diastolic volume (LVEDV) and LVEDP are relatively high; during *tachycardia,* wedge pressure, LVEDV, and LVEDP are relatively low.

Effects of changes in intrathoracic pressure   Clinically, pulmonary vascular pressures are measured with respect to atmospheric pressure rather than to intrathoracic pressure. Consequently, changes in intrathoracic pressure are superimposed on pulmonary vascular pressures. In normal individuals who are free of obstructive airway disease and are not undergoing positive pressure ventilation, the intrathoracic pressure at end-expiration returns virtually to atmospheric pressure. Therefore, measurement of pulmonary arterial pressure at end-expiration provides not only a measure of pulmonary arterial luminal pressure, i.e., with respect to atmospheric

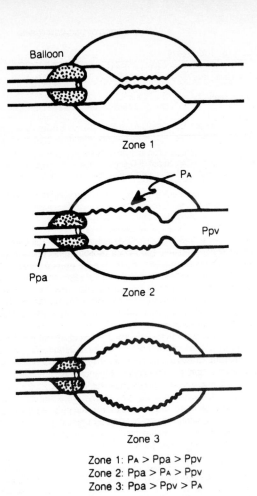

Zone 1: $P_A > Ppa > Ppv$
Zone 2: $Ppa > P_A > Ppv$
Zone 3: $Ppa > Ppv > P_A$

FIG. 53-2 Effect of the location of the tip of the pulmonary artery catheter with respect to vascular and aveolar pressures. In zones 1 and 2 the alveolar pressure (P_A) exceeds the pulmonary venous pressure (Ppv) interrupting the column of blood from the catheter to the left heart; pulmonary wedge pressure will reflect alveolar and not pulmonary venous/left heart pressures. Only in zone 3, where pulmonary arterial pressure (Ppa) and Ppv are greater than P_A will the wedge pressure represent vascular pressure accurately.
SOURCE: Palevsky HI, Fishman AP: Hemodynamic Monitoring in acute respiratory failure. *Pulmonary Diseases and Disorders*, 1988, p 2355.

pressure, but also of the pulmonary arterial pressure with respect to intrathoracic pressure (distending or transmural).

In diseases in which intrathoracic pressures undergo inordinate swings during the respiratory cycle, e.g., obstructive airway disease, or in which the lungs may be noncompliant and breathing is rapid and shallow, e.g., widespread interstitial disease, measurements of pulmonary arterial pressures that are made in the conventional clinical way, i.e., with respect to atmospheric pressure, should be made at end-expiration when pleural pressures most closely approximate atmospheric pressure. However, even this approximation is often inaccurate during severe tachypnea or in obstructive airway disease, e.g., in asthma; in the latter, high intrathoracic pressures persist even at end-expiration. It is possible (but rarely done) to obtain an estimate of intrathoracic pressure by using an esophageal balloon.

The imposition of PEEP during mechanical ventilation also increases intrathoracic pressure which remains positive at end-expiration; it induces a proportional increment in pulmonary arterial pressure measured with respect to atmospheric pressure (luminal pressure). Although it might seem desirable to interrupt PEEP for the sake of determining accurately the luminal pulmonary vascular pressures, there are several reasons why this should not be done: (1) the unstable hemodynamic values which are obtained immediately after discontinuation of PEEP and mechanical ventilation are difficult to interpret; (2) the abrupt decrease in intrathoracic pressure after PEEP is discontinued causes an acute increase in venous return, in effect, an autotransfusion; and (3) the arterial hypoxemia that often follows the discontinuance of PEEP can persist for a long while after PEEP is reinstituted.

For clinical purposes, it is worth remembering that PEEP decreases transmural left ventricular forces and increases the wedge pressure. Also, during PEEP, *consecutive* changes in wedge pressures are more helpful than is any single determination of pulmonary vascular pressure in following the course of the patient and the effects of therapeutic interventions.

Cardiac output: thermodilution In normal individuals, the thermodilution technique provides accurate and reproducible measurements of cardiac output. However, in certain diseases, the validity of cardiac outputs determined in this way can be seriously compromised: (1) a low cardiac output; (2) tricuspid regurgitation, pulmonic regurgitation, or shunts; and (3) large respiratory variations in intrathoracic pressure, and the accompanying fluctuations in venous return and cardiac output unless determinations are made at a preset point in the respiratory cycle. Not only accuracy, but also reproducibility, can be a problem in cardiopulmonary disorders. In practice, variability in the results obtained by the thermodilution techniques has been decreased by averaging the results of three consecutive determinations that vary by no more than 15 percent and that are obtained at similar points in the respiratory cycle.

Mixed venous oxygenation and cardiac output by the Fick principle
A catheter in the pulmonary artery also makes it possible to sample mixed venous blood for determinations of O_2 content and partial pressures (Po_2). The mixed venous blood samples can be used in conjunction with systemic arterial samples to determine cardiac output by the Fick principle (see Table 53-5); oxygen consumption, i.e., the numerator of the equation, is either measured directly or, more often, estimated on the basis of prediction formulae.

Every now and then for the past 50 years, it has been proposed that the O_2 saturation of mixed venous blood can suffice not only as an index of the cardiac output, but also for assessing the adequacy of tissue oxygenation. However, this practice has proved to be unreliable in a multitude of clinical states, e.g., ARDS, sepsis, and after cardiac surgery. At least part of the unreliability is associated with increased sympathetic activity or alterations in the distribution of blood flow to systemic tissues and organs. In brief, the mixed venous oxygenation is only one element in the Fick equation and cannot be reliably substituted for the entire equation either for the determination of the cardiac output or as a reflection of the adequacy of tissue oxygenation.

Calculations of vascular resistance Hemodynamic measurements that have proved useful in a variety of clinical circumstances are shown in Table 53-5. One of these is vascular resistance. The same generic elements enter into the calculation of systemic and pulmonary vascular resistance. Although the denominator (cardiac output) is the same in both, the components of the numerator (the inflow and outflow pressures) are different.

Calculation of vascular resistance is essential for managing patients with abnormal vascular pressures and blood flows and for guiding interventions. For example, raising systemic arterial blood pressure by using vasopressors gains little if the systemic vascular resistance is already high; in this circumstance, increasing the circulating blood volume or reducing cardiac afterload by administering vasodilators is apt to be of greater benefit.

BIBLIOGRAPHY

For a more detailed discussion, see Palevsky HI, Fishman AP: Hemodynamic monitoring in acute respiratory failure, in Fishman AP (ed), Pulmonary Diseases and Disorders, 2d ed. New York, McGraw-Hill, 1988, pp 2347–2360.

Iberti TJ, Fischer EP, Leibowitz AB, Panacek EA, Silverstein JH, Alberson TE, and the Pulmonary Artery Catheter Study Group: A multicenter study of physicians' knowledge of the pulmonary artery catheter. JAMA 264:2928–2932, 1990.

Marino PL (ed): Invasive hemodynamic monitoring, section III, in *The ICU Book*. Malvern PA, Lea and Febiger, 1991, pp 98–128.

Ornato JP: Hemodynamic monitoring during CPR. Ann Emerg Med 22:289–295, 1993.

Nutritional Therapy in Acute Respiratory Failure

Alfred P. Fishman

Individuals who are chronically short of breath, e.g., patients with chronic obstructive pulmonary disease (COPD), tend to be chronically malnourished. Should such individuals have to undergo surgery, preoperative feeding will strikingly reduce the frequency of respiratory complications. Even worse off with respect to nutrition is the critically ill patient in the intensive care setting where the patient is being mechanically ventilated while undergoing life-sustaining interventions. These patients are often malnourished not only because of diminished food intake, but also because of an increased turnover of fats, proteins, and carbohydrates that results in a catabolic state.

Biologically active mediators released during injury and stress aggravate the metabolic derangements. Increased gluconeogenesis, hyperglycemia, and hyperinsulinemia are also part of the imbalances created by critical illness. One threat arising from the malnutrition and metabolic upset is weakness of the respiratory muscles which, in turn, paves the way to respiratory failure and promotes dependency on assisted ventilation. The aim of nutritional support is to satisfy the caloric and protein needs of the body while avoiding serious negative nitrogen imbalance.

However, one major pitfall in the attempt to restore metabolic balances by nutritional support is overfeeding which, by increasing CO_2 production, automatically increases the need for a greater minute ventilation by a respiratory apparatus that is always overtaxed.

NUTRITIONAL THERAPY IN RESPIRATORY FAILURE

Nutritional support has become commonplace in hospitalized patients. As a rule, it is supervised by specialists and tailored to the particular disease and its pathophysiologic mechanisms, e.g., chronic renal failure, diabetes mellitus, and others. A supplement that is nutritionally complete includes sources of calories, protein, and micronutrients, e.g., minerals and vitamins. In many critically ill patients, energy (caloric) expenditure is considerably increased. This increase is manifested by an increase in oxygen consumption and carbon dioxide production which, in turn, increase the ventilatory drive and the work of breathing. The risk posed by an intrinsic increase in carbon dioxide production must be kept in mind when formulating nutritional support for the patient in respiratory failure.

ESTIMATION OF NUTRITIONAL REQUIREMENTS

Predictive formulas for nutritional needs are much more reliable for normal, healthy adults than for critically ill patients. Although energy needs can be estimated from measurements of O_2 uptake and CO_2 production, it is rarely practical to make such measurements in the intensive care setting. Quantitative guides, such as indirect calorimetry (for energy needs) and nitrogen balance studies (for protein balance), are usually impractical in the critical care setting. Nor are certain popular clinical indices, such as the thickness of skin folds or daily weights, apt to be helpful because they may reflect fluid balance rather than nutritional status. In contrast, a total lymphocyte count < $1200/m^3$ suggests a poor nutritional status.

Nonetheless, nutritional support can be provided using empirical guidelines rather than precise measurements. Although different clinics use somewhat different guidelines, the following generalizations may be helpful in dealing with nutritional support in the critically ill patient who is verging on respiratory failure. (1) Total caloric needs are estimated as the sum of baseline energy requirements, plus an estimated increment in calories attributable to the clinical state of the patient. For example, based on the estimate that the critically ill patient requires caloric intake to satisfy twice the baseline energy expenditure, 3000 kcal per day might be administered. (2) To avoid an inordinate increase in CO_2 production resulting from the nutritional support, the ratio of carbohydrates to fats can be kept at about 50:50, i.e., an increase in the fat content of conventional formulas at the expense of carbohydrates. (3) Since proteins do not enter into the calculation of energy balance, they are dealt with separately. The amount of proteins administered per day is based on the estimated degree of negative protein balance. For a previously healthy adult without inordinate protein loss, a reasonable estimate would be about 0.75 to 1.0 g/kg per day. (4) Adjustments to the protein component of the formula can be made on subsequent days by determining levels of short-lived circulating proteins, i.e., those with half-lives of hours rather than days. Two proteins that are useful in this regard are thyroxine-binding globulin and retinol-binding protein. Levels of serum albumin or transferrin are of little help because the turnover rate of albumin is slow.

STARTING NUTRITIONAL SUPPORT IN RESPIRATORY FAILURE

The Start of Nutritional Support

Nutritional support is generally begun within 24 to 48 h after the start of a critical illness that is expected to last for more than a few days. Feeding may be enteral or parenteral, depending on the circumstances. A variety of commercial products are available as nutritional supplements.

Enteral feeding, even if used only for partial nutritional support, is preferable whenever possible. It entails the introduction of a nasogastric tube (weighted, polymeric, silicone) so that the tip is in the duodenum or jejunum; to minimize the threat of aspiration, the tip is not left in the stomach. In the mechanically ventilated patient, fluoroscopic guidance of the tube (containing a stylus) is used to avoid entering the lung or pleura.

Parenteral feeding is used when enteral feeding is impractical. For this purpose, total parenteral nutrition is administered via a central venous catheter. The basic solution used for parenteral nutrition consists of a mixture of amino acids and dextrose; lipids are usually infused separately but are sometimes incorporated into the amino acid-dextrose solution. Other ingredients, such as vitamins and trace elements, are added in accord with the patient's needs. Overfeeding should be zealously avoided. The possible complications of central venous catheterization always have to be kept in mind: pneumothorax, air embolism, hemothorax, and myocardial perforation.

COMPLICATIONS OF NUTRITIONAL MISALIGNMENTS IN RESPIRATORY FAILURE

Caution is required to avoid certain side effects that are of particular concern in patients with acute respiratory failure. (1) As noted above, excessive carbohydrates engender the risk of inordinate increments in CO_2 production in a patient in whom CO_2 production is already high because of the increased work of breathing. Also as noted, the likelihood of this complication can be minimized by increasing the proportion of fats at the expense of carbohydrates. (2) Administration of excess fluid entails the risk of heart failure and pulmonary edema. To avoid fluid overload, more concentrated solutions are often preferable. For example, depending on the patient's age and clinical state, a formula that provides 2 cal/ml may be preferable to more dilute preparations. (3) The likelihood of tracheobronchial aspiration in the patient who is being fed enterally can be reduced by elevating the head of the bed for at least 2 h after a bolus feeding. Aspiration is a continuing threat during enteral feeding. For example, aspiration can still occur after duodenogastric reflux—even if the tube ports are in the duodenum.

In addition to these particular complications of nutritional therapy in the patient in respiratory failure, the patient is vulnerable to other side effects that are inherent in nutritional support by either the enteral or parenteral routes. Among these are hyperglycemia and hyperosmolality, electrolyte disturbances, e.g., hypophosphatemia, deficiency of vitamins and trace minerals, and azotemia.

BIBLIOGRAPHY

For a more detailed discussion, see Askanazi J, Mullen JL: Nutrition and acute respiratory failure, in Fishman AP (ed), *Pulmonary Diseases and Disorders,* 2d ed. New York, McGraw-Hill, 1988, pp 2387–2396.

Bursztein S, D'Attellis NP, Askanazi J: Nutrition and the respiratory system, in Hall JB, Schmidt GA, Wood LD (eds), *Principles of Critical Care.* New York, McGraw-Hill, 1992, pp 1093–1097.

Gonzalez-Huix F, Fernandez-Banares F, Esteve-Comas M, Abad-Lacruz A, Cabre E, Acero D, et al: Enteral versus parenteral nutrition as adjunct therapy in acute ulcerative colitis. Am J Gastroenterol 88:227–232, 1993.

Richard Schwab

GENERAL

Trauma is the third leading cause of death in the United States, and chest trauma accounts for 25 percent of these deaths. Most cases of blunt chest trauma are secondary to motor vehicle accidents or falls. Penetrating chest injuries, usually secondary to a gunshot or stab wound, have a lower mortality than blunt chest injuries and are less likely to have multisystem involvement.

The initial treatment of any patient with chest trauma requires basic resuscitative management, i.e., the ABCs—airway, bleeding, and circulation. The airway needs to be carefully evaluated because it can be obstructed at any point between the lips and bronchi. Trauma patients may develop respiratory failure requiring mechanical ventilation secondary to compromise of the chest wall (flail chest) or pulmonary parenchyma (lung contusion or aspiration). Tube thoracostomy should be performed in all patients with a hemothorax or pneumothorax. Adequate intravascular volume must be maintained with blood, colloid, or crystalloid.

PENETRATING CHEST WALL INJURIES

Penetrating chest injuries usually result from gunshot or stab wounds. Over 85 percent of these wounds result in peripheral pulmonary injuries that can be managed conservatively using chest tubes and volume replacement. Surgical intervention is necessary only if one of the following conditions exists: (1) persistent hemorrhage from the lung; (2) esophageal perforation; (3) cardiac and/or great vessel perforation; and (4) tracheobronchial rupture. If the injury (either gunshot or stab wound) entered or exited below the tip of the scapula or the nipple, injury to intra-abdominal viscera must be considered. In these situations laparotomy or peritoneal lavage should be performed.

CHEST WALL FRACTURES

Rib fractures Rib fractures are common in victims of blunt trauma. In general, rib fractures involve the fourth through ninth ribs along the posterior axillary line, most often on the left. The diagnosis usually can be made with a standard chest radiograph but occasionally rib films are required.

Approximately two thirds of patients with blunt chest trauma and rib fractures have accompanying injuries, most commonly pneumothorax or hemothorax. Upper rib fractures are associated with aortic, tracheobronchial, or pulmonary parenchymal injuries, whereas lower rib fractures are more apt to be associated with lacerations of the kidney, spleen, and liver. However, even isolated rib fractures can cause significant mortality and morbidity, particularly in elderly patients and those with underlying pulmonary disease. Atelectasis, pneumonia, and respiratory failure can result from the pain, splinting, and ineffective cough associated with rib fractures.

Management of rib fractures involves minimizing the pain and splinting, while promoting good pulmonary toilet. Strapping the chest with adhesive bandages to reduce pain from rib fractures may hinder ventilation and worsen atelectasis. Moderate to severe chest pain can be treated with local injection of long-acting anesthetic agents to block the associated intercostal nerves. Certain types of rib fractures result in specific complications, as detailed below.

First rib fractures The first rib is difficult to fracture because it is short, wide, and well protected. Because a large amount of force is required to fracture this rib, first rib fractures are frequently accompanied by flail chest, pneumothorax, hemothorax, pulmonary contusion, and aortic injuries. Although management of first rib fractures is similar to that of other rib fractures, vigilance is required for associated injuries because these may warrant additional interventions.

Flail chest A flail chest occurs when multiple rib fractures free a section of the chest wall. It commonly occurs after steering wheel injuries in which the first six ribs are fractured. The diagnosis is indicated by paradoxical motion of the flail segment of the chest wall during respiration; during inspiration, the flail segment is sucked inward rather than moving up and out like the rest of the chest wall. Pain and splinting can result in pneumonia and atelectasis in patients. Underlying pulmonary contusion may lead to hypoxemic respiratory failure.

It usually takes 7 to 10 days for the flail segment to stabilize. In the interim, the patient should be medicated for pain and undergo pulmonary toilet. Early institution of mechanical ventilation should be considered in any patient with *severe* flail chest (eight or more rib fractures), respiratory failure, or significant accompanying injuries. Surgical intervention is occasionally needed to stabilize the chest wall, usually in patients who have become difficult to ventilate mechanically or in whom thoracotomy is being performed for another reason.

Sternal fractures Sternal fractures are usually secondary to steering wheel injuries in motor vehicle accidents. These fractures do not require surgical treatment unless they are displaced. The possibility of cardiac contusion and injury to the great vessels must be considered in all patients with sternal fractures. Therefore, in the patient with a sternal fracture, an electrocardiogram or echo-cardiogram (or both) is often indicated. Also, if the aorta is wide on a chest radiograph taken in the upright position, an aortogram or a computed tomography (CT) scan may be helpful in identifying aortic dissection or bleeding.

PNEUMOTHORAX

Pneumothorax is a common complication of chest trauma. Etiologies of blunt traumatic pneumothoraces include (1) disrupted alveoli resulting in pulmonary interstitial emphysema (which subsequently can rupture through the mediastinal pleura and cause a pneumothorax); (2) laceration of the pleura from a broken rib or from the sheering forces transmitted through the chest at the time of the trauma; and (3) fracture of the tracheobronchial tree.

Diagnosis

Patients with a pneumothorax usually present with dyspnea and chest pain. Hyperresonance on percussion and diminished breath sounds on the affected side suggest a pneumothorax. Marked dyspnea, hypotension, distended neck veins, and tracheal shift away from the affected side suggest a tension pneumothorax. The diagnosis can usually be made with an upright chest radiograph. Unfortunately, severely traumatized patients frequently cannot be radiographed in the erect position and pneumothoraces may be difficult to visualize on a supine chest radiograph. On a supine chest radiograph, pleural air collects in the least dependent portions of the lung, i.e., anteromedial area (above or below the hilum adjacent to the vascular structures of the mediastinum or cardiac border) and subpulmonic area. A chest CT scan is more sensitive for the detection of pneumothoraces in trauma patients and is particularly helpful if an upright radiograph cannot be obtained.

Management

A traumatic pneumothorax almost always requires the insertion of a chest tube which also provides information about the presence of a hemothorax. Patients with a tension pneumothorax require immediate needle thoracentesis (second intercostal space in the midclavicular line) or tube thoracostomy to alleviate the increased pleural pressure and hemodynamic compromise. Following tube thoracostomy, wall suction is needed to re-expand the lung. A persistent large air leak suggests a tracheobronchial injury or a large pulmonary parenchymal tear.

HEMOTHORAX

Hemothorax is defined as blood in the pleural space (hematocrit of the pleural fluid at least 50 percent of the peripheral blood hematocrit). Hemothorax occurs in 25 percent of patients with significant blunt chest trauma. Bleeding is most commonly secondary to parenchymal lung injuries but can also occur from the chest wall, diaphragm, or mediastinum. Hemothorax is generally self-limited unless the bleeding is from a major vessel.

Diagnosis

Patients with a hemothorax usually have dullness to percussion and decreased breath sounds on the affected side. An upright chest radiograph should be diagnostic of an effusion if more than 300 ml blood is present. A large hemorrhage may deviate the trachea away from the involved side.

Management

Unless the hemothorax is very small (only blunting of the costophrenic angle on the chest radiograph), it should be managed with a large-bore chest tube. Chest tube thoracotomy permits evacuation of the blood and quantification of the amount of blood loss; it may decrease the likelihood of subsequent fibrothorax. Approximately 10 to 20 percent of patients with a hemothorax require a thoracotomy. Guidelines for immediate or early thoracotomy include (1) > 1500 to 2000 ml blood evacuated from the chest; (2) chest tube drainage in excess of 400 ml over 2 to 3 h; or (3) hemodynamic compromise attributable to the hemothorax.

Empyema is an important complication of traumatic hemothorax. The incidence in patients with traumatic hemothorax is 4 to 10 percent. Risk factors for development of empyema include shock or gross pleural contamination at the time of the initial injury, prolonged chest tube drainage, accompanying abdominal injuries, and pneumonia. How to handle blood remaining in the pleural space after chest tube thoracostomy is still being debated. Early studies had suggested that residual hemothorax after chest tube thoracostomy was a risk factor for the subsequent development of empyema, whereas a more recent review of more than 400 patients with traumatic hemothorax found no difference in the incidence of secondary empyema between those patients with and without residual blood in the pleural space. In some centers, "prophylactic" thoracotomy is done only if the residual hemothorax occupies one third or more of the hemithorax or results in persistent lobar atelectasis. Management of a complicating empyema consists of the combination of effective antibiotics and drainage of the infected pleural space. If adequate drainage cannot be achieved with one or more chest tubes, the patient should be taken to the operating room for open drainage and decortication.

Fibrothorax, the development of a thick, fibrous peel around the lung, is a relatively uncommon complication of hemothorax with an incidence of about 1 percent. This complication occurs weeks to months after the initial injury and can seriously compromise pulmonary function because of restriction of the underlying lung. The definitive treatment of fibrothorax is decortication.

TRACHEOBRONCHIAL INJURIES

Tracheobronchial injuries are uncommon but are associated with considerable mortality. Tracheobronchial fracture occurs more often after blunt chest or neck injury rather than after a penetrating wound. The three most common types of tracheobronchial disruption from blunt trauma include (1) a longitudinal separation of the membranous and cartilaginous trachea; (2) a spiral or straddle injury of the mainstem bronchus near the carina; and (3) a transverse laceration of the trachea.

Diagnosis

Patients with tracheobronchial injury usually complain of dyspnea, cough, and localized chest pain. Hoarseness or dysphagia suggests laryngeal or cervical tracheal injury. The diagnosis of tracheobronchial fracture is suggested by mediastinal or cervical emphysema, hemoptysis, recurrent pneumothorax, massive air leak despite adequate chest tube drainage, or persistent lobar atelectasis. The chest radiograph may demonstrate subcutaneous emphysema, pneumothorax, or pneumomediastinum. The diagnosis is confirmed by flexible bronchoscopy; the tear is usually within 2 cm of the carina. If suspicion of a tracheobronchial injury remains high after two negative bronchoscopies, a rigid bronchoscopy is in order. If a bronchial injury is present, positive pressure ventilation (especially positive end-expiratory pressure) can be catastrophic; it should only be attempted if well-functioning chest tubes are in place.

Management

Management of tracheobronchial injuries consists of antibiotics, maintenance of adequate ventilation, and prompt surgical repair. Complications of an untreated tracheobronchial tear include mediastinitis, pneumonia, and bronchial stenosis.

PULMONARY CONTUSION

Pulmonary contusion is a frequent complication of blunt chest trauma. It is often associated with rib fractures and flail chest.

Pulmonary laceration appears to be largely responsible for lung contusion by causing interstitial and alveolar extravasation of blood.

Diagnosis

Patients present with dyspnea, hypoxemia (increased physiological shunting), and hemoptysis. The chest radiograph usually shows a homogeneous infiltrate adjacent to the site of trauma although infiltrates can also occur as a result of contrecoup injury. The radiographic infiltrate caused by the contusion becomes evident within 6 h of the injury and usually resolves within 2 to 5 days. The infiltrate or opacity is localized but not confined to segmental or lobar boundaries. The lack of conformation to anatomic boundaries and the time course of the infiltrate (its evolution and resolution) help to differentiate a lung contusion from pneumonia, pulmonary embolism, aspiration, and atelectasis. CT scanning is more sensitive than chest radiography in diagnosing a pulmonary contusion.

Management

Management relies heavily on providing adequate ventilation and good pulmonary toilet. In patients with extensive pulmonary contusion, fluids have to be administered sparingly because overzealous fluid administration may increase leakage from the damaged microcirculation.

ESOPHAGEAL INJURIES

Esophageal perforation can occur with blunt or penetrating external injury. The proximal two thirds of the intrathoracic esophagus is adjacent to the right pleura, and the distal third is adjacent to the left pleura. Therefore, upper esophageal injuries manifest as a right pleural process, whereas distal esophageal injuries manifest on the opposite side. Acute purulent mediastinitis, due to mediastinal contamination by saliva and gastric contents, develops rapidly and is the major cause of morbidity and mortality.

Diagnosis

Patients with esophageal injuries are acutely ill with substernal chest pain, fever, and shock. The chest radiograph reveals a pleural effusion or hydropneumothorax, pneumomediastinum, and evidence of subcutaneous air. Thoracentesis often reveals sanguineous fluid with food particles, an elevated white count, a pH < 6.0, and a markedly elevated amylase level. Gastrografin or thin barium taken by mouth confirms the diagnosis by entering the mediastinum or pleural space.

Management

Early surgical drainage of the mediastinum and pleural space and repair of the esophagus are essential. Delay in recognition and surgical intervention beyond 24 h increases mortality dramatically. If surgical intervention is delayed beyond 24 h, it is recommended that primary repair of the esophageal tear not be attempted. Instead, as a temporary measure, a diverting cervical esophagostomy is performed, and the lower esophagus is isolated and stapled.

DIAPHRAGMATIC INJURIES

Diaphragmatic injuries are most commonly seen in patients with penetrating injury to the chest or abdomen. They also occur in about 5 percent of patients who sustain blunt trauma to the chest, likely as a result of an abrupt increase in intra-abdominal pressure. Ninety percent of diaphragmatic ruptures occur on the left, presumably because the liver protects the right hemidiaphragm.

Diagnosis

The diagnosis of diaphragmatic injury after blunt chest trauma can be difficult to establish. Patients may be asymptomatic or may complain of gastrointestinal symptoms (abdominal pain, nausea and vomiting, postprandial discomfort), shortness of breath, or shoulder pain. Physical examination may reveal bowel sounds in the chest. Chest radiography may show one or more of the following: (1) abdominal viscera above the diaphragm; (2) an elevated hemidiaphragm or loss of its normal contour; (3) a fresh pleural effusion; (4) basilar atelectasis or infiltrates; and (5) a mediastinal shift away from the affected side. Placement of a radiopaque nasogastric tube in the stomach is helpful in demonstrating herniation of the stomach across the left hemidiaphragm. Other diagnostic tests include abdominal CT scans, peritoneal lavage, and upper gastrointestinal series with contrast media. Unfortunately, the diagnosis of a ruptured diaphragm is often made more difficult by the concomitant presence of other injuries such as a fractured pelvis or head trauma which draw attention away from a diaphragmatic injury. The possibility of diaphragmatic injury should be considered in *all* patients with significant thoracoabdominal trauma, especially if there is a compatible chest radiograph. Herniation of viscera can occur months to years after the initial injury if the diaphragm is not repaired.

Management

Once the diagnosis is made, surgical repair should be undertaken expeditiously.

MYOCARDIAL CONTUSION

Blunt injury to the heart can damage the heart in a variety of ways, including myocardial contusion, myocardial necrosis with ventricular rupture, valvular damage, ventricular aneurysm, and pericardial injury or tamponade. Among these, cardiac contusion is the most common. Because the diagnosis is difficult to establish, cardiac contusion often goes unrecognized.

Diagnosis

There is no "gold standard" for the diagnosis of myocardial contusion. The diagnosis is inferred from the appropriate clinical setting and supportive diagnostic tests. Myocardial contusion usually occurs as a result of a decelerating injury to the thorax. Commonly, there is accompanying evidence of chest wall injury. Patients with myocardial contusion may be asymptomatic or have anginal symptoms. Physical examination may reveal a friction rub, arrhythmia, or unexplained tachycardia.

Electrocardiogram Q waves, ST segment, or T wave changes on the electrocardiogram are characteristic but can be delayed for 24 to 48 h after presentation. Ventricular or atrial arrhythmias (especially in a euvolemic nonhypoxic patient) or the development of a new bundle branch block are suggestive of the diagnosis. Serial electrocardiograms should be taken during the 48 h after injury.

Cardiac enzymes The levels of creative phosphokinase (CPK) and aspartate aminotransferase (AST) can be increased in any patient with blunt chest trauma because of injury to chest muscles. Increase in the MB isoenzyme fraction of CPK to > 5 percent is a more specific test of myocardial injury. Unfortunately, CPK and the MB isoenzyme fraction of CPK correlate poorly with clinical findings in patients with myocardial contusions.

Radiographic studies Radionuclide angiography, echocardiography, thallium scanning, and technetium pyrophosphate scanning have all been used in attempts to diagnose myocardial contusion. However, none of these studies is exceedingly sensitive or specific. Two-dimensional echocardiography may be the best adjunctive test because it can detect focal wall motion abnormalities that are characteristic of myocardial contusions. Additionally, echocardiography may be helpful in detecting concomitant pericardial effusions, valvular disruption, or ventricular thrombi.

Management

Patients with suspected myocardial contusion should be admitted to an intensive care unit or telemetry unit for electrocardiographic monitoring. Lidocaine can be used to control significant ventricular arrhythmias. If surgery is required in a patient with a myocardial contusion, hemodynamic monitoring with a Swan-Ganz catheter is recommended.

AORTIC INJURY

Approximately 10 percent of patients involved in a severe motor vehicle accident or deceleration injury will experience aortic injury. Ten to 20 percent of these patients survive to reach the hospital. The site of the aortic rupture is usually adjacent to the ligamentum arteriosum, slightly distal to the take-off of the left subclavian artery. Aortic injuries are often accompanied by other injuries including disruption of the tracheobronchial tree and fractures of the clavicle or the first two ribs.

Diagnosis

Patients with aortic injury generally complain of retrosternal chest pain. The diagnosis should be considered in all patients with a blunt chest injury who manifest a widened mediastinum on the chest radiograph or an appreciable difference in blood pressure and pulse amplitude between the upper and lower extremities (upper extremity hypertension and lower extremity hypotension). The typical radiographic finding indicative of aortic injury is widening of the superior mediastinum near the aortic knob. Other characteristic radiographic features include blurring of the aortic knob and arch, left hemothorax, deviation of the trachea to the right, esophageal deviation to the right, downward displacement of the left mainstem bronchus, and a left apical cap. It is critical to obtain an upright chest radiograph because the mediastinum can normally look wide on a supine chest film. If the superior mediastinum is wider than 8 cm on an upright chest radiograph in a trauma patient, aortography should be performed. Serial chest radiography over 6 to 12 h should be obtained after severe chest or abdominal trauma because the radiographic finding of an aortic tear may be delayed several hours. Although CT scanning is useful for evaluating the aorta and mediastinum in less urgent situations, it has only a limited role in the emergency setting.

Aortography is the "gold standard" for making the diagnosis of an aortic tear. However, if the patient is in shock and suspicion of an aortic rupture is high, forgo aortography and take the patient immediately to the operating room.

Management

If aortic injury is suspected, maneuvers which increase blood pressure (such as insertion of a nasogastric tube) should be avoided.

Once a diagnosis of aortic rupture is made, the patient should be taken immediately to the operating room for surgical repair.

BIBLIOGRAPHY

For a more detailed discussion, see Trinkle JK, Harman PK, Grover FL: Chest trauma, in Fishman AP (ed), *Pulmonary Diseases and Disorders,* 2d ed. New York, McGraw-Hill, 1988, pp 2443–2458.

Calhoon JH, Grover FL, Trinkle JK: Chest trauma. Clin Chest Med 13:55–67, 1992.

Dee PM: The radiology of chest trauma. Radiol Clin North Am 30:291–306, 1992.

Feliciano DV: The diagnostic and therapeutic approach to chest trauma. Semin Thorac Cardiovasc Surg 4:156–162, 1992.

Maddern IR, Goodman LR, Almassi GH, Haasler GB, McManus RP, Olinger GN: CT after reconstructive repair of the sternum and chest wall. Radiology 186:665–670, 1993.

INDEX

INDEX

Page numbers followed by the letter f *indicate figures. Page numbers followed by the letter* t *indicate tables.*

NOTES

NOTES

NOTES

NOTES

NOTES

NOTES

NOTES

NOTES